Memoirs of a Neurosurgeon

—A PERSPECTIVE FROM THE "LUCKY FEW" GENERATION

By James D. Geissinger, Jr., M. D., F. A. C. S.

Lightning Source Printed Edition

Published by James D. Geissinger

Paperback version
ISBN 978-0-615-54454-0

Hardcover version
ISBN 978-0-9847418-0-9

CreateSpace Printed Edition

Published by James D. Geissinger

ISBN 978-0-9847418-1-6

To all of my teachers

Contents

~~~
~~~

Preface

~~~

In his book entitled "The Lucky Few," Elwood Carlson discusses the demographic factors which might be important in the lives of individuals born between 1929 and 1945. This generation was immediately preceded by two generations collectively harboring a great depression, embraced by two world wars. Immediately following Tom Brokaw's "The Greatest Generation," the "Lucky Few" generation is unique in many ways. For instance, it has been characterized by both a low birth rate and hence a smaller member population. When coupled with high postwar employment, greater job opportunities, and the highest education rate seen thus far in our country, it has allowed its members to enter a unique period in our country's history. Like the two preceding generations, the "Lucky Few" generation possessed strong family values and low material aspirations, grounding them to enjoy a period of time in which individuals could anticipate a longer life expectancy and a nation entering into its longest economic boom (5). Those of us born as members of the "Lucky Few" generation have witnessed explosive corporate growth and prodigious technological advancement during the latter half of the 20th century. As a representative of the neurosurgeons born within this fortunate generation, I would like to reflect on my experiences of the time.

My daughter, Kim, once said, "Dad, there are things you could write about in a book that I have never known about you." Similarly, my attorney, after finding out about my intentions to write my memoirs, was openly elated when saying, "Every individual life contains important events that many others would find very interesting." Finally, a close friend recently asked, "To whom will you be addressing this book?"

The initial intent, in sharing with others the unique life of a neurosurgeon during this period, was to use it as a source of inspiration for the young student in high school or college who might be interested in the practice of medicine. In presenting an image with which they
~~~

could clearly identify, the early chapters are written as I remember them— first as a child and later as a highly motivated young adult. During the early formative years of school, the student often questions why he must learn what seems at the time to be extraneous material. As a means of encouragement, I have attempted to point out the relevance of such study (e.g., in physics) by showing its practical application later in life, in fact during actual medical practice. Also, the ability to remain focused and motivated in achieving one's goals— yet flexible and adaptable at times of adversity— remains a theme throughout the book.

A few years ago I became inspired to discuss in detail the specialty of neurological surgery in this book after having delivered a lecture on that subject to a special interest group in neurology within the sophomore medical class at the Florida State University College of Medicine. The students appeared quite attentive in hearing me speak about several different subjects, one of which related to the diagnosis and treatment of tumors of the pituitary gland. Because of the lasting positive feedback I received after that lecture, I thought perhaps a book might serve as a motivator to those who might be entertaining a career in some aspect of neuroscience. Not long after that lecture, while attending a spring graduation supper, one of the senior medical students displayed a genuine interest in my memoirs when stating— "There are not that many books out there recently written by doctors."

We are a sophisticated society in which descriptions of complex scientific endeavor and medical phenomena are commonplace in the newspapers and on television. In the same context, people of all ages have curiously asked me questions such as: How does one go about entering the skull during an operation, or how is a tumor safely removed from deep within the delicate brain? Certainly, as a neurosurgeon I would be remiss in having the reader come away not knowing the nature and treatment of such common entities as a "herniated disc," concussion or intracranial hemorrhage. In particular, coaches may find especially informative the sections on spinal and cranial injury. Finally, while there has been little written about the surgery of the nervous system, there has been even less concerning the reflective thoughts and personal experiences of the neurosurgeon himself.

In essence, I hope that this chronicle recording my life will reach out to many who might aspire to enter the field of medicine in general or neurological surgery in particular. Some may find the rather detailed descriptions of the surgical techniques and newer medical apparatus informative, but to the others who find these excerpts too complex, I must apologize. In that regard a glossary has been provided to assist with the medical terminology. Along the way I also hope to leave a trail of neurosurgical history as I experienced it for almost three decades. In doing so I shall pay tribute to a number of distinguished individuals, who not only were important in my personal education but instrumental in advancing various aspects of medicine and surgery as well. I would also like to reflect on some of the important innovations of our day and the ever-changing approaches to the diagnosis and operative treatment of neurosurgical disorders. To accomplish this, I will cite selective experiences from our personal surgical practice, hoping to emphasize specific technical points. Allow me to emphasize that the cases described throughout the book are merely representative of those done by the average neurological surgeon in practice, and not intended in any way to elevate my own above the rest. And finally, some cases are presented as important vehicles of education reflecting surgical ideology and philosophy.

There are few parents who would not be proud of a son or daughter entering the practice of medicine. Moreover, virtually everyone at some time in his or her life will require the services of a physician. It is for those parents and potential patients that I am also writing this book. It is important for everyone to be fully aware not only of the arduous task of becoming a doctor, but the multiples of adversity confronting the physician long after graduation, and indeed throughout his professional life. The various professional medical specialties and organizations are cognizant of the problems facing medicine today, and are working within the private and government sectors to arrive at reasonable solutions to the satisfaction of all, but the public has basically remained uninformed as to the nature of those problems.

After contracting an unexpected illness later in my career, I was forced to lay down the scalpel. While ranching had always been a childhood dream, it necessarily became a second vocation. The reader is thus vicariously transitioned from an academic stream of thought in following the hospital-based life of a neurosurgeon to the life of a professional cattleman, meeting the daily problems posed by nature and the business world. One of my younger medical colleagues recently expressed a genuine interest in reading about those forces driving the life of a man who, after having been a neurosurgeon, later accepted the many challenges facing a cattle rancher.

Because these pages contain my life's story, they necessarily involve many other aspects of my varied experiences aside from the practice of surgery; I can only hope that the reader enjoys finding some of these topics both informative and in some instances even entertaining. Thus, in answer to my friend's question— I hope a broad readership will find this memoir an educational experience both within and beyond the field of neurosurgery.

Very few of us get through life without major life-changing events, such as separation from one's family, the loss of a loved one or a career-changing illness. Perhaps my experience in dealing with these matters will also serve as an inspiration to others encumbered by them, showing that life offers many roads leading from despair to further achievement and happiness.

The final chapters concern my view as to how medicine is currently being practiced, and how it relates to the proposed healthcare reform. These opinions are my own and are not intended to necessarily reflect those of other members of the Tallahassee Neurological Clinic. I was privileged to have practiced during the "golden years" of medicine when landmark scientific innovations were commonplace, and patients could call a doctor their own— day or night, routine care or emergencies. As seen from my particular perspective as a physician from the "Lucky Few" generation, I yearn for those days of the past, hoping that the younger generations of physicians will return to them.

James D. Geissinger, Jr., M. D., F. A. C. S.
Tallahassee, Florida
December, 2011

Foreword

~~~

Having read more than "a few" medical memoirs, histories, and biographies, it is a pleasure to consider this autobiography exceptional. Grant that Harvey Cushing, M.D., that very great star of American neurosurgery— indeed the founding Father of that difficult specialty— wrote a biography of Sir William Osler, that other great star of North American medicine; and for it won the Pulitzer Prize in 1926. Grant that biographies of Dr. Cushing, containing the high drama of all that he achieved, rivet the attention of readers. Grant further that there are countless famous physicians and surgeons who have put to paper the extraordinary events of their fascinating professional lives and discoveries. All of these are the background of what is, even so, generally missing.

The drama, excitement, and glamour of Harvey Cushing's surgical interventions into the human brain would be very nearly irrelevant were it not for those who followed in his footsteps, those who dutifully and doggedly applied day in and day out what he taught, their greatest reward being little of fame, but rather the simple perfection of their own judgment and techniques. But by that they give to their patients a second chance for hope, love, and life itself. Such practitioners of any profession are the silent intermediaries who stand between us in need and those icons who had the grit and genius to enter the unknown and boldly reveal the opportunities that lay within. Dr. Geissinger is one of those intermediaries who may never be known for his "discoveries," but who in the highest tradition of his kind gave hope and life to thousands. In any case, I have never read the life of "a small town neurosurgeon." How, one might well wonder, does a person like that actually spend his days? We all know the cliché that defines the "rocket scientist" as that very perfect paradigm of intellectual achievement. So also, and equally commonly defined is the neurosurgeon, as in "it ain't brain surgery!" And, perhaps even more than the "rocket scientist," the neurosurgeon embodies attributes not only intellectual (this is the brain, after all!) but
~~~

a special moral and physical stamina combined with a delicacy of judgment that cannot waiver even under the most critical pressure. So we believe; and so grant the neurosurgeon our awe and adulation. But in the midst of our admiring exclamations, how little we know of what, in fact, the neurosurgeon is and really does. You assume they sleep at night; but maybe not much. They eat now and again, surely. They doubtless fall in love, for we have seen that on soap operas. You assume that they might fret over their patients, but in what manner and to what degree we are not certain. Capable of going no further, we must be content with our trust that the neurosurgeon stands forth as one of those *beaux idéals* of human potential. In my estimation, few among the professions stand higher. And Dr. Jim Geissinger is "high" among the few.

In his autobiography, Dr. Geissinger tells us with concision what it is like to become, and then be, a neurosurgeon. He describes first the appreciation of the fact that he would want to become a physician. He captures the intensity of a neurosurgeon's training and the demands placed on the body, mind, and soul— the toll those demands take. Beyond these points, in themselves so inextricably a part of our "idea" of what it must be to be a neurosurgeon, Dr. Geissinger provides us with numerous case studies. Never talking "down" to his reader, he nonetheless brings an articulate clarity of detail to his descriptions of the patients and surgeries he so eloquently remembers. He explains to us the intricacies of planning a neurosurgical procedure; the care with which each step must be individually considered; and the sometimes scathing doubts as the risks are weighed and then come to terms with by both him and his patients.

In his career, which stretched from the end of what might be called "the heroic years" of neurosurgery into these latter days of more exquisite refinement, we see him grow with his experience. He explains to us the near magical benefits of the new technologies, wherein CT scans, MRIs, stereotactic techniques, and laser surgeries become the norm. And then, at the very peak of his ability, he finds himself struck down, and cast away from all he has so brilliantly grown to know and love. And so... he must deal with that as well.

He does. This book is a part of that "dealing," a poignant sharing of both fact and feeling, so that by its end you will not only have some real idea of what it means to be a practicing neurosurgeon, but be glad to know, also, a great human being.

Charles E. Moore, M.D.

ONE

The Early Years

~~~

My life's story began in Pueblo, a town in southern Colorado, where my grandparents settled in the early 1900s. The town was the second largest city in the state at the time, being located 43 miles south of Colorado Springs and 20 miles east of the Rocky Mountains. Through it runs the Arkansas River which had caused a flood disaster in 1921. Having been geologically positioned near coal fields, it was one of the nation's largest steel production centers (Colorado Fuel and Iron Corporation) during the war, often being referred to as the “Pittsburgh of the West.”

To write about any life should reasonably begin with a description of one’s grandparents, for it is from them that we derive our defining genetic and often social constitution. Mine were all of good stock having endured the rough, stressful times of the Great Depression and the two world wars.

My maternal grandmother was the academic member of the group, having been first raised during hard times on the dry-lands of Kansas, and later having been graduated from Kansas University as one of its proud Jayhawks. She married my grandfather who had been reared on a farm, as many Americans were in those days. Having been case-hardened through the rigors of Missouri farm life and the cold winters of the mid-west, he was graduated with a teaching degree from the state university. Together they moved further westward, and settled in Pueblo where they taught school. While both were on the faculty at Central High, she taught business skills and he was the headmaster of the industrial arts department. I remember my grandmother as a very sophisticated, articulate, gentle lady. She was also a strong advocate of
~~~

the educational process as evidenced by her having returned to school to receive her Master's degree at the age of 52.

My grandfather, on the other hand, was very gifted in the use of his hands as exemplified by his abilities not only to design and build houses, but also to teach high school students the art of constructing attractive articles of fine furniture. Even as a child I appreciated the beautifully figured walnut constituting the exquisite pieces of furniture which he had so elegantly crafted for our home. He not only served as an everlasting source of inspiration to me regarding his woodworking skills, but I shall always be profoundly indebted to him for his having passed on to me those inherent mechanical attributes so critical for my success later in life — a point to be emphasized in this book.

My paternal grandfather was also raised on a farm, but in Iowa, and often said that he worked very hard in school to "get away from it." After matriculating through college, he entered medical school at Northwestern University in Chicago. Upon graduating in 1907, he became a family doctor, whose practice was heavily weighted in obstetrics and pediatrics. After marrying my grandmother, a farm girl of Swedish descent, they also eventually moved to Pueblo to settle into their family life.

I remember my father's mother as a very active, self-confident woman with unlimited household skills and boundless energy. With regard to the latter, she could put out the daily work of a man and was "tough as nails." In emphasizing her endurance, years later she hired me one hot summer to paint her white stucco house. She not only helped me paint all day in the blistering sun, but stopped just early enough to bake a couple of fruit pies in preparation of a family dinner for a dozen people. And there were no microwave ovens or automatic dishwashers in those days. While having achieved only an eighth grade education herself, she was not only a strong advocate of higher education, but was always one of my most ardent supporters.

In further describing my granddad, he could have easily been the centerpiece of one of Norman Rockwell's paintings in that he was a bespectacled, stately, kind-appearing man, often toting a black bag; and almost never to be seen in public without wearing a three-piece suit with the customary watch fob dangling from his vest. He was the epitome of Pueblo's medical community having originated one of its most prestigious clinics, been a highly respected physician in both of its hospitals, and a foremost obstetrician in delivering many of its babies.

Not only was I fortunate to have been born a member of the "Lucky Few" generation, but was also extremely privileged to have had such motivated and gifted grandparents. I owe much of any success which I have had in life to each of them.

~~~

On February 23, 1937 I was the first of three sons born to James and Ruth Geissinger of Pueblo, Colorado. My father was, at the time, assistant district attorney in that small town; and my mother, an artist and musician, remained a homemaker — customary in those days. Four years later the Japanese bombed Pearl Harbor, propelling us into World War II. Our home, like so many others, became disrupted when my father, an officer in the Navy, was deployed to Guam. For reasons never clear to me, there were two years during which my mother was nowhere to be seen, and, as a result, failed to care for me and my little brother, Richard. Richard recalls having spent two years with a poor immigrant family living in a bad district on the south side of Pueblo. I was fortunate to have spent 1944 with my paternal grandparents and 1945 with those on my mother's side. The "fears and uncertainties" of the war hung like a dark cloud over everyone, as stories of slaughter reached the home front. My grandparents not only assuaged any stress I might have had from the absence of parents during the world war, but gave me both security and encouragement. Richard, on the other hand, suffered immense feelings of neglect from the absence of our parents.

In 1945 my little classmates elected me president of the third-grade class; even today I can recall the strong sense of patriotism when leading them in the Pledge of Allegiance and the Lord's Prayer each morning. I consider myself fortunate to have developed a positive self-identity and confidence at such an early age.

Several other events occurring during those two years with my grandparents engendered what would become lifelong interests. Foremost was the intriguing black bag from which my physician grandfather produced an assortment of items like rabbits from a hat. He seemed to have a different light for each orifice of my head. And then there were those two small rubber hoses attached to a long narrow bell which he applied to my chest; and, while intently listening, I could sense concentration in his deep blue eyes. I was also in awe of his office with the big, sturdy examining table covered with white paper and the glass
~~~

cabinet full of bottles, syringes and needles. I recall my first smallpox vaccination with the multiple needle pricks on my shoulder and the associated aroma of alcohol used to sterilize the skin. Then, there was that awful gagging triggered by the wooden tongue depressor seemingly slid far down into my throat; whereupon, he would sternly say, "Now say, — ah ah ah." Needless to say I was absolutely terrified to ever return, vividly bearing in mind not only the wretched tongue blades but all of those strange instruments in the glass cabinet. But with time, I learned to develop a genuine trust in this kind man, who would, years later, be a major influence in my becoming a doctor. Soon those tongue blades no longer frightened the little kid.

When I was with my schoolteacher grandparents, several inspirational events transpired. There was a neighbor boy my age whose father worked for the local power company, and, at a very young age, he had learned the basics of electricity and magnetism which he in turn taught to me. His dad also had a large bandsaw in his basement which became a lasting fascination as well. Even now, I remember watching in awe the long blade rotating on those large wheels as it effortlessly cut through thick pieces of wood.

Then one day my skillful woodworker grandfather took me down to his high school workshop. It appeared to that eight-year-old as an enormous expanse with a painted gray cement floor supporting a myriad of gigantic, shiny, cast-iron machines studded with various-sized chrome-plated knobs and wheels, accented in orange and black, and many housing a different type of blade. The odor of freshly cut wood permeated the air. The sight and smell of that spectacular shop remains etched into my brain well over 65 years later.

Another lasting memory was encoded in the summer of 1945 when my mother picked us up from my grandparents, and hastened us off to stay for the summer with a farm family at the base of the Rocky Mountains. I was intrigued by the panorama of the beautiful far-reaching fields, animals, and the smell of hay that summer, and dreamed of perhaps having a farm of my own someday.

~~~

On September 2, 1945, on behalf of the Allies, General Douglas MacArthur accepted the surrender of Japan on the USS Missouri, ending World War II.
~~~

After the war my father safely returned home, my mom reappeared to enter our lives, and for reasons never clear to me, we left Pueblo permanently for Denver in 1946.

The postwar years were tough. My father, while basically starting over in the law business, initially accepted a very low-paying state job as an attorney. We lived in a small old house, had no car; and, not infrequently, I can recall going away from the table hungry. Tensions were always high around the place, and there was constant bickering over money. My dad was an aggressive lawyer (formerly a prosecutor in Pueblo) by profession, and a tough disciplinarian at home, cutting no one any slack. My only recourse was to stay busy and out of his way.

Although by no means intended to gain any sympathy, now is the appropriate time to discuss some relevant points regarding my early childhood. Make no mistake — my home, although it could have been much worse, was not that depicted by the classic Ozzie Nelson family. Perhaps it was torn because of the personal and financial consequences of the war, or perhaps it was simply a case of two frustrated, unhappy individuals trying to make a go of it. My mother was inherently a loving person, but also a very severe depressive. More often than not when coming home from school in the afternoon, I would find her lying on the living room couch in a darkened room, still in her nightclothes and frequently unkempt. She was often mute, showed no emotion, and despite my best efforts to cheer her up, she could scarcely ever begin to generate any hint of a smile.

My father, as already noted, was someone to avoid. But let me give him the benefit of the doubt — financial times were tough, he was struggling to rise in his profession, and my mother was a very negative force in his life. He, in turn, was totally unpredictable. It takes but a few fingers to count the total number of times that he was truly affable where we were concerned; he was more often negative and at times tyrannical. He would explode over trivial matters and, in so doing, would transform into a Mr. Hyde persona who would make even the strongest of men quiver. Together my parents were simply a bad mix. Our home was a turbulent, unpredictable place with plenty of emotional and physical abuse to go around.

Yet there was an irony in all of this— as a child I thought my home was perfectly normal! When I would spend a weekend night with a friend, and sat at a quiet dinner table among considerate, compassionate adults, I would often think to myself —"something is wrong here."

Several weeks each summer I took refuge with my aunt Rosemary and uncle Dub in Pueblo. They had a nice place out at the edge of town with some acreage and a barn. As a child I loved spending time on this small "farm," and I always considered these folks as second parents—people in whom I could confide as a child. Fondly, I can recall a number of long fishing trips into Southwest Colorado, where, as a nine-year-old boy, I learned from Dub the art of fly-fishing in the south fork of the Rio Grande River.

I consider this background information important, for it serves to explain my early childhood independence and accounts for many of my life's future decisions. I credit much of my strength to my paternal grandmother who later once said, "Jimmy, despite the outlandish behavior exhibited by your parents, you must not let that destroy you — keep looking ahead and you will become a successful man when you grow up!"

Years later I told others that neither the most callous of professors nor the most aggressive of attorneys could intimidate me, for I had been aptly conditioned as a child. Furthermore, I had realized at a very early age that in order to escape that unpleasant household, I needed to firmly set my goals as to what I was going to do with my life. It didn't take me long to appreciate the value and security of an education, beginning as early as elementary school. Nor can I emphasize enough the importance of both sports and those physical survival skills that I later learned in scouting. These are very important elements in building confidence and self-esteem in spite of a suppressive, suffocating home environment. For those young people who can identify with this snippet, I hope that you find in it words of encouragement.

When we first moved into the old house, it was heated with a coal-burning furnace. My parents soon got tired of shoveling the filthy stuff and converted to electric heat. I worked out a deal with my dad, whereby, if I cleaned out the coal bin I could use it for my own workshop. Although being only nine years old, I was highly motivated to have my own space. It was a nasty job, but I worked diligently to clean up the bin, paint it, and do my own electrical wiring. Grandpa built me a workbench and a wooden toolbox, stuffed with a nice assortment of hand tools (all of which I have in my possession to this day). For Christmas, the family all chipped in to buy me a little bench-type jigsaw. While I didn't really ever build anything of significance, I was constantly trying to cut out and make things from wood. Also, my attempts at wiring motors, circuits and magnets revealed my early fascination with electricity.

During the first two school years in Denver, I recall having been more interested in sports than in class work, and, as another extracurricular activity, I focused on the Cub Scouts. In so doing I not only gained many new friends but also nurtured an interest in constructing projects requiring the use of both hand and mind.

1949 was the year the light came on in my brain —"Perhaps I should become a doctor like my grandfather!" After all… being a highly respected figure in the community, he possessed the virtues of honesty, kindness, empathy and a dedicated work ethic, all typifying the physicians of that time. Even at that early age, I was cognizant of his past professional success which, when coupled with a strong spiritual belief, had provided security for his family during those very difficult times.

But oddly enough he was not the trigger event in my final decision. It occurred one day when I was visiting him in Pueblo and picked up from his coffee table the well-known and highly acclaimed book—*Microbe Hunters* by Paul De Kruif (8). It was riveting to me, as a twelve-year-old, to read the exciting discoveries of Koch, Pasteur, Antony Leeuenhoek and others. Leeuenhoek, a Dutch lens-grinder who invented the microscope and was the first to visualize and draw microorganisms, is considered the father of bacteriology. Little did I realize as a child that some day when making observations through my own microscope, I would often think of Leeuenhoek. As for the book itself, it was the first totally scientific book to sell one million copies, and is credited for stimulating a generation of biological scientists into research.

Thus began my curiosity for medicine, and my grandfather happily encouraged me. Years later, I asked him what he felt was the greatest breakthrough in medicine during his lifetime, thinking that he would probably cite Fleming's discovery of penicillin. Without hesitation he replied, "The discovery of Diphtheria toxoid." He then went on to elaborate on the end of a scourge during which he had helplessly witnessed the loss of life of countless babies and young children.

~~~
~~~

In 1949 it was off to junior high school where most of us felt that we were now really growing up. No longer were we stuck in a single classroom like little kids, but were trusted to move from one room to another with each 50-minute ringing of the bell. While wood shop was my favorite subject (where I first learned to use a lathe in turning a lamp), my appetite for medical phenomenon was heightened in the general science course. When Mr. Parsons began speaking about digestion with the enzymatic breakdown and assimilation of foodstuffs I began to comprehend, for the first time, how the body really worked. A lasting interest in physiology was sparked in that eighth-grade class, and I couldn't learn enough about it.

Sports were a big thing in my school, and, like many boys— I loved them all. Besides the three major sports, I participated in both track and the wrestling tournament all three years, later becoming interested in golf as well. I have extremely fond memories of those years at Smiley Junior High.

In seventh grade I met a friend whose parents had a stately, modern home on one of Denver's major boulevards across from a golf course. A group of us consistently gathered in Jim's driveway night after night, weather permitting, to play basketball. While I knew his dad was a doctor, I didn't know just what kind of doctor he really was. Then one day in the headlines of the *Denver Post*, it was revealed that some school kid in town had been running with a mechanical pencil in hand when, upon falling down, he tragically drove the instrument deep into his chest and heart. It was Jim's dad, I soon came to find out, who was the chest surgeon who saved the child's life by removing the object in a Denver hospital. Suddenly my interest in Jim's driveway exceeded that of playing basketball; I hoped merely to catch a glimpse of the man driving toward us who could perform such a miraculous feat. Indeed, I did meet him one day, and my image of a surgeon was cast. Here was a highly respected man with the surgical skills to save lives; yet, he was an affable, down-to-earth, human being who just happened to drive a nice car and live in a magnificent house. Could I ever hope to achieve such an enviable status in my lifetime?

Dreaming about carrying a black bag, synthesizing a vaccine, or saving lives in the operating room is one thing, but realizing those dreams is an entirely different matter. The young boy soon discovered what it would take, and it wasn't going to be easy!

My seventh grade English teacher, Betty Welch, was a petite, attractive, no-nonsense lady whose job was to see that we learned the

English language. I recall spending hours in the classroom learning the parts of speech and the mechanics of diagramming sentences. To this day I am ever so grateful to Ms. Welch. English today is often not emphasized enough, and there has been criticism that even many college graduates do not possess an adequate command of it. It was once said that in approaching a scientific problem, one must first be able to understand it (English); he must possess the tools with which to analyze it (mathematics); and only then can he solve the problem itself (e.g., physics). Language has been considered by many scholars to be the "instrument of thought and expression of the human mind."

Another subject I was advised to take by my father was Latin, and the first teacher introducing me to it was Mr. Spencer. He was short, balding, dapper, and a very proper man who spoke in a whisper, and who veritably defined the word "perfectionist." Always immaculately dressed in suit and tie, he would stroll around the classroom while carrying a small deck of cards, each marked with a student's name. After shuffling the cards, he would deftly draw one from the top and ask the identified student a question. It could vary anywhere between a single vocabulary word to the translation of an entire sentence from Latin to English or vice-versa; worse yet, one might even have to step up to the blackboard in a moment of terror. After the student's response Mr. Spencer would quietly enter a grade on the card, and would then move to the next. The respondents were seated from best to worst in the classroom, so that everyone always had a chance to move forward (or backward). He demanded absolute perfection in the answers, and no word could have either an improper ending or be out of order in the sentence. The competition for advancement was intense, and the kids needed steady nerves. In those days, Mr. Spencer did not hand out consolation "smiley faces" to those in the back-row seats. Their only "reward" was the opportunity to work harder and move forward. My father once told me early on that Latin was a good discipline in orderly thinking, and I soon found out that he was right. Moreover, as a bonus, it was later very helpful knowing the roots of medical terms.

In the ninth grade we were introduced to algebra. The concepts were new and at times baffling. Once mastered, it almost became fun. For the prospective student, it is imperative that this subject be learned well, because it is a major tool needed in complex mathematics and science. For the eventual physician, it is used in the calculation of medications and fluid doses, the statistical analyses of medical data, and in the formulas used for radiation therapy — much else depends upon it. Even as an older adult I use algebra in solving occasional day-to-day problems.

With the passage of time, as I matriculated through junior high school, it became more and more evident how difficult, if not impossible, it would be to become a doctor— whether one like my granddad or Jim's dad, the chest surgeon.

As a positive influence in my character development during those pre-adolescent years, I pursued scouting and later received the Eagle award. It was an achievement attained by many of our generals in the armed forces, and I was proud to have earned it. Furthermore, it taught me lifelong skills that many never learn; skills that I have been able to pass on not only to my children but to friends alike.

Another important facet of my young life was having been a newspaper carrier for the *Denver Post*. Getting up at 4 A.M. on a Sunday morning, folding those heavy 100- page newspapers, and filling the canvas bags on the handlebars of my bicycle, taught me what it meant to be responsible to others. Delivering the papers through biting winds and blinding blizzards was a duty to my customers. Furthermore, in collecting my monthly fees, I found myself to be a "boy in business." Because society is replete with those who do injustice to children— just as they often do to adults— I learned early to be tenacious and firm, yet diplomatic in getting the job done.

But the good people far outnumbered the bad. I recall a Mr. Kibbie on my paper route, who just happened to be the vice president of the largest cemetery in Denver. Later, when I entered high school and needed a full-time summer job, I turned to Mr. Kibbie. Because I had always been timely with the paper, and threw it on his porch out of the rain, he offered me a job at the graveyard. The early lesson learned was that in order to acquire a record of good referrals, it always paid to do a good job.

The cemetery work for three years during the summers was hot and monotonous, mowing around literally thousands of tombstones. I was the only kid in a group of older men cutting grass with a hand-pushed mower for 10 hours a day, six days a week at eighty cents an hour. Many of them were elderly, tobacco-chewing, veterans from World War I, and I'll never forget that we all drank water out of the same corked, heavily soiled, canvas water bag. It was a good lesson in telling me exactly what I did not want to do for the rest of my life. But it did allow me to buy my first car. It was a recently painted, black 1941 Ford club coupe with chartreuse and black leather upholstery, wide white sidewall tires and dual mufflers that my friends said "purred like a kitty". Despite having always been on the lookout, I've never seen anything quite like it since.

My last three years of high school were tumultuous. Because my father, by then a prominent attorney, was given an appointment by the Eisenhower administration as Deputy Solicitor in the Department of Interior, we moved to Virginia, just outside of Washington, D.C. Indeed, this was an impressive place, surrounded by history, to spend a year in high school. Each weekend our family would spend time visiting an important government building, monument or battlefield. In addition, while lettering as a member of the golf team, I was privileged to play competitive golf on the many beautiful golf courses in the Washington, D. C., area, including the well-known Congressional course, the future site of the U.S. Open.

With the arrival of spring in 1954 the excitement of major league baseball began to fill the air. Several of my friends and I would frequent Griffith Stadium on those cool Saturday evenings to watch the Washington Senators take the field. Having been a child growing up far out West, the closest I had ever gotten to the big-name teams was intently listening to a famous sports broadcaster, Bill Stern, talk about baseball as I crouched by the radio. Now the mystique surrounding many of the great athletes in the sport was turning into reality, as we gathered by the tall chain-link fence where the players exited after the game. I cherished the autographs of such Yankee greats as Mickey Mantle, Yogi Berra and manager Casey Stengel. When the Boston Red Sox rolled into town for a weekend series with Washington, I even managed to get the signature of the legendary Ted Williams in my book. Such was this memorable period in baseball history and in my young impressionable life as well.

Not to be excluded was the medical museum at the Smithsonian Institute, which, at that time, was one of a kind. There were extensive shelves upon which rested thick, heavy, glass bottles containing preserved human organs, many exhibiting rare and unusual diseases. Unfortunately for more recent generations that particular museum has since been disassembled.

On the down side for me the temporary move to Virginia resulted in three different high schools in each of the three years. While I made many friends it created problems with both participation in sports and satisfying the course requirements for college entrance. For example, when we returned one year later to Denver, we lived in a school district that did not provide advanced mathematics or physics. After a great deal of uncertainty and frustration, I was finally able to attend a high school in another district where I could complete my college preparatory work.

Throughout high school I had friends often question why they had to take specific courses for which they could see no future application; quite frankly, there were times when I often wondered that myself. In retrospect there was usually a good reason for most subjects. For example, the study of Euclidean geometry in solving theorems serves to tune up the mind both in logic and in spatial relationships. Similarly the concepts learned in physics will be useful to the doctor throughout the rest of his life, not only in medicine but in the world outside of it. I shall refer back to these and other important related subjects as the book unfolds.

By the end of high school, my life's goal was well defined. With a high level of motivation and surrounded by a ringside of family supporters, I was off to college for my pre-medical education. And, to no one's surprise, I was going to attend Northwestern University, where my grandfather had received his medical degree forty-eight years previously.

TWO

The Journey into Medicine

~~~

One day late in the summer of 1955, a car occupied by three college upperclassman from the west coast pulled up in front of my Denver home. With belongings in hand, I piled into the car with them, and we were soon off to Northwestern University in Evanston, Illinois. With her eyes clouding up my mother waved goodbye realizing, like many parents, that I was probably permanently leaving home to strike out on my own.

Chicago was a magnificent place to this eager, young lad from the West. I thought I was on a different planet the first night I stepped off of the noisy, elevated train in the center of "the loop," downtown. With the gusty cool wind blowing through my hair while standing amidst hordes of impersonal pedestrians briskly walking by me in every direction, I cranked my head far back in looking straight up through the bright lights to the tops of the towering buildings. And the Evanston campus on Lake Michigan was like a dream come true. Within days I was involved in fraternity "rush-week," and soon thereafter joined Phi Gama Delta, establishing treasured lifelong friendships.

Registration into the pre-medical curriculum at the University soon followed, and within no time I felt comfortable in my new surroundings.

The first year was an eye-opener for a number of reasons. Although novel and fun, the fraternity was quite demanding of my time. Despite the university rule which required all freshmen to reside in university housing that first year, it seemed that I spent most of my non-sleeping hours at the fraternity house. Anyone who is knowledgeable about Greek life knows exactly what it entails. I did, however, enjoy my experiences in the intramural athletics program, and the opportunity as a
~~~

freshman to perform as a clown diver in the well-publicized university water show.

The academic side of things understandably was much different from high school. It didn't take me long to realize that I was in the midst of a group of premedical students who were my equal or greater in intelligence; furthermore, any lack of motivation wasn't inherent in any of them. Standing foremost in my memory was that first year of chemistry, complete with its new concepts, lengthy formulas and extensive calculations; and least to be forgotten were the long afternoon labs that let out into the darkness of those blustery, frigid, winter nights along Lake Michigan.

Speaking of chemistry, it was often fashionable in the fraternity to pull an "all- nighter," wherein the brothers would cram for the ensuing day's examination in a smoke-filled room, the ill effects of tobacco yet to be recognized. On one such occasion, three of us together churned through the night, stuffing ashtrays with cigarette butts, and consuming several pots of black coffee while balancing and memorizing a formidable list of chemical equations.

Early the next morning we took our seats in the spacious amphitheater of the engineering building, and at eight o'clock the blue books for the examination were distributed. The last thing that I remembered was having written my name on the front of the book. An hour later, as if awakening from a surgical anesthetic, I felt a tap on my shoulder, and heard a voice quietly say… "Son, it's time to hand in your examination." After that overwhelming, deep sleep, my totally blank book was handed forth. Any future chance of my getting into medical school suddenly appeared to vanish. After dejectedly leaving the building, I immediately called my dad in Denver to tell him that I was all washed up. But always having been my strongest advocate and totally imperturbable, he brushed it aside by saying, "Things like that at times seem to happen to everyone. Learn from your mistake, and keep focused on working hard." With those encouraging words having been said, my future suddenly again became brighter. Incidentally, I never again stayed up all night studying for an examination.

During my sophomore year I moved into the fraternity house, and obtained a board job there (working in the kitchen and dining room), helping to defray my college expenses. Again, it was enjoyable living in a five-story building with the brothers, but it also had its disadvantages, primarily from the distracting, time-consuming, noisy, extracurricular activities. In addition, I was elected intramural sports chairman, and given the responsibility for the entire year of assembling participants for each sport— both individual and team. Because I usually played the sport as well, little time remained overall for study.

On the academic front, it was organic chemistry that first began to take its toll on the premedical group. Understandably, with each passing year the courses generally became tougher, the time to digest the increasing volume of material relatively shorter, and the competition for good grades more intense. People began to drop by the wayside. When I was visiting my aging grandma Geissinger in Pueblo during Christmas vacation, she earnestly warned me about distractions such as alcohol, parties and girls. She said with strong conviction, "Keep your mind focused, and if you continue to study hard and use your time wisely, there is no doubt that you will succeed in becoming a doctor."

Summers were spent doing hard work and saving every penny to supplement what my dad provided for me. As indicated previously, in my generation higher education was affordable to most Americans, and the "Lucky Few" men had the benefit of the greatest schooling improvement of the century.

During the first summer after my freshman year I belonged to a pipefitters' union. Among other things, my job entailed mechanically hoisting red-hot, sand-filled, steel pipes from a furnace, and helping to bend them on a large water-cooled steel bending slab. As a lasting benefit from those days in the "pipe shop," I became proficient with a cutting torch and developed welding skills which I have maintained and found useful to this day.

Subsequent summers were spent in the Rocky Mountains working for the National Park Service. I was on a mountain-climbing crew that was on the slopes all day spraying for the fungus, "Blister-Rust," a disease destroying white pine trees. Because we were in good shape from constant daily hiking at high altitudes, my crew was trained as the fire and rescue team as well. What a unique experience that proved to be. As if yesterday, I recall one serious event in which a lady tourist from the eastern U.S. fell far to her death while traversing the top of a glacier. Upon receiving word of her accident early that evening, we assembled a rescue party and departed in the early morning darkness to climb the mountain before daybreak. After finding her badly broken body in a boulder field far below the glacier, the entire day was then spent hand-carrying the litter with her lifeless body down a ravine from the 10,000-foot peak. It was a very solemn life-lesson from which we energetic, bold, young men suddenly began to realize our own mortality.

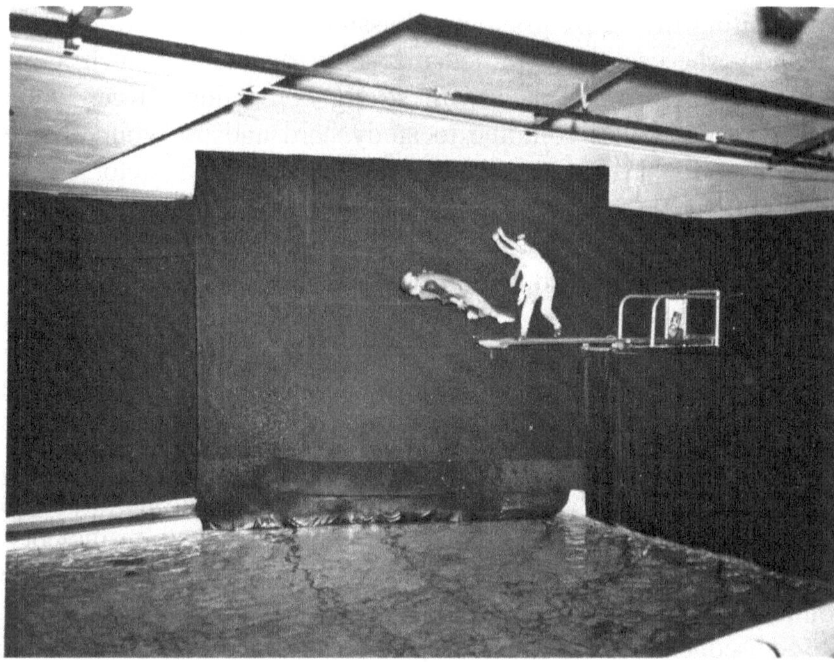

The Student and Sportsman

The author as a clown diver while executing a back-flip off of the 3-meter board in the Northwestern University Water Show in 1955.

My junior and senior years at the undergraduate school were spent living "off- campus." Because the extracurricular activities associated with the fraternity were damaging my grade-point average, I needed to bear down on my advanced mathematics, physics, and comparative anatomy courses. As a bit of levity regarding the latter, we maintained a cat skeleton in our apartment, and kept freshly dissected feline body parts reeking of formaldehyde in an ice cream cup in the refrigerator— only dedicated premedical students would dare such a thing.

During the beginning of the senior year I moved into the top floor of a boarding house with a good friend and fraternity brother, Bob Doherty. Bob was also a premedical student at Northwestern at the time, and someone I always considered one of the brightest of my friends. Not only as a junior was he elected president of the French club at Northwestern, but as a senior I remember his reading for the first time the night before the final exam a very thick literary work in advanced French— only to receive an "A" in the course. Bob and I both worked board jobs, his at a sorority house and mine at a freshman woman's dormitory, thus enabling us to get our meals free. It also afforded us the opportunity to meet and date attractive young women. Before leaving the latter subject, I must mention a long road trip which Bob, I and another friend, Carl, took to Florida during spring break in 1959. We drove all the way to Key West from Chicago, and hopped a plane to Havana, Cuba, for a few days. That was shortly after Fidel Castro had taken over. Fifty years later, we were to reminisce over the vivid memories of our exploits during that trip.

With the approaching senior year, the time finally arrived to apply for admission into medical school. I remember the day when a group of us took the medical aptitude test at Loyola University in Chicago. We were "shell-shocked" when we walked out of the building after the test, wondering how they expected us to know all of those "extraneous" facts. I comforted myself that we were all in the same boat and so dismissed any concern. We had come too far to worry at that point.

For medical school I had decided I wanted to return home to the University of Colorado; consequently, it was the only school to which I applied. I subsequently had an interview with Dr. Fitch, the dean, when I was home for Christmas in 1958. He appeared to be a very intuitive man, and seemed at the time to sense my strong desire for a medical education. The application process was complete by early 1959, and I was supposed to receive the university's decision regarding my application later in the spring.

That final spring quarter at Northwestern seemed to move slowly and, among other things, my studies focused heavily on aspects of electricity and magnetism in the challenging physics course. In addition my friend, Bob, has since been quick to remind me that I took Spanish that last quarter in college, having become interested by our recent encounters with the beautiful Hispanic girls in Cuba— a motivating factor that led me to an "A" in the course.

Then came the day I received a letter from Dean Fitch informing me that the fall freshman medical class at the University of Colorado had preferentially been filled by the premedical undergraduates from that school. He assured me, however, that I had been placed on the alternate list in the event that a slot would later open up. After so many years of aspiring to become a doctor, my hopes were suddenly dashed, and I had to cope with the deflating letdown.

But human beings by nature are tough and resilient, and I soon began sifting through alternative vocational goals. Again, I thought of the *Microbe Hunters* which I had read when twelve years old. Perhaps a place might exist for me in the remarkable field of microbiology, which had been further explored by the likes of Metchnikoff, Bruce, and Walter Reed.

Applications were thus sent out to several different postgraduate schools. I was accepted into its postgraduate program in biological science at the University of Illinois in Champaign-Urbana and so began refocusing on a purely scientific career. It was an exciting field of endeavor, a field that one of my pre-medical fraternity brothers, Don Cox, had decided to pursue years previously. Don later became a successful research virologist.

After having received my BA degree from Northwestern in June 1959, I again returned to work in Rocky Mountain National Park for the summer, anticipating with enthusiasm entering graduate school at the University of Illinois in September.

~~~

Late one Friday afternoon in August 1959, after returning to my cabin from work, I received a life-changing phone message from Dr. Fitch at Colorado's medical school. He informed me that he had just received a call from his friend, Dr. Walter Hard, dean of the medical school at the University of South Dakota. Dr. Hard had told Dr. Fitch
~~~

that there had been an unexpected slot which had opened up in the freshman class, inquiring whether he was aware of any immediate good prospects. When the Colorado dean recommended me, Dr. Hard agreed to my acceptance with the provision that I be present in his office at the medical school on Monday morning, three days later, in Vermillion, S.D. My fate as a doctor had rested in the hands of two influential men who believed in my potential, and I shall be forever grateful to them.

In those days the University of South Dakota School of Medicine was a two-year medical school in the basic sciences. Upon graduating with a Bachelor of Science degree in medicine, the students would then transfer to a four-year school for the remaining two years, culminating in the M.D. degree.

Given the greatest opportunity of my life to that point, I wasted no time in gathering up my belongings that night, and driving down those dark, narrow, winding roads out of the mountains en route to Denver. On Saturday I packed, took care of my finances, and fueled up my 1952 Ford in preparation for an early Sunday morning departure heading northeast through the tall, green Nebraska cornfields to South Dakota. The last thing I did before leaving Denver, out of respect to my recently deceased and closest childhood friend, Bill Berry, was to call his mom. I simply said, "Bess, I'm finally going to be a doctor!"

As I drove into Vermillion at about dusk on Sunday evening, I thought I was entering a small town out of an old Western movie. It was very rustic, having very few business establishments fronting the narrow, raised sidewalks. The main (and only) "drag" couldn't have been more than three blocks long. As I recall, there were no more than three places in which to eat. It was hot, dusty and, because of the nearby Missouri River, extremely humid. Insects of all kinds abounded, and I clearly remember a swarm of tiny aphids landing in my milkshake at MacDonald's. But as a Westerner with humble beginnings I felt right at home in Vermillion.

On Monday morning promptly at 8 A.M., I met Dr. Hard in his office. He was an imposing figure in his long white lab coat, standing well over 6 feet tall. He was gray and balding, and spoke with a deep authoritative voice while peering sternly over his dark rimmed glasses. There was little question who was in charge here. But as I shook his hand I sensed both a compassion and fairness; i.e., providing that this tough game of medical education was played strictly by his rules.

After a brief introduction into the structure of the curriculum at the medical school, he told me where I could immediately procure my microscope, white lab coats, and of course— the symbolic black bag with all of its contents.

He had even prearranged for me to live in a little room on the second floor of Matilda Gephardt's boarding house. That elderly lady lived two doors down from the Dean himself and had three upper-story rooms always occupied by medical students. We all shared an adjoining half-bath on the top floor but bathed in the basement, where a rather crude shower head projected down toward the cement floor from a pipe that was also rigged with a circular shower curtain. It was indeed a cold affair in the South Dakota winters. Furthermore, in order to get to the basement from our rooms, we had to parade down the stairs in our bathrobes and were highly visible to any family members or guests sitting at the dining room table by the staircase.

When I met my two upperclassman roommates, they wasted no time telling me how tough things were at the school, and how many didn't make it. Above all they emphasized: When you have to leave the house, always carry the largest book you have visibly tucked under your right arm. Remember, you are always being scrutinized by the Dean who lives but a few feet away, and who expects us to study all of the time. "Let him think you're going to the library— even if you're not!"

On Tuesday morning the freshman students met for the first time in the large class room. Everyone appeared a bit apprehensive as Dr. Hard entered the room to welcome us and to explain what was expected. At the onset, he made it quite clear that we were not going to be "spoon-fed" anatomy. "Given a copy of Gray's anatomy, a dissecting kit and a cadaver— you are expected to learn, in the utmost detail, the entire human body," he solemnly told us.

With regard to the cadavers there were to be four of us to each one, two students working on either side. The Dean warned us that first day that we were not to remove any body parts from the laboratory, and that the cadavers were to be treated with respect. He went on to elaborate: "These individuals have donated their bodies so that you students may learn anatomy; in so doing, they will probably make a greater contribution to humanity than any of the rest of us will ever make." Thus, one begins to gain some insight regarding the high moral plane of functioning of this man— Dr. Walter Hard.

Furthermore, in living up to his name, Dr. Hard admitted that the school was going to be demanding. Only those who were proficient would be allowed to graduate. The medical school had an excellent national reputation for turning out well trained medical scientists ready for transfer to other institutions for the final two years of clinical medicine. As a point of emphasis, he was frank in stating that although we had 44 incoming freshmen, the bus taking us to Sioux Falls for clinical work at the beginning of the sophomore year had only 36 seats — and they have never had to get a larger bus!

The professors wasted no time getting us started in the subject of gross anatomy, this course being the largest (five credit-hours) in medical school. Each morning, five days a week, we would convene in the anatomy laboratory in the basement of the medical school where, from eight until noon, we meticulously dissected and studied the human body. Other major courses studied that first semester were histology and neuroanatomy in addition to several other smaller courses.

The workload was enormous, much more so than college. But in contrast to college, this is what I wanted to do for my life's work, and that was motivation enough for me to become obsessive in my studying. Worthy of emphasis: Because it was so interesting learning the very fabric of the human body—to me it did not seem like work at all. What's more, I found a particular interest in the study of neuroanatomy. If one learns the central nervous system in the expected detail, with all of its intersecting nerves and tracts, a lesion placed almost anywhere within it can be localized upon careful examination of the patient. To be emphasized later, few areas of medicine offer the physician such a road map to the diagnosis. This was a fascinating subject which was taught by Dean Hard, himself a neuroanatomist.

After having been at USD for two weeks, I again heard from Dean Fitch at Colorado's medical school. Apparently they had recently had a student drop out, and the Dean offered me the opportunity of coming back to the University of Colorado School of Medicine after all. I graciously thanked him but declined the offer, while telling him that I was well pleased with South Dakota's medical school.

As the semester progressed it seemed like we were expected to learn an ever-increasing, inordinate volume of material within the allotted time frame. There was literally no time for anything else.

As we became more involved in the coursework, the escalating stress of the forthcoming examinations began to affect us all; unfortunately, not everyone passed when the posted grades began to appear on the Dean's door. In addition to the written tests, oral examinations were given in the dissecting laboratory, whereby each student would move from one cadaver to another while answering questions concerning the identification of various structures and their anatomic relationships. I recall one student who would consistently smoke several cigarettes in the hallway, and would often vomit prior to each oral examination. During the course of questioning he would visibly tremble, sweat and stammer while trying to grope for the correct answer. That unfortunate fellow ended up failing the entire year.

We adjourned for Christmas for an extended holiday vacation allowing me the much needed opportunity to be with my family in Denver. I soon found, however, that I couldn't sleep at night because of incessant worrying about school. Final examinations were scheduled for mid-January. In the meantime we not only had to review the entire human body (including the brain and spinal cord), but also had to dissect out and learn the lower extremities on the cadaver as well. The mere thought of the enormity of the task at hand was enough to launch me into the Ford and back to Vermillion one week early.

Despite the pace being torrid and the material voluminous, I saw it as doable. I knew very well that what was being learned provided me with the tools with which I was going to practice medicine. And when the workload began to obscure my purpose, I would fetch my black bag from the corner of the closet and examine the bright new instruments. With renewed enthusiasm and a resurgence of motivation, I would then return to my Gray's anatomy.

At semester's end I clearly recall several of us timidly walking up to the Dean's door to observe the posted final grades. Upon seeing my class standing, I felt an immense sense of relief and accomplishment. While saying nothing, I quietly strolled away with an enhanced confidence to succeed, humbly aware that I had not let those down who had given me this unique opportunity.

During the second semester, even though the subject matter was different, it was just as demanding. Biochemistry raised concern not because it was particularly difficult, but because it was so voluminous. I have spoken with colleagues in later years who were quick to concur. One could ill-afford to miss a single lecture, for if he did— there was simply no time to make it up! The next day the professor would expose us to an equally imposing amount of new material.

When summer arrived, it was back to work saving money for the next year. It was refreshing to savor the fresh fragrance and beauty of the mountains adorned with pine and aspen, while crowned with contrasting glaciers and rock-faces. I certainly appreciated the break from the monotony of studying, but by the time the fall came, I was anxious to tackle the second year.

The sophomore year was extremely interesting, as we were exposed to the study of disease (pathology) and its treatment (pharmacology), along with a host of other subjects.

As a sidelight, on May 5, 1961, while we were in the middle of a written examination in clinical pathology, Dr. Hard entered the room to proudly announce: Alan B. Shepard had just been successfully recovered from the sea as America's first astronaut to have traveled in space after having made a sub-orbital flight in his Mercury capsule. While the Dean was cognizant that we were all in deep concentration, I saw this as the act of a proud and patriotic American, sharing important breaking news with his students.

The final month of the second year was to be spent with a family doctor (preceptor) in one of South Dakota's towns. Mine was spent with Dr. John Rodine in Aberdeen, a town not far from the North Dakota border. He was a solo general practitioner with a solid surgical background. After first settling down in a rooming house, I found myself constantly on-call and was expected to tag along with him, either to his office or in surgery at the hospital. I will never forget the first night there, when I was startled by my ringing bedside phone about 3:00 A.M. I was instructed by the operator to meet Dr. Rodine immediately at the hospital for the anticipated birth of a baby. I hurriedly dressed and was on my way in the old Ford, fully realizing for the first time what it was really like to be a doctor. Upon entering the delivery suite I was tersely greeted by a nurse who instructed me to scrub my hands with a brush, and then don sterile gown and gloves. My sleep- deprived mind became muddled when I left the sink, only to have the nurses begin rudely shouting that I had scrubbed my hands neither correctly nor long enough. After repeating the scrubbing process, I again returned to the operating room only to have them scream at me even louder… to hold up my arms, not touch anything, etc. While Dr. Rodine was busy delivering the baby, I felt positively stupid, humiliated by my ignorance of sterile technique in front of all of those nurses, young and old alike. But suddenly finding oneself in this "boot-camp" like situation was merely the beginning of learning the strict discipline of the operating room.

Dr. Rodine, like my grandfather, was the prototype of whom one would envision as a dedicated, hard working, caring family physician. After that Aberdeen experience I decided that by entering a future residency in general surgery, I could still work with my hands, and also enjoy a general practice like Dr. Rodine's. That man has since remained ingrained in my mind as both an exemplary mentor and a strong inspiration.

Earlier in the spring, the time had arrived for me to decide where I would prefer to spend my last two years of medical school. I had been told that I could go wherever I chose. After serious thought I elected to return to Northwestern University in Chicago, a highly regarded institution, and located in an area with which I was familiar. When my letter of acceptance arrived, I was very pleased and eager to begin my clinical years at the Chicago campus after another summer of mountain work.

~~~

As an introduction to the final two years of medical school during which the medical student is consistently engaged in seeing patients, I would like to cite an often quoted passage by Sir William Osler: "To study the phenomena of disease without books is to sail an uncharted sea, while to study books without patients is not to go to sea at all." (15).

The journey back to Chicago was full of great expectations as I entered those clinical years. I won't bother the reader with all of the required courses presented to the student of medicine but will highlight a few memorable experiences.

Noteworthy was my three-month surgical clerkship, as a junior, which was spent at the famous Cook County Hospital, at one time considered not only the largest such facility in the U.S., but also one of the largest in the world. It was within those same walls that my grandfather had completed his postgraduate internship training in 1908.

One morning during my rotation within that gigantic old facility, several of my classmates and I were required to observe Dr. Robert Freeark, professor of surgery at Northwestern and chief of surgery at Cook County Hospital, perform an ablation of an aneurysm of the hepatic artery. At about 8 A.M., I remember entering that old antiquated operating room with its prominent skylights as we gathered around to observe the surgeon who, in deep concentration, began meticulously dissecting the aneurysmal sac. We later had to depart for surgical rounds and lectures. Finally, after having had lunch, we returned at about noon to the operating room where we found Dr. Freeark still bent over the patient in the same position, having hardly moved his feet, while continuing to work fervently on the aneurysm. I wondered to myself how
~~~

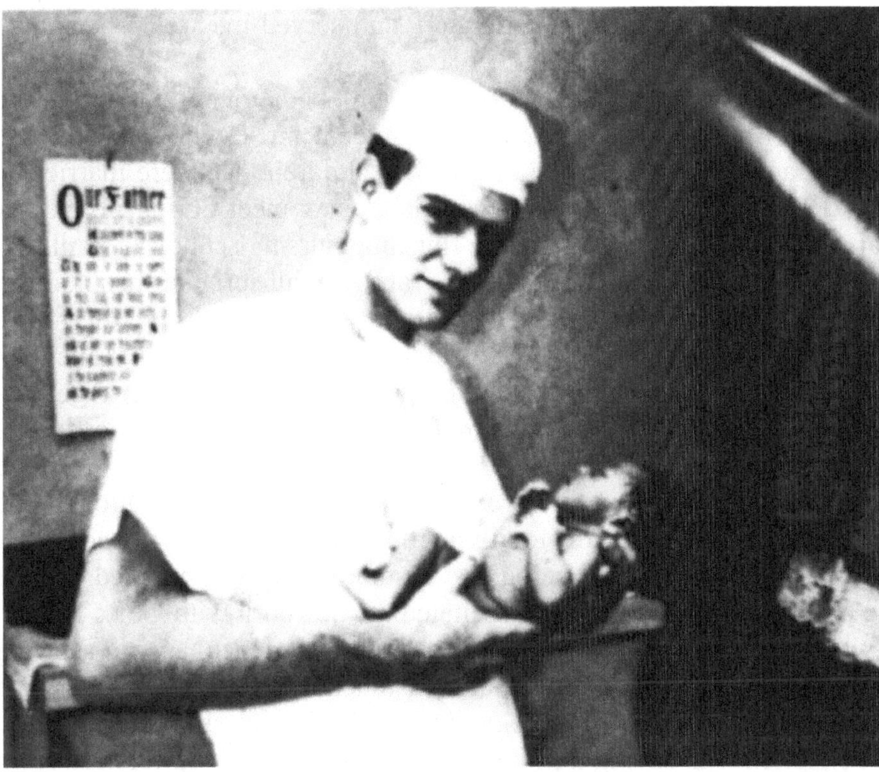

The Medical Student

an individual could possibly generate the mental and physical stamina to endure such a daunting task. That was my first exposure to a long and difficult surgical procedure. Dr. Freeark later became the ever more prestigious chairman of the department of surgery at Loyola University, and was considered one of America's foremost trauma surgeons of the time. As an early mentor in surgery, his bedside teaching techniques were exemplary, never to be forgotten, and served me well in teaching others in the years to follow.

During that junior year, while on my pediatrics rotation at the Children's Memorial Hospital, I met a student nurse who later became my wife and the mother-to-be of our four children. We were married in June, 1962, in Chicago. In order to make ends meet during my senior year, she worked extra hours while finishing nursing school; I, similarly, "moonlighted" by delivering babies at a small private hospital on Chicago's North Shore Drive.

During a stint at that small hospital, I recall one particular incident occurring in the middle of the night when I was assisting a general practitioner. He had just delivered a very large, deeply cyanotic, unresponsive baby. After several unsuccessful attempts to initiate spontaneous breathing with the customary slapping of the buttocks, the doctor panicked and became totally ineffective. He literally did not know what to do next. Despite being just a student, I felt compelled to take over, much to his relief, and resuscitated the newborn with CPR. To date it was my most exciting and rewarding experience as an aspiring physician when the little guy sputtered mucous, and burst forth with a loud cry, the pink hue of life beginning to glow in his skin. This was my first experience in saving a life; certainly, it was a big step forward from the textbooks.

During my senior year I had a three-month elective quarter in which I chose a clinical clerkship in neurology. Because of my previous fascination with neuroanatomy, I thought it prudent to look closely at that specialty. It was fascinating following the professor around as he examined patients with various interesting maladies, thereafter clearly setting forth a very academic differential diagnosis on each. While on that service I also first became acquainted with neuropharmacology. To cite a relevant example: In those days migraine headache was thought to consist of two phases of activity involving the smooth muscle of the blood vessels to the head. The initial component was a vasoconstrictive phase, restricting blood flow, and causing visual disturbance with blind spots and shimmering lights. This was followed by a vasodilatory phase which produced the headache itself. A drug appeared on the market named Cafergot, which contained both caffeine and ergotomine, drugs that caused therapeutic dilatation and constriction, respectively, of the affected intracranial arteries; hence, it treated both phases of the migraine attack. Recalling the physiology laboratory as a freshman medical student in which we witnessed contraction and relaxation of arterial smooth muscle, I now saw a practical application in treating a disease. The information learned in the physiology laboratory was now being carried to the patient's bedside. Something as straight-forward as this made a great deal of sense and dramatically heightened my interest in neurology. I even contemplated it as a future specialty after that rotation. But with the passage of time, it seemed that I developed keen interests in several specialties after ensuing clerkships. To be honest, I considered at least half a dozen areas of medical practice in which I could have achieved self-fulfillment. However, general surgery remained foremost. It not only provided the opportunity to work with my hands, but also offered the prospect of an immediate therapeutic result.

Several months after that neurology experience, another major trigger event occurred in directing my future. One afternoon I was sitting in the auditorium at the well-recognized Chicago Children's Memorial Hospital listening to a lecture on contrast myelography given by Dr. Anthony J. Raimondi, a pediatric neurosurgeon on the faculty. Dr. Raimondi stood at the blackboard drawing the contrast-filled spinal canal in both the frontal and the lateral geometric planes, beautifully demonstrating the relationship of the spinal cord shadow to an intraspinal tumor. It was a masterful presentation which had me on the very edge of my seat, something I related to him years later. While on the way driving back to our apartment, I thought to myself, "Why not combine surgery with neurology?" Upon arriving at home that night I told my wife that I should seriously consider becoming a neurological surgeon. Both the wherewithal to diagnose neurological disease, combined with the surgical expertise to treat it, offered me the best of what I wanted from both worlds. That decision was soon final, and I never looked back!

Northwestern was unusual, in-so-far, as it had two neurosurgical residency programs in those days. One was at Passavant Memorial Hospital under the directorship of Dr. Loyal Davis. I first contacted Dr. Nicholas Wetzel, who was Dr. Davis's partner and expressed an interest in neurological surgery. He later invited me into the operating room one day, when he and Dr. Davis were removing a tumor from within the spinal cord. After donning a mask and gown, I caught my first glimpse of that remarkable structure covered with its veil of tiny vessels, pulsating in its glistening bath of cerebrospinal fluid. Just to have been invited to observe that organ with a diameter smaller than a dime— yet able to control every movement of our extremities— was a privilege few ever enjoy.

Subsequently, after further interviews and after having examined my record, a future position in Dr. Davis's neurosurgical residency program was offered to me along with one of my classmates, Leonard Kranzler. Our appointments were provisional with one stipulation— they were contingent upon our spending both the postgraduate year of internship and also the required first year of general surgical residency at Passavant Hospital under the watchful eye of Dr. Davis. Among many other things, Dr. Loyal Davis had also been the chairman of the department of surgery at Northwestern's medical school for 30 years, had edited Christopher's famous textbook of surgery, and was an instrumental figure in the function of the American College of Surgeons. Furthermore, he not only had personally trained under Harvey Cushing, the father of neurological surgery, but was also the father-in-law of the governor of California at the time— Ronald Reagan. What a wonderful opportunity it was to enter into this very demanding specialty, still in its infancy, under the tutelage of such a prominent surgeon and educator.

When June 1963 arrived, I proudly received my M.D. degree from Northwestern University and the realization of my childhood dream. Like so many parents around our country, my mother and father were very proud of their son who had finally become a doctor of medicine.

~~~
~~~

THREE

The Molding of a Neurosurgeon

~~~

My mixed medical internship at Passavant hospital began in June 1963. Now was the time to begin taking full responsibility for the patient, and, in so doing, to apply the knowledge gathered from the books over so many years. At that time the only state in the U.S. not requiring a year of internship out of medical school prior to licensure was Mississippi. Of course we always worked under the supervision of the residents and medical staff, but, for the most part, the intern made the initial "call" in the management of such complex illnesses as diabetes, hypertension and heart disease. Moreover, I was even to get paid $200 a month! It wasn't much, but for the first time in the educational process, money began to flow in my direction.

Let me cite one disease entity illustrating the magnitude of the intern's responsibility: I can recall several occasions when I, along with the nighttime nursing supervisor, was called to treat patients with massive upper gastrointestinal hemorrhage from ruptured esophageal varices (distended veins) due to the end-stage liver disease (cirrhosis) of chronic alcoholism. The sight and smell of a terrified patient vomiting and choking to death on his own blood, as it spewed forth from his mouth all over the bed clothes, is something never to be forgotten. The patient's life depended not only upon the speed with which we could insert an intravenous line to begin transfusing fluids and blood but also upon creation of a tamponade to stop the bleeding by passage of a large inflatable tube (Blakemore) down the esophagus of the struggling person in peril. Today that nightmare can largely be averted using modern fiber-optic diagnosis and treatment.

A high point in the year was the month spent on the renal-dialysis unit with Dr. Francisco Del Greco, a brilliant internist and renal
~~~

physiologist. Each morning at 7 o'clock we would plan and chart out the fluid and nutritional management for the ensuing 24 hours for each of the gravely ill patients plagued by loss of kidney function. Some were in such dire straits that their fluid and electrolyte requirements had to be meticulously calculated daily on a milliliter / milliequivalent basis respectively prior to peritoneal dialysis. I recall one poor, sallow middle-aged man whose heart and kidneys had been ravaged by rheumatic fever, a serious complication of streptococcal infection. His renal output was nil, his heart always on the brink of congestive failure, and his lungs in a potential state of pulmonary edema from excessive fluid accumulation. He lay there with a hopeless look, as if he all too clearly realized death was imminent, yet yearning for a mere sip of water; something not allowed lest this delicate balance between life and death be wrongly tipped. We had to put chains and padlocks on the faucets in his room to prevent the man from killing himself with a drink. Although not satisfying his thirst, any fluid given to this pitiful soul had to be delivered intravenously in conformity with our careful calculations. But we kept him alive to see the sunrise each day, always hoping that we could at some time deliver him a kidney through transplantation, a procedure in its infancy in our hospital. Such was his status at the time that I departed from the service. Dr. Del Greco outwardly encouraged me to specialize in this challenging branch of medicine, and I did give it strong consideration.

In moving on to an entirely different subject: It had always been customary for the surgical residents to cover the emergency room at Passavant hospital. One night, without informing the senior medical staff, one of them signed out to one of my intern colleagues. When Dr. Davis got word of the switch, he was absolutely livid, mandating thereafter that the interns— not the residents— would cover the emergency room. Furthermore, each would have that duty by himself for one month straight, day and night— the only relief being from 8 P.M. Sunday evenings until 7 A.M. Monday. The intern alone was to see, examine and recommend treatment for each and every patient during that entire month.

While it was a marvelous experience from a medical point of view, it was an absolutely brutal one. The days and nights began to blend together as one, the only distinction not being related to changing sunlight (there were no windows) but rather to the greater extent of the day-time patient load. The single consistency during that month was a prolonged state of sleep deprivation. I remember late one night about two weeks into this marathon, when the hospital telephone operator awakened me in my quarters from a deep sleep, instructing me to go to the emergency room immediately. Hastily I got up, dressed, and scurried down, only to find the emergency department totally vacant. A surprised nurse asked me, "Doctor, why are you here? I didn't call you." Only at that moment did I realize that my sleep had been interrupted by an auditory hallucination, the result of extended sleep disturbance.

During that emergency room stint I had another disconcerting experience. One night a very obese, bull-necked man experienced a massive stroke from a deep brain hemorrhage. They wheeled him in on a gurney in a comatose state, his face suffused and plethoric. He was deeply cyanotic, and he labored to breathe with deep, stertorous respirations from an airway obstructed by a large swollen tongue clenched firmly between his teeth. With a compromised airway, death was imminent unless a tracheotomy could be performed. The nurse tried frantically to summon the surgical resident to the ER to assist me with the procedure, but it was to no avail — he did not answer his page. With great apprehension I stood watching this man die before my very eyes. Soon realizing there was no other recourse than to perform my first unsupervised tracheotomy— I proceeded. Although the procedure was successful in saving the man's life, the next day both the surgical resident and I found ourselves in serious trouble with the medical staff. It was like going before a military tribunal as they disciplined us. But from my standpoint, it had been a judgment call under the most dire of circumstances; I knew underneath it all that I had done the right thing.

On November 22, 1963, while making afternoon chart rounds with the junior resident in internal medicine, we were stunned as the nurse informed us that President John F. Kennedy had just been assassinated. The sorrow and emptiness of that tragic event loomed heavily over our hospital, as it did over the entire nation.

When rotating on the neurosurgical service as an intern, time after time I would witness patients dying from ruptured aneurysms, brain tumors and head injuries. I began to think that my chosen field of neurosurgery was a dismal, rather hopeless field of medicine. Then, on one particular occasion while trying to comfort a patient whose life was fading from an end-stage metastatic intracranial tumor, I had a rather sudden, sobering revelation. It occurred to me that because the mortality rate appeared so high in many of these conditions at that point in our history, things could hardly get any worse— only better. Anything that I, as an individual, could provide in the future to enhance survival would be an improvement. I had nothing to lose; there was much to gain.

The year was a very long one, and the on-call schedule demanded 36 hours working straight and then off for 12. One night I recall having come home exhausted after the end of a stint, and collapsed into a deep sleep before even eating dinner. Almost immediately the telephone rang. On the other end was the medical resident who, in a very demeaning tone, barked out, "Where are you, Jim? You are supposed to be taking two consecutive on-call rotations, and you are needed over here right away!"

Such was the year of the internship. It was the year in which material from the textbooks was applied directly to the patients on a daily basis. The aspiring young physician not only reinforced all of those many important facts that had been learned in medical school, but tried to become proficient in implementing them as well. There were no electronic devices to aid in proposing a differential diagnoses or in choosing a drug for immediate treatment. In those days our tools were diligence, persistent study and reliance on our memory. The end result was to gain in confidence as we developed our skills in patient management. We were no longer students in school, but doctors of medicine.

~~~

The second year out of medical school was spent in general surgery. One year of a general surgery residency was a prerequisite for most surgical subspecialties. In my case it was the first of a five-year program in neurological surgery. Dr. Loyal Davis was a strong proponent of that year in preparation for neurosurgery, feeling that in order to become a good neurological surgeon the candidate must first be a good general surgeon. That is to say: He must be well grounded not only in basic operative techniques, but also in metabolism, wound-healing, postoperative care, trauma, etc. This meant intensive general study and also preparation both to observe, and serve as first assistant on a great variety of surgical procedures. We residents had our own cadaver preserved in a tank across the street at the medical school building. Not infrequently at night in preparation for the ensuing day's operation, I would dissect the cadaver to review the pertinent surgical anatomy.

Another learning tool was the preparation of cases for the Surgical Grand Rounds, which was held Saturday mornings in the hospital auditorium. The presenting resident ran the conference for the entire
~~~

hospital surgical staff. This meant not only bringing the patient out on the stage and delivering the history and findings, but also citing pertinent information from the current medical literature as well. To gain an appreciation for the value of these large conferences, I will describe one of my teaching cases: a middle-aged man who had undergone a bowel resection for an intestinal disorder termed regional ileitis (Crohn's disease). To his misfortune, he developed a life-threatening abdominal infection (peritonitis), which necessitated his having to receive a large constellation of different antibiotics over several weeks. In those days we were limited as to the number of antibiotics even available, and because of the serious nature of the infection we were forced to administer very potent, if not potentially toxic, drugs in order to preserve his life. The focal point of that particular conference concerned the fact that he had developed a number of complications from many of the antibiotics received, some of which were extremely serious. They included: total kidney failure, loss of the use of his legs from peripheral neuropathy (nerve damage) and aplastic anemia (inability to make red blood cells) just to name the serious ones. One doesn't forget such a disastrous outcome, for this patient eventually died from the complications of his treatment rather than the primary illness.

During the year I rotated through three surgical services, each comprised of several different specialties, and each lasting four months. My total exposure covered everything from anal-rectal surgery to neurosurgery and almost everything in between.

I was responsible for all of the patients coming in on my service, usually having an intern and two medical students whom I would teach in return for their assistance with the workload. A typical day would consist of: rounds at 6 A.M., surgery all day and often well into the night, the late-day workup and preparation for the ensuing day's surgery of all newly admitted patients, and finally ending the day with late rounds. I had night call every third night, but usually wasn't home before 10 P.M. on my nights off.

The year, though at times quite arduous, was invaluable in molding me into becoming a surgeon. While mastering good surgical technique was an important part of that experience, learning good surgical judgment was equally important. When discussing judgment, we are speaking of evaluating a disease and deciding treatment in the best interest of a favorable outcome; namely, whether or not to operate, and if so, to remain within one's level of competence. Let me cite an illustrative case.

One day I was assisting one of the general surgeons, a full professor at Northwestern, who was tackling a cancer of the lower bowel. The tumor was located very high within the rectum. In a laudable effort to preserve the man's voluntary rectal function, the surgeon attempted a new procedure to remove the entire cancer from below rather than through the abdomen. The latter would have necessitated an inconvenient, diversionary colostomy. For what seemed like countless hours, he labored to remove the cancer; but the further he proceeded, the more hopeless it became. As his frustration level rose he began to perspire, his face became flushed. Soon thereafter he became totally ineffective. Completely exhausted, and desperate at that point, he said, "Jim, call Dr. Laufman to see if he can help us out." To me that was a courageous use of good judgment by humbly admitting defeat in front of the entire operating room staff, while seeking assistance for the good of the patient. Moreover, the patient ultimately did well, for Dr. Harold Laufman came in and immediately solved what had been an impasse.

Historically, Sir William Osler emphasized imperturbability or "cheerful" equanimity (aequanimitas) at times of either great success or disaster. In so doing the physician not only calms the patient, but retains his trust (15). A relevant example is cited:

Shortly after midnight, when adverse events so often seem to occur, the floor nurse summoned me to see a patient on whom we had performed an extensive abdominal operation for cancer earlier that day. She reported that he had suddenly begun to experience excruciating abdominal pain. Upon my arrival into his private room, I found an apprehensive, groaning man with a rapid, thready pulse and pale, moist skin. Upon gently pulling the bed sheets aside to examine his abdomen, I was aghast! He had experienced a total wound disruption, and there were at least twelve feet of small intestine piled up on his abdomen. As I quickly replaced the sheet, my pupils surely dilated and my heart "racing" in reaction to this frightful, first-time experience, I somehow was able to remain calm and vividly remember saying to him… "Sir, now just relax and everything is going to be okay. We are going to need to take you back to the operating room and fix you up a little bit." After the second procedure in which we closed the abdomen with stainless steel wire, he recovered. Sadly, he lived for only a few months before later succumbing to residual cancer. However, I don't think that patient ever did know what had actually transpired under those sheets that frightful night.

As a general surgical resident rotating through Dr. Davis's service in neurosurgery, I had a neurosurgical resident supervising me. Absolute perfection was expected of us at all times from this man who had studied under the master himself, Dr. Harvey Cushing. Every night I was expected to personally call Dr. Davis at home to update him on the status of all of his patients. If he wasn't there, he instructed me to report to his wife, Edie.

On a much lighter note, one Sunday morning when I was making early morning rounds with Dr. Davis, he informed me that he had two extra tickets in his pocket for the Bears vs. Packers football game that day at Wrigley Field. He invited my wife and me to join him and Edie in their box-seats. At the time I felt it was a privilege, even without realizing what the future would hold. In retrospect, it was a bright focal point in my life to have been able to enjoy a football game with the in-laws of the future president of the United States — Ronald Reagan.

November 21, 1964, was an exciting day for Robbie and me. It was the day our first child was born — Kim Dorinda Geissinger. My mother, who had given birth only to sons, was absolutely thrilled to have a granddaughter, and she flew to Chicago from Denver to be there at the time of her arrival.

At year's end Lenny Kranzler and I were told we had made the grade and were formally accepted by Dr. Davis as, what ultimately proved to be, his last two neurosurgical residents before his retirement.

Meanwhile, the nation was at war in Vietnam, and it looked certain that I would be drafted in the middle of my surgical training. However, an opportunity to voluntarily enlist in the armed forces arose in what was known as the Berry Plan. This option, as opposed to getting drafted in the middle of the year, had been introduced by Dr. Frank B. Berry. It basically guaranteed me my choice of the following: branch of service, the geographic area in which I would serve, and the opportunity to practice general surgery, that is, providing I enlisted and passed the physical at that time. I would then enter the armed service at the end of that year of the general surgery residency with a future service commitment for two years.

Luckily it worked out well for us. I received a letter in the spring of 1965 asking me to report to duty in July at Turner Air Force Base; Albany, Georgia, where I would be classified as a general surgeon with the rank of captain. The base itself was part of the Strategic Air Command, comprised of a B-52 bomber wing and a KC-135 Stratotanker refueling squadron.

~~~

My wife, baby daughter, Kim, and I drove from the cool, breezy Midwest to the warm, humid southeast, much relieved to get a respite from the demands of residency training.

Within a few days at Turner Field, I was clothed in Air Force blue, had been indoctrinated by the medical commander, and was settled in a large new three-bedroom house on a corner lot. My duties were to be those of a general surgeon with responsibility for the care of not only those active military personnel on the base but also all retired service personnel and their dependents in the entire area. The estimated total patient population was 39,000. The surgical responsibilities were to be shared with another young surgeon from Vanderbilt, who had also completed one year of general surgical training.

The hospital was an old, raised, wooden, multi-winged cantonment structure reminiscent of those during World War II with a 75-bed capacity, plus all of the ancillary support facilities such as x-ray, pharmacy, outpatient clinic and emergency room.

I recollect the first day of transition, when the departing, fully trained general surgeon took me on hospital ward rounds. Upon entering one of the long, narrow, multiple-bed wards, we immediately encountered a very pungent, nauseating odor. In the last bed at the far end was an elderly, retired, World War II submarine torpedoman with an infected, weeping, gangrenous leg. Severe diabetic vascular disease was the culprit. The despondent, unshaven veteran looked up at me with hope in his eyes as the departing surgeon tersely said, "I hate to leave you with this problem, but I have not been able to get him well without surgery."

After rounding on the poor old man for several days it became clearly evident that the leg was not viable. I so advised him that we should proceed with an amputation. He literally begged me to take the leg off, for he was non-ambulatory and failing fast. I performed a below-the-knee amputation on him, and he was subsequently fitted with a prosthesis, thereafter learning to walk again. Several weeks after the operation, on the day of his departure from the hospital en route to Atlanta for further rehabilitation, he thanked me time and time again for intervening to give him back a functional life. The tears welled up in his eyes as he handed to me an inspirational book which he had purchased for me as a gift. He was a most grateful patient, indeed.
~~~

That first year I spent intently studying and practicing general surgery. My partner, J.T., and I assisted each other on every major case, and we were fortunate to have exercised the judgment, surgical technique and postoperative care necessary for optimal results. Most of our work entailed the common problems generally seen in young airman such as hernias and hemorrhoids. For the latter we even administered our own epidural anesthesia.

The surgical experience was invaluable. To cite an example: By the time of discharge from the service I had personally performed over 100 appendectomies, having encountered just about every pathological type, position, and complication of that illness. Included were some appendices which had ruptured days before arriving under our care, already exhibiting fulminant, life-threatening peritonitis or abdominal abscess formation. Other times, the organ proved to be necrotic and friable, literally falling apart upon removal. Always to be remembered was the graphic case of appendiceal gangrene in which the organ was black and the size of a large sausage. I always felt that I should have written a small, descriptive monograph on my 24-month experience with appendicitis.

Other more radical cancer operations involving the neck, breast and abdomen were performed as well, thus, not only providing the necessary care for our large patient population, but also firmly grounding both of us in general surgery. To this day I am indebted to the Air Force for having given me that experience.

During that first year at the air base I learned that back in Chicago Dr. Loyal Davis was going to retire. As mentioned earlier, Northwestern had two neurosurgical training programs, one at Passavant Memorial hospital, and the other across the street at Chicago Wesley Memorial Hospital. Len Kranzler and I were now given the opportunity to transfer to the other Northwestern program. The latter was headed by Dr. Paul C. Bucy, also a preeminent neurosurgeon who was well-recognized the world over. Dr. Bucy had studied under the legendary Percival Bailey, himself a student of Harvey Cushing, and later the head of the Department of Neurosurgery at the University of Chicago. Dr. Bucy was board-certified not only in neurosurgery but also in neurology, and was well recognized as having taught many prominent neurosurgeons throughout the country. The Air Force sent me to a national neurosurgical meeting (then known as the Harvey Cushing Society) in St. Louis, where I met Dr. Bucy for the first time, and discussed my future training with him. The program consisted of four additional years beyond general surgery. One of those years was designated as an elective to be spent either in laboratory research or in one of the basic sciences. For my elective, I selected clinical neurology. Later, after having submitted my application, I was accepted at the University of Iowa under the chairmanship of the world preeminent neurologist, Dr. Adolf Sahs.

The nights and weekends of the second year at the air base were spent in preparation for that forthcoming year in neurology. This included reading in its entirety Crosby's textbook of *Correlative Anatomy of the Nervous System* (a book then commonly used in doctorate programs). Other basic textbooks read included those in neurology, neurophysiology, and cerebral angiography. Based upon past experience I knew there would be insufficient time in the rigorous grind of a residency program to read everything I would need to become proficient. Also, while in the Air Force, I was afforded the time to begin subscribing to the *Journal of Neurosurgery* (JNS). It seemed that I soon became riveted to virtually every article, especially, those on operative techniques.

In the JNS there commenced a series of articles on spontaneous subarachnoid hemorrhage, an entity often due to the rupture of intracranial aneurysms. Because that was the time when I first became interested in aneurysms, I will take this opportunity to enlighten the reader on this serious disease.

There are many of us who are familiar with the sudden death of either a national celebrity or a local citizen with a “stroke,” later attributed to the rupture of an aneurysm. Such a lesion is formed from the bulging and thinning out of an arterial blood vessel wall, such that it takes on a geometric configuration much like a miniscule light bulb; i.e., with a neck and a dome. Given enough time they have a propensity to rupture at the dome, resulting in a hemorrhage. The articles in the JNS on this condition were derived from a large multi-center university study and were based on thousands of cases of hemorrhage. From this data we gained much needed early insight into the pathology and natural history of these potentially deadly lesions. We learned, for example, that they may rupture during either wakefulness or sleep, and may hemorrhage irrespective of whether the victim is either straining or in repose. Both early and late mortality rates from the first hemorrhage were discussed. Should the patient survive the first hemorrhage, when might a second occur? Finally, the treatment options offering the best chance of survival were discussed. The general consensus out of this landmark study was that these unfortunate victims all needed some form of treatment. And if it could be safely done, probably the optimal therapy was surgical obliteration of the aneurysm neck.

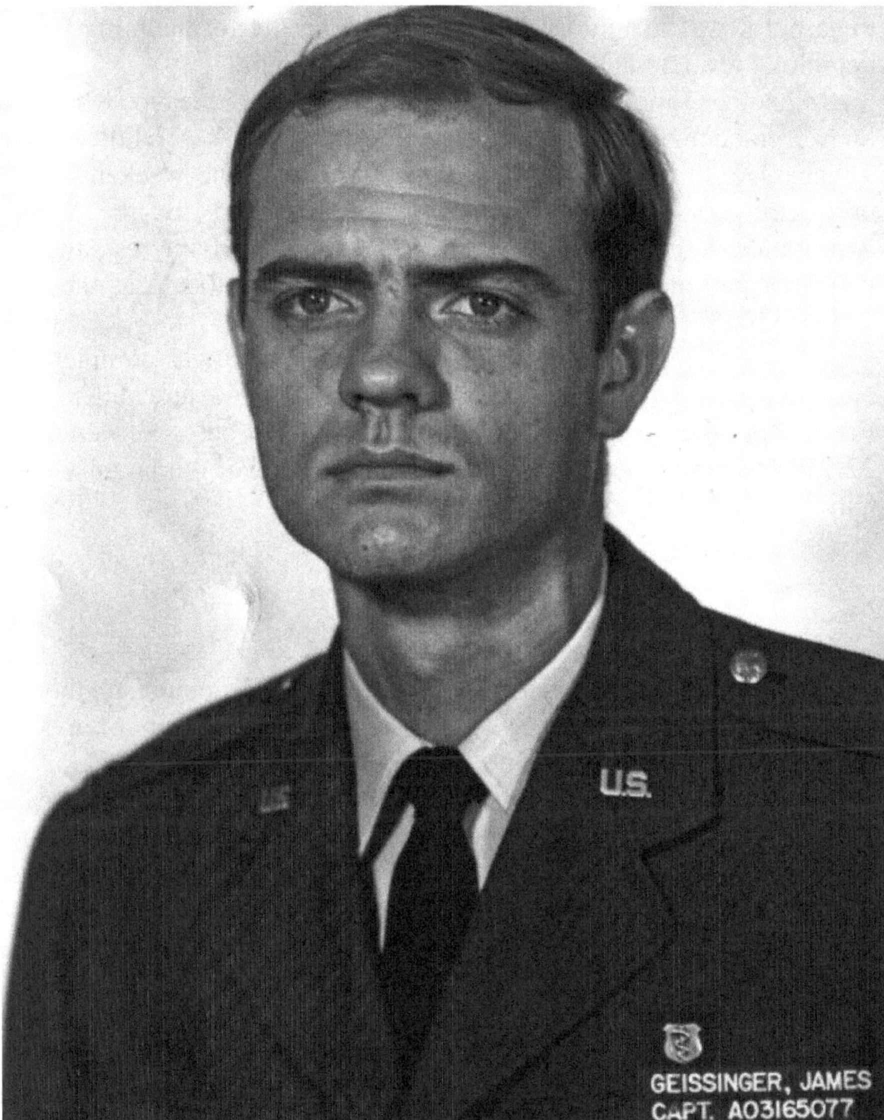

Captain USAF

Much to my surprise, the center of the study collecting and preparing for publication of all of these data on aneurysms was at the University of Iowa under the direction of Dr. A.L. Sahs. Not only was I intrigued by the series of articles on this disease which someday I would be asked to treat, but it was fortuitous that I would spend my forthcoming year as a neurology resident at the Cooperative Study center.

In another timely happenstance a friend from Chicago, who was by then a practicing radiologist 90 miles south of the Air Force Base in Tallahassee, Florida, invited us down for a visit one weekend. We not only enjoyed that trip but were also intrigued by the attractive appearance of both the town and the hospital. Of interest, there was neither a neurologist nor a neurosurgeon in that locale at the time—serious food for thought, indeed.

In June 1967 my tour of duty in the Air Force was completed, and after two very fruitful and enjoyable years, we bid farewell to Turner Field. My wife, daughter; and son, Jeff, who had been born on October 22, 1966, all left Georgia en route to the heartland of our country— Iowa City.

~~~

Dr. Adolph Sahs, co-author of one of the foremost textbooks in neurology at the time and the well-respected chairman of a leading neurology residency program, was now my mentor. The University Hospitals at Iowa City drew patients from a wide geographic area, and was a literal museum of both common and unusual neurological disorders. On the day of my arrival the senior neurology resident said, "Jim, by the time you leave here at the end of the year, there will be very few neurological diseases of which you haven't seen at least one example."

Every day of the week, including weekends and all holidays (not to exclude Christmas morning at 8 A.M.), either Dr. Sahs or his associate, Dr. Maurice Van Allen, would hold a "check clinic." The resident on-call the previous night would present each case admitted, whereupon the professor would examine the patient and would elegantly lay out a differential diagnosis on the blackboard. We learned directly by observing the master, not unlike the old European schools in which demonstrations were performed in an amphitheater.
~~~

I observed first-hand both adult and pediatric neurological disorders that I hadn't known even existed. For example, one day they pushed in a wheelchair in which sat a frighteningly ghoulish-appearing, albeit pitiful, blind man with a tall pointed head called turmschädel (tower skull). Also noted were his markedly protruding, horribly crossed, blood-shot eyes, and a persistent drooling from his mouth. His outward appearance depicted someone without any sense, whatsoever. By having had a premature fusion of multiple cranial sutures during infancy, his skull had grown tall and grotesque, but, as we soon learned, the brain was spared the ravages of pressure. Much to our surprise, when he was asked a question he responded in a very fluent, well-modulated, articulate manner— obviously a bright man, indeed. Interestingly, he was an accomplished individual in his chosen profession of journalism. He was reminiscent of the central character portrayed in the movie, *The Elephant Man* (1980 — starring Anthony Hopkins). The important difference was our patient's non-prejudicial acceptance into our society as a highly regarded talented human being despite his disturbing appearance.

Another very fascinating disease gaining worldwide attention, during my tenure at Iowa, was a condition termed normal pressure hydrocephalus (NPH). Just two years previously (1965), this treatable cause for dementia was reported in the *New England Journal of Medicine*, and we had the opportunity of observing several such cases. These were patients with a syndrome of urinary incontinence, gait disturbance and progressive (at times profound) dementia resembling Alzheimer's disease. Air ventriculography revealed enlarged fluid chambers (ventricles) within the brain, which were under normal pressure as directly measured with a spinal manometer. However, the enlarged ventricles were exerting a compressive force against adjacent brain tissue, leading to the symptoms—which could be reversed by surgically shunting the fluid. The enlarged ventricles (despite normal measured pressure) can be explained by Pascal's Law, $F = pa$; where F represents the total force within the ventricles, and "p" and "a" represent pressure and surface area, respectively. The enlarged brain-compressing chambers are likened to large tractor tires which have much lower measured pressure than thin racing bicycle tires, even though the total force within them is much greater (the pressure multiplied by the extensive surface area within the tire). This explains why the former support a much greater weight. I have just reintroduced a concept learned in high school physics class that can be applied not only to the basics of hydraulics but also medically to the human body.

Parenthetically, six months after having left Iowa, I had the pleasure of meeting one of the co-authors of that 1965 paper, Dr. William Sweet, chairman of neurosurgery at Harvard. Despite my only being a resident at the time, he shared his experiences of NPH with me at a national meeting in 1968 at the Broadmoor Hotel in Colorado Springs. I have fond memories of that evening conversation in which we enjoyed a mutual enthusiasm in discussing this very interesting condition. Worthy of emphasis is the fact that this is a curable form of dementia, the important message being that many people presenting as Alzheimer's disease may indeed have this reversible condition instead.

In terms of pathology at Iowa, we studied a multitude of disease entities including: genetic and metabolic disorders causing mental deficiency, various demyelinating diseases such as multiple sclerosis, neuromuscular disorders, cases of meningitis, encephalitis, strokes, and a wide spectrum of tumors. Equally important to the academic exposure to a host of diseases, many of them unfamiliar to the majority of doctors, was our instruction as to how to recognize them, namely, implementing the all-important history and a meticulous neurological examination.

Another highlight in the program consisted of a weekly conference presented by one of the neurology residents. He would research and write a paper on some recent development in neurology, thereafter presenting it to the entire group. In consonance with my aforementioned interest in neurochemistry as a medical student, I delivered a paper on catecholamine metabolism (neurotransmitters) — work done by Julius Axelrod for which he later received the Nobel Prize in 1970. I mention this only to emphasize that neurological surgeons often have an interest in all aspects of the nervous system and not merely the surgery thereof.

Dr. Bucy always emphasized that to become a good neurosurgeon means to have first been a good neurologist. Indeed, my experience at the University of Iowa was an indispensable part of my education, and one that I learned to appreciate even more over the course of time. A sound background in neurology allows the neurological surgeon to be able to readily differentiate between neurological conditions requiring surgery from those to be treated medically. Examples might include distinguishing brain symptoms due to a shunt obstruction from those due to a convulsion, or for him to be able to differentiate the symptoms of Lou Gehrig's disease from compressive cervical spondylotic myelopathy (spinal arthritis). Similarly, it is equally important that the medical neurologist recognize surgical conditions such as a spinal cord tumor, and not err with a diagnosis of multiple sclerosis. Although we have all missed a diagnosis from time to time, the probability of doing so is much reduced if one is well-versed in all aspects of neurological illness.

At year's end, I felt well prepared as both a neurologist and a general surgeon to enter the final phase of my training—neurosurgery itself. In July 1968, the family climbed into our black Volkswagen beetle, and headed back to Chicago for the final three years of neurosurgical training.

~~~

My last day on the neurology rotation fell on a Saturday, and the first day of neurosurgery was scheduled to begin Monday morning at the Evanston Hospital, a day's drive over into Illinois. Northwestern University had provided us with a beautiful apartment at the medical center in downtown Chicago, my wife and children already going ahead of me with the movers to have things set up.

I drove over to Chicago on Sunday in anticipation of work the following day. Sometime around 10 o'clock Sunday evening, I received a frantic phone call from an intensive-care nurse at the Evanston Hospital, after she had received word that I was the new neurosurgical resident scheduled to begin work on Monday. It seems that they had an emergency, and couldn't reach the physician whom I was replacing. Expectantly, they had been observing a patient who, two days previously, had undergone removal of her pituitary gland. Several hours prior to the phone call, the patient had suddenly experienced an excessive and continuous loss of water through her kidneys— a condition known as diabetes insipidus (DI). This is a hormonal deficient condition in which the kidneys are unable to reabsorb water filtering through them, the urine output often becoming dangerously voluminous. Moreover, if left untreated it can rapidly lead to dehydration with a fall in blood pressure— potentially resulting in shock or even death. While I had never even seen a case of DI, let alone treated one, I told the nurse to turn up the intravenous fluids to match the urine output, and I would be there as soon as possible. Thus, the stresses of a neurosurgical resident had begun two hours before I was even scheduled to start the job. My heart raced as I drove 15 miles up Lakeshore Drive in the middle of the night, trying to anticipate what I might find and how I would handle it. Shortly after my arrival, we fortunately not only managed to get the
~~~

patient stabilized with medication, but I had passed my first real test as the new (and only) neurosurgical resident in the entire hospital.

The next morning I met my two mentors: Dr. Joe Tarkington, himself a former trainee of Dr. Loyal Davis and thus a disciple of the strict, meticulous Cushing way of doing things, and his younger associate, Dr. Ivan Ciric, who was equally compulsive and a recent protégé of Dr. Paul Bucy's program. Therefore, I was privileged to have the good fortune of being the recipient of both lines of neurosurgical teaching— especially regarding surgical techniques.

No time was wasted in showing me around the hospital, and explaining my role on the service. I would be the sole neurosurgical resident in the facility for six straight months, was to be on-call 24 hours a day the entire time; and was expected to examine every neurosurgical patient whether they were routine admissions, consults, or emergency room cases. In addition, I was to run my own charity clinic, thus directly benefiting from hands-on surgery (under close supervision) when indicated.

There was, however, an immediate problem: It was mandatory that I reside strictly on the hospital premises for six months, and my family was currently living 15 miles away in Chicago. After nearly making a federal case out of it, the administration arranged for a tiny studio apartment on the hospital grounds to house my family. Robbie and I slept on a badly worn, pull-out sofa in the middle of the hot, linoleum-covered central living space. The only source of ventilation and cooling was through an open transom above the door to the hallway through which a bright light shined directly down upon us throughout the night. But at least I had my family with me.

In those days radiological imaging of the brain and spinal cord had to be provided by some form of contrast injection, the reason being a plain x-ray only reveals the bone and not the soft tissues. In the case of the brain, opaque contrast material was injected by direct puncture of the carotid artery in the neck or the brachial artery in the arm (angiography); alternatively, air could be injected into the ventricular chambers of the brain (pneumoencephalography or PEG).

In visualizing intraspinal structures, positive contrast oil was injected into the spinal canal through a lumbar puncture (myelography). It was critical to inject this material directly into the subarachnoid space, for not doing so would not only negate the results of the study, but could also cause serious irritation of the spinal nerves. In the literature, there had been isolated reports of arachnoiditis — a condition resulting in severe inflammation and scarring of the nerve roots leading to persistent pain and neurological disability. Each of these radiological procedures was like a "mini" operation in itself, and had to be a learned, precise skill—lest something go awry. Even in the best of hands, an incorrect needle placement could result in the extravasation of contrast material into the surrounding tissues, resulting in a failed study. This could become critical if radiographs were urgently needed in a life-or-death situation such as an intracranial hemorrhage. My mentors taught me well, and soon after becoming proficient in these techniques I was entrusted to work on their private patients.

Intracranial aneurysms were encountered from time to time, and the outcome in any given case was unpredictable. A few patients didn't even survive long enough for surgery, while others left the hospital in reasonably good condition. Some, however, despite meticulous, very skilled operative technique by the staff surgeons did not fare well. Everyone in the operating room invariably felt the extreme tension as the surgeon carefully dissected the neck of the aneurysm, at times for hours, in preparation for ligature. Sometimes the dome would rupture, flooding the operative field with blood, and obscuring the surgical site. On occasion there were instances when the patient either didn't fully awaken after surgery, or might regain consciousness, only to remain in a state of akinetic mutism. Other times they did awaken to a full sense of awareness but had major neurological deficit. I can distinctly remember after one such case when Dr. Tarkington, who was a meticulous surgical technician, said that he was at the point that he didn't believe he could tolerate another bad outcome from an aneurysm operation. And as I will point out later, he was far from being the only neurosurgeon in the country who was discouraged by the results.

These senior staff surgeons are credited with having been the first to show me fundamental surgical techniques in cranial and spinal surgery. In the case of the brain, I was taught the basics in approaching aneurysms and complicated tumors. In the process of being taught spinal intervertebral disc surgery, it was emphasized that the offending disc fragment compressing the nerve root should be removed in a relatively bloodless manner. This minimizes future scar formation—a common cause of the "failed back syndrome." And in the case of the cervical spine, depending upon the nature and location of the pathology involved, it could be approached from either the front or back side of the patient.

As an illustrative example of operative procedure, Dr. Ciric methodically instructed me in the technique of exposing the intracranial contents while properly removing a portion of the skull. I remember so vividly that first cranial procedure which I performed alone on one of my charity patients. It was a young boy who had a large brain cyst, which presented as a large skull deformity. The operation served as a prelude for my chosen field. Technically speaking it was not only successful but very rewarding when he later left the hospital with a childish grin spreading ear to ear.

With regard to the treatment of pain, it is now of historical interest that Dr. Ciric instructed me in the technique of percutaneous, radio-frequency (RF) cordotomy. In this procedure, a needle electrode is passed under x-ray control into a precise anatomical target within the spinal cord to ablate the pain-conducting fibers. The flow of current between two concentric metal conductors, separated by an insulator, causes a controlled, destructive heat lesion in the cord tissue. This can be done without any paralysis to the patient. The operation is a splendid example of clearly demonstrating the application of the neuroanatomy taught to me in the classroom many years previously by Dr. Hard.

The emergency room, while not as demanding as some in which I have worked, nonetheless bridled me both day and night for the entire six months. It also was a valuable learning experience, for it was a great source of thought-provoking, often interesting cases, which would appear unannounced, and demanding an immediate decision. Such examples might include the patient convulsing with a grand mal seizure, or an accident victim spiraling into a coma from a rapidly expanding intracranial hemorrhage.

The innovative nature of neurosurgery at the Evanston Hospital, then a satellite hospital in the Northwestern University system, is illustrated no better than in employing the technique of transsphenoidal hypophysectomy. This entails a procedure in which the pituitary gland, a tiny structure at the base of the brain, may be removed either in part or totally by an approach through the nasal cavity and skull base. While the operation was popularized by Cushing many decades earlier, it had since evolved into a high level of sophistication through the use of lateral fluoroscopic real-time x-ray imaging of the head, the surgical microscope, and the development of small, precision instruments. The patient preparation and technical setup alone took two hours before the incision was even made. Understandably, the list of orderly steps to be taken was quite extensive. I shall never forget the first such operation that I performed on my own. When it came time to setting up the microscope, I had difficulty recalling which of the several lenses had the appropriate focal length which, when attached to the microscope, would allow me adequate working depth of field. Dr. Tarkington gruffly shouted at me, "Jim, you were not paying attention when I did the operation!" In my own defense, it had been several weeks previously and, needless to say, I had been preoccupied with many other important aspects of the procedure. Such is the existence of a neurosurgical resident, who must work tirelessly and digest an endless amount of material while under the constant, critical scrutiny and demands of his superiors. One learns quickly to eat lots of humble pie.

To further amplify on the latter point, I shall end the discussion of the grueling, yet invaluable Evanston experience with the following story: I had been working there literally day and night for several months, when Dr. Tarkington approached me one Saturday morning and, with his hand on my shoulder, acknowledged what a good job I had done. He benevolently said that I had earned a well-deserved break. Later that day the University of Southern California football team with a running back by the name of O. J. Simpson was going to play Northwestern at Dyche Stadium— only a few blocks from the hospital. Dr. T. handed me a ticket, telling me to take the afternoon off, and to go over to the stadium and watch the game. He then qualified it by saying… "And while you're at it, be certain to sit in the west side stands." The doctor then further elaborated, "Jim, incidentally, before you leave for the stadium, first notify the nurses in the emergency department where you will be. In the event of an emergency, they will hang a large white sheet out of the fourth story window of the hospital. You must be on the lookout for the sheet, and will have no difficulty spotting it from the west side of the stadium. If that should occur, you must quickly get back to the hospital. Now go enjoy the game."

~~~

January, 1969, saw me back downtown at Chicago Wesley Memorial Hospital. Dr. Paul C. Bucy was not only our chief and our teacher but took a personal interest in those of us who were fortunate enough to have been his neurosurgical residents. Described as a man of extraordinary intellect and creativity, he was indeed a neurosurgical giant of the 20th century. Dr. Bucy was one of the true pioneers in neurological surgery
~~~

and was well-recognized worldwide. He was also a member of the original group which incorporated the American Board of Neurological Surgery in 1940. By virtue of his extensive laboratory and clinical experience, he had published nearly 200 scientific articles, and co-authored several textbooks in his field of expertise. In addition, he was formerly director of publications of the *Journal of Neurosurgery*, and, after his retirement, he created a new journal—*Surgical Neurology*. Finally, he was a superb teacher not only of medical students and neurosurgical residents in the United States but was also responsible for training foreign surgeons who would return to their native countries as the first to practice our specialty; e.g., in Malaysia and Thailand.

Early teaching rounds each day saw an entourage of residents, interns and medical students following the chief from one patient's bedside to another as he directed questions to each of us, always keeping an important academic point in mind. I vividly recall one such day shortly after my arrival on the service, when, after we had examined a patient with a visual disturbance, he asked me for my diagnosis. After I had confidently delivered my response, he then followed by asking, "What else, Jim?" Before the session ended he had extracted eight or nine possibilities out of me as to what the diagnosis might possibly have been. Thus was his method of teaching — never demeaning but thought-provoking, interesting and always instructive.

The surgical load at Wesley hospital was heavy by virtue of an abundance of patients with neurological disorders from the Chicago area; everyone was always busy. It was the responsibility of the current junior and senior residents assigned to the operating room at any one time to finish rounds and report to the surgical suite promptly at 6:30 A.M. Following the induction of anesthesia, we then shaved the patient's head with a straight-edge razor in preparation for cranial surgery, and, after positioning and draping him, we prepared to open up the cranium. The old time-honored procedure used for opening up the skull first consisted of marking out a curvilinear incision on the scalp, grossly based upon the estimated location of the underlying brain pathology. After reflecting the scalp, four or more spaced burr holes were bored using the hand trephine while following the same circumferential path of the skin incision. The underlying tough, fibrous dura mater covering the brain was then separated from the interior of the skull, and a heavy cutting wire (Gigli) drawn under the bone between any two adjacent holes. By attaching a handle to each end of the wire saw, the skull is then easily cut linearly between the burr holes. A series of such cuts then allows the bone plate to be totally removed. Although air driven drills and saws were available at the time, Dr. Bucy insisted that we perform all craniotomies in the same manner as our predecessors, namely, by using hand tools only. Wisely, he emphasized that power-driven instruments have a habit of failing at critical times, and the surgeon must not be thwarted at a time when the patient's life is at stake. After the residents had finished opening up the cranium, Dr. Bucy would then enter the operative theater and commence performing the main portion of the operation. When finished he would then exit, and we would close the wound.

I have herein attempted to give the reader some insight into the making of a neurosurgeon. The resident physician is technically involved from the onset, but stands aside as the master-teacher appears and executes the main phase of the procedure— his assistants always at his side, constantly benefitting from his skill and experience. This sequence is then repeated time after time during subsequent operations.

Most of the operations proceeded uneventfully, but one learns equally well from those which don't. I will describe two such cases.

The first incident occurred one morning when I was assisting the senior resident perform a craniectomy at the skull base with the patient in the sitting position. Upon trephining a burr hole into the skull, a frightful event suddenly occurred when he inadvertently entered a major venous sinus, cataclysmically resulting in a profuse, unrelenting hemorrhage. Unable to control the torrential bleeding, he asked the nurse to quickly summon Dr. Edir Sequeira, Dr.Bucy's young assistant, who was meanwhile making rounds in the hospital. As we desperately attempted to hold pressure over the deluge, Ed was at our side minutes later, and promptly controlled what was a potential life-threatening nightmare. He not only showed us how to manage this unforeseen surgical complication, but also manifested calm and composure in doing so. Later during my professional career, I would encounter similar unpredictable catastrophic events from time to time, and always managed to navigate through them, often asking myself — now what would Ed do under these circumstances?

As a beginning junior resident with relatively little neurosurgical experience, I was asked by Dr. Bear, one of the older attending staff neurosurgeons, to assist him on a craniotomy. It concerned a young, neurologically intact woman who had a very large avascular tumor mass beneath the brain's right occipital lobe. Angiographically, it was suspected that the mass was "extra-axial"; specifically, it appeared to originate outside of the brain substance, and invaginated into it. A strong consideration in the diagnosis was a large dermoid cyst attached to the tentorium below (dural layer covering the cerebellum). After we raised the occipital bone flap, the dura mater appeared only modestly tense. Once the underlying brain was exposed, Dr. Bear began carefully dissecting between the occipital lobe and the dural lining of the skull base, looking for the underlying mass. At that point in time, I sensed that the brain seemed to be swelling more than usual. Once well beneath the brain, Dr. Bear did indeed encounter the capsule of a benign dermoid cyst. My vantage point was poor as I stood holding the brain retractor, precluding my appreciation of what the doctor had to do in incising the cyst's capsule, and gutting out its contents. Nor could I appreciate any difficulties he might have had in controlling hemorrhage. However, I was soon to become aware of an alarming further increase in brain swelling. This rendered my retraction more difficult, resulting in an ever-decreasing size of the opening through which Dr. Bear was working to decompress the tumor. Minutes later, what was previously noted as severe brain swelling, suddenly escalated into what we term malignant brain edema. Large beads of perspiration drenched the professor's face as he desperately tried to access the tumor through a portal which was now rapidly closing shut. Then, within moments the brain began to actually extrude itself out of the cranial vault, and became strangulated by cutting off its own venous drainage. Soon to follow was brainstem failure, catastrophically resulting in the patient's death. This horrific, seemingly unavoidable and untreatable event was terrifying to everyone in the operating room. Needless to say, Dr. Bear was devastated beyond description. And I, as a prospective young neurosurgeon, was to keep this case indelibly in my mind for the rest of my professional career.

All neurosurgeons at some time face dire situations such as those just described. Nowhere is this better illustrated than in the case of General Leonard Wood, Dr. Harvey Cushing's most famous patient. After having lost the General after a second operation for an intracranial tumor, he basically never got over it. To quote the renowned neurophysiologist, John Fulton, who wrote Cushing's first biography…"He continues to talk about bad surgical judgment and remarked to Cairns the other day that the only thing he had accomplished since coming back from Europe was to kill an important person. Except for his son's death… I have never seen him so deeply affected by a disappointment" (2).

Throughout the book I will continue to cite instances in which the surgeon must shoulder the responsibility for a poor outcome, often resulting in self-deprecation of one's judgment at the time while trying to absolve guilt and lift the clouds of melancholy. It is the very nature of our difficult and challenging specialty. Despite using our best judgment, and the utmost care and skill, things do not always turn out favorably. While it is important to be self-critical in order to improve, persistently dwelling on an adverse result may lead to despondency and ineffectiveness. Relevant to what has just been written, and out of the greatest respect for my surgical colleagues, I would like to quote the following excerpt —"The Man in the Arena" by Theodore Roosevelt from his world-famous speech entitled, "Citizenship in a Republic" (April 23, 1910, at the Sorbonne in Paris).

> "It is not the critic who counts, not the man who points out how the strong man stumbles or where the doer of deeds could have done better. The credit belongs to the man who is actually in the arena, whose face is marred by dust and sweat and blood, who strives valiantly, who errs and comes up short again and again, because there is no effort without error or shortcoming, but who knows the great enthusiasms, the great devotions, who spends himself for worthy cause; who, at the best, knows, in the end, the triumph of high achievement, and who, at the worst, if he fails, at least he fails while daring greatly, so that his place shall never be with those cold and timid souls who know neither victory nor defeat." (43).

~~~

Aside from the practical experience of learning neurosurgical judgment and technique, another point of erudition afforded itself in Dr. Bucy's program. The atmosphere was replete with opportunities for both laboratory and clinical research. With regard to the latter, it was then that I first became introduced into writing scientific papers, two of which were presented at meetings of the Chicago Neurological Society.

Another important, well attended, biannual meeting in Chicago was the Central Neurosurgical Society. Neurosurgeons, many of them professors at universities, from all over the Midwest and Canada would attend, and the program was always excellent. Not infrequently, the
~~~

subject of intracranial aneurysms would appear on the program. Aneurysms seemed to be the plight of most neurosurgeons at the time, and as one of the visiting professors once said, "The surgical treatment of an aneurysm is the king of neurosurgical operations." At these Central Neurosurgical meetings, one aneurysm surgeon always seemed to stand above the rest. He was Dr. Charles Drake from London Ontario, Canada. Dr. Drake's superior surgical results established him as an early pioneer in this field, and this modest man commanded the utmost respect of neurosurgeons from both here and abroad. Impressive was the remarkable silence and attentiveness of the entire group as Dr. Drake would project his slides, and describe his technical methods of treating difficult cases. Following his presentations there was always an informal session, encompassing well directed questions from outstanding neurosurgeons— attempting to gain insight into Dr. Drake's early mastery over this killer disease.

The constant exposure to clinical research, writing papers and attending these meetings provided a sense of academia which I never seemed to lose during the ensuing professional years of my life.

A major highlight in the Bucy program consisted of monthly visits by neurosurgeons of prominence, not only from the United States but also from foreign countries around the globe such as England, France, the USSR, and Japan. The guest would arrive on Tuesday in preparation for Wednesday ward rounds in the morning and a formal presentation in the auditorium in the afternoon. On Tuesday evening the residents would dine alone with him in the small, elegant, dimly lit doctor's dining room with a white tablecloth and fine glassware. It afforded us the unique opportunity to ask him questions of neurosurgical relevance within an informal, relaxed setting. Dr. Bucy would intentionally abstain from the event, not wanting to interfere in any way with our interaction with the visiting professors.

Dr. Loyal Davis came out of retirement to join us on one such occasion, telling us about the time he spent studying under Dr. Cushing. We were fascinated to listen as Dr. Davis graphically described his first-hand experiences with the father of neurological surgery. Understandably, Dr. Cushing had to have been compulsive and obsessively meticulous in his neurosurgical technique as evidenced by his remarkable results very early in the 20th century— at a time in medical history without the benefit of contrast x-ray imaging, magnification, modern fine instrumentation or antibiotics! As one might surmise, he expected nothing but perfection from his assistants, thus establishing an early reputation not only as a surgeon beyond reproach but as a very stern taskmaster as well.

Another memorable resident dinner experience was with Dr. Edgar Kahn, professor of neurosurgery at the University of Michigan. When asked what had been his greatest neurosurgical challenge during his lifetime, Dr. Kahn replied that it was the intracranial removal of the craniopharygioma (congenital tumor in the region of the pituitary at the base of the brain). But he was then quick to add that the most rewarding operation was the release of the median nerve in the carpal tunnel syndrome. He had pioneered a surgical approach through the palm of the hand— as opposed to the wrist—this later becoming the standard approach used even to this day. Dr. Kahn was not only considered a gifted teacher and talented neurosurgeon, but also a quiet, humble, good human being. An interesting side-light is the fact that he was the neurosurgeon who served as the inspiration for the classic novel, *Magnificent Obsession*, by Lloyd Douglas. Dr. Kahn was played by actor Rock Hudson in the movie.

A memorable historical experience that year entailed Dr. Bucy's arranging for several of us to visit over afternoon tea with the then elderly and ailing Dr. Percival Bailey and his wife in their Chicago area home. Dr. Bailey was also an assistant under Cushing in the early part of the century, and together they described the microscopic characteristics and biological behavior of the gliomas (primary tumors) of the brain—a pathological classification still in use many decades later. Our group of neurosurgical residents was indeed humbled with this unique opportunity of visiting with one of the lasting legends of our specialty.

Collectively, these fireside-like sessions provided the residents with even greater insight into our profession. When listening to the younger of the professors from around the country/ world, we learned, firsthand, of ongoing research and newer techniques being developed outside of our own institution. And when attentive to those older men of neurosurgical prominence, we not only were given historical vignettes of alternative ways of doing things, but gleaned much from their experience and wisdom as well. We recognized that both they and their predecessors were the pillars of our neurosurgical heritage, and we appreciated the short time spent with each of them. It is unfortunate that for many in the succeeding generations of neurological surgeons, this respect for the wisdom and surgical heritage of our past seems to have largely been lost.

~~~

1969 was a memorable year in many respects, not only for me personally in my study of neurological surgery and my association with all of those outstanding mentors who contributed to it, but it was also an important year for our country: On July 20, 1969, Neil Armstrong was the first human being to set foot on the moon during the Apollo II mission, declaring it… "One small leap for a man, one giant step for mankind."

~~~

In January of 1970 my residency rotation again shifted; this time it sent me across Chicago to Children's Memorial Hospital (CMH) for six months of pediatric neurosurgery.

My professor at that institution was Dr. Anthony J. Raimondi, the man alluded to previously as having been a major figure in redirecting my life's course from general surgery into the neurological field. Years later, after Dr. Bucy's retirement, Dr. Raimondi became chairman of the division of neurological surgery at Northwestern University.

The case load at CMH was substantial, consisting primarily of newborns with hydrocephalus, spina bifida and craniosynostosis. Childhood trauma and craniospinal tumors encompassed much of the remainder.

At this juncture a brief description of hydrocephalus is in order because we shall be referring to it throughout the book. This is a condition resulting from either an obstruction to the circulation or a failure of absorption of cerebrospinal fluid (CSF), fluid produced in the ventricular chambers of the brain. If unchecked, it may lead to an increase in pressure and enlargement of those chambers— usually translating into subsequent head enlargement. Left untreated, the brain may fail to develop normally which can result in mental sub-normality. In advanced untreated cases, enormous head enlargement and severe brain destruction may ensue. In the 1950s the valve-regulated shunts, still in use today, were developed to divert the fluid into various body compartments, and by reducing pressure they allow for more normal brain development. Our mission at CMH was the early diagnosis and treatment of this condition in an effort to ensure normal brain growth and maturation.

Our pediatric neurosurgical staff consisted of me and my cohort, Marshall Cushman, serving as the only two junior residents; the senior resident and, of course, the staff neurosurgeons. On a weekly basis, either Marshall or I was scheduled to spend each day performing either arteriography or ventriculography in the x-ray department. In those days, we had to rely on these indirect contrast modalities of visualizing the intracranial contents. While we have previously discussed both procedures, things become much more complicated and difficult in babies. Not only are the blood vessels themselves miniscule compared to an adult's (therefore, being much more difficult to puncture), but also one is dealing with uncooperative, squirming, tiny newborns and infants who require some degree of sedation and restraint. These problems not only make it more difficult to obtain decent radiographs, but also increase the hazard of the procedures.

The second junior resident, alternating with his cohort, would spend his week in the operating room. In addition, we were each on-call alone at the hospital every other night for six months. Furthermore, the man on radiology for that week had to spend his nights off at home drawing diagrams of each radiographic contrast study done by him during that day.

The six months were grueling, and Marshall and I both— while harboring intense feelings of imprisonment—literally counted the days until it was over. One's routine would consist of early morning rounds, working in either the operating room or the radiology department all day every day, working up new patients and consultations later in the afternoon and early evening; and finally, checking all of the intravenous needle placements and fluids in the intensive care unit before retiring at night. Of course the man on-call any given night had to deal with any emergencies that might arise. There was little time for sleep, and no time for one's family.

As the days, nights and weeks all seemed to blend together, we began to lose perspective as to either the good which we were accomplishing at the time or the importance of pediatric neurosurgery in general. At one point Marshall even went to his program director at his parent university, trying to get relieved of the demanding pediatric rotation, but later told me…"Jim, I could not quit and conscientiously leave you here by yourself."

But the experience was invaluable, only to be realized in later years. Of paramount importance, we learned in great detail the various techniques of the abdominal and cardiac shunting procedures, having installed 65 of them in the first two months alone. Also, we became well-versed in the technique of performing multilayer, watertight closures for myelomeningoceles (congenital "bubble-like" sacks containing neural elements on babies' spines). Finally, it was important that we learned how to repair skulls where the sutures had prematurely fused, thereafter leading to future normal, and cosmetically-pleasing head growth. The overall pediatric experience, however, went much further than work done in the x-ray department and the operating room. In order to become a pediatric neurosurgeon, it is equally important to learn such fundamentals as the delicate handling of fragile tissues, the pediatric calculations of fluids and pharmacologic agents, and precise estimates of blood loss and replacement during hemorrhage in newborns and infants. While a hemorrhagic loss of 90 ml (3oz.) of blood is inconsequential in an adult, it could be fatal to a newborn.

In essence, that rigorous, intense period of pediatric training prepared me well for any infant or childhood neurosurgical problem that I might encounter in the future, enabling me to assist in providing an important service in medical care to our community.

Speaking of children, a personal human interest story will end my discussion of CMH. On May 4, 1970, I was in deep concentration trying to puncture the carotid artery of a newborn, the vessel being not much larger than a matchstick, when the telephone began to ring. The nurse picked up, and relayed to me that my wife had gone into labor with our third child. While excited and trying to maintain a steady hand, yet realizing that time was of the essence; I did finish the arteriogram. I then quickly drove part way across Chicago, and was able to get my wife to the hospital in time to see our second baby daughter, Gretchen, take her first breath.

~~~

On June 17, 1970 at the annual meeting of the American Neurological Association (ANA) in Atlantic City, New Jersey, Dr. Bucy and I had been asked to present a clinical research paper which we had co-authored on a particular childhood brain tumor —the cerebellar astrocytoma.
~~~

Two events occurred earlier in the day on which I had been scheduled to take the podium before this large, prestigious group: Foremost, Dr. Bucy had been voted president-elect of the ANA for the ensuing year; and secondly, he had just been summoned to Washington, D.C., to appear as an adviser before a committee at the National Institute of Health. Because of abruptly having to leave, he called me aside, telling me that I was going to have to carry the ball alone in presenting our paper.

While only a junior resident, and with my mentor and their next president being absent, I felt an immense pressure to do well in presenting a landmark manuscript before this critical group of world renowned neurologists. Certainly, I cannot recall a more important professional event in my life.

~~~

The final year of a neurosurgical residency is always spent as senior resident at one of the teaching hospitals as designated by the program director. In my case it was at the Veterans Administration Research Hospital (VARH) in Chicago.

Included with me on the house staff were a general surgical resident and a junior neurosurgical resident. Collectively, we were responsible for each patient's evaluation and work up including x-ray contrast studies, any indicated surgery, and all postoperative follow-up during the time remaining in the year. There were two attending faculty neurosurgeons, Dr. Nicholas Wetzel and Dr. Daniel Ruge, to oversee our service, but we were basically entrusted to accomplish the work on our own. For the board certification process, I was required to manage all activities on the neurosurgical service, and to be the primary operating surgeon.

The first craniotomy that I solely performed that year involving a brain tumor has remained an indelible signature case in my mind. The patient was a young man who had slowly become blind (could discern minimal light only) in his right eye. His subsequent work-up revealed a tumor involving the right optic nerve, and was thought to represent an optic nerve glioma. Realizing that we could not restore the lost vision in the right eye, but could possibly prevent extension of the lesion into the left optic nerve through the optic chiasm, we elected to operate. The approach used was through a right frontal craniotomy. An osteoplastic
~~~

bone flap was first reflected, after which the right cerebral hemisphere was carefully retracted. We next entered the right orbital cavity through the skull base. Out of concerns for safety and because of the long working distance, I elected to use a six-inch extension on the hand brace (trepan) to begin that phase of the operation. Once the trephination was completed, a portion of the orbital roof was then removed with a *rongeur*, thus exposing the intra-orbital contents. The tumor, an astrocytoma inextricably involving the optic nerve, was then removed in its entirety. By having correctly made the diagnosis, and orchestrated the procedure successfully, I found the removal of this man's tumor to be a pivotal case in my training. Extirpating that tumor represented the culmination of many years of study, sacrifice and hard work. The challenge and satisfaction of having accomplished this operation assured me that I had indeed chosen the right field of medicine.

We were fortunate to have had a good cross-section of case material at the VA hospital that year. It proved representative of the more common cases one might expect in the private practice of neurological surgery, plus some of the more unusual cases as well. Allow me to discuss one such rare encounter.

I was asked to consult on a man whose symptoms consisted of neck pain, tingling of his hands and feet, and of nearly blacking out each time he would attempt to rotate his head to the left upon entering a motor expressway. A plain x-ray of his neck suggested a tumor smoothly eroding three of the cervical vertebrae. His work up corroborated a spinal tumor which had totally occluded the left vertebral artery supplying his brain. When turning his head, he would partially block the contralateral or normal right artery, basically shutting down the blood flow to the hindbrain. We were able to totally extirpate this benign neoplasm, a neurofibroma, and cure him while concurrently relieving his symptoms of pain and tingling. However, he was instructed to forever be cautious of extreme rotational movements of his head, lest he could still black out. In totally removing his tumor, we had to sacrifice the compressed artery which was completely encased and destroyed by the neoplasm.

We later published this unusual case in one of the British medical journals in 1972. Of historical interest is the fact that one of the co-authors of this paper, Dr. Daniel Ruge, subsequently was appointed President Ronald Reagan's personal physician. This was a position which Dr. Ruge was holding on March 30, 1981, the day of the assassination attempt on the president's life by John Hinckley Jr.

Other important events occurred during that last year of residency training, but none more important than a job offer in Tallahassee, Florida, the town we had visited while in the Air Force several years previously. It seems that a neurosurgeon and a neurologist had set up a neurological clinic in Tallahassee 18 months after we had visited there in early 1967. By the time I was ready to finish my training in Chicago, they badly needed a third man to help with the heavy patient load; hence, they extended me an offer to join them. After two subsequent trips down south, I committed to the clinic, purchased a lot, and even hired a contractor to build my first house. Several months later I traveled again to Florida, that time to Jacksonville, where I was to sit for the lengthy state board examination for medical licensure. Even though I was a Diplomat of the National Board of Medical Examiners, Florida unfortunately did not recognize reciprocity with them. The state mandated that all applicants for licensure pass the difficult, comprehensive, two-day Florida examination. After having taken the test I was supposed to receive the results within four weeks. Well over two months passed and I still hadn't heard a word. So very much was predicated upon my passing that single examination: My family, a future medical partner, and a building contractor were all depending upon me. In essence, my future in Florida was held in balance, and I began anguishing daily over the possibility that I had perhaps failed. The entire set of circumstances surrounding that Florida Board experience caused more consternation, I believe, than anything I might have encountered up to that point in my life. At long last…the only remaining obstacle separating 29 years of diligent study and my future as a practicing neurosurgeon was removed— I finally received word that I had passed that pressing state board examination!

When June, 1971, rolled around, we were finally ready to bid farewell to Chicago and set out driving to the land of sunshine, an enviable place to practice medicine and raise a family.

~~~
~~~

FOUR

Ascending the Mountain of Experience

~~~

Throughout the years people have often asked me why I chose Tallahassee, Florida, as a place to practice neurosurgery. My first consideration necessarily had to answer the question of the community's need for another neurosurgeon. What type of population base would require such a specialty? When Dr. James Lyerly, the first neurosurgeon in Florida, began practicing in Jacksonville, I understand he provided service to a total referral area of at least 500,000 people. He then became so busy that he called my chief in Chicago, Dr. Paul Bucy, asking whether he knew of someone who could join him. Of course, those were the days when the scope of neurosurgery was somewhat limited. But with the advent of newer techniques and innovations, the neurosurgeon could subsequently provide a broader spectrum of services unthinkable years before; as a result, the extent of the total population-in-need had become smaller. The figure highlighted when I entered into practice was one neurosurgeon per 100,000 people. Since our county (Leon) totaled 150,000, and our geographic referral area extended as far as Gainesville to the southeast and Pensacola to the west, while reaching well above Moultrie, Georgia to the north — we well exceeded the support limit.

A second consideration was the scope of neurosurgery to be practiced. I had previously been offered an opportunity to practice solo in a small town out west, but immediately recognized that my practice would have been weighted heavily on the trauma side, the more complicated and interesting cases fleeting past my hospital en route to a nearby university medical center. To the contrary, my future partner in Tallahassee, Dr. Frank Davis, after having been in practice for two years,
~~~

assured me that we would have a wide variety of cases which would prove both interesting and challenging.

Another major criterion concerned the town itself. Tallahassee is a very picturesque small city, situated roughly at the junction of Florida's Panhandle with the peninsula, and is located 26 miles from the Gulf of Mexico. The greater area is laden with forests, rivers and lakes, and abounds with wildlife, beautiful flowers, and trees. Large towering oaks with Spanish moss draping from their limbs stand proudly to form canopies over many of the roadways emanating from the center of the city like the spokes of a wheel. Of historical interest is the fact that 36 square miles of land within Leon County had been a township granted by Congress in 1824 — 1825 to the Marquis de Lafayette in honor of his gallant and invaluable services during the American Revolution. The city is currently the seat of the state capital of Florida and the home of a community college and two state universities. The environmental landscape presents itself as a paradise for the outdoor sportsman, and there also exists a source of rich fulfillment in the cultural arts at Florida State University. Although basically there is no industry in Tallahassee, it is an economically stable area by virtue of the state government and university system. Furthermore, I was also told that Tallahassee was a splendid place in which to raise a family with all of its amenities and opportunities, both educational and recreational. In addition, because of the geographical location it offers a change of seasons— enough so that the fireplace can be stoked up in the wintertime. This is in contradistinction to South Florida which remains warm the year around.

When we settled in there was basically one hospital, Tallahassee Memorial, consisting of approximately 250 beds at the time. We had 152 doctors on the medical staff, with many, yet not all, specialties being represented. Even though it was small, the medical staff was a splendid one; its members freely exchanged medical information with one another, while exercising the wisdom and medical expertise necessary to provide optimal medical care.

Despite what has been said thus far, things were by no means perfect in those days. While difficult to believe, our ambulance service was provided by a funeral home! And then there were problems in the operating room: Although the nurse anesthetists provided a competent service, we had to carry out our complicated neurosurgical procedures without physician anesthesiologists. What's more, the "old guard" of elder surgeons, together with the operating room supervisor, were not about to let the young, upstart, neurosurgeons have any priority on early surgical starting times. The fact that many of our cases were long, tedious, and complex in nature was of little relevance. Furthermore, they only begrudgingly endorsed expenditures for much needed neurosurgical equipment. That was all to change in due time.

My neurosurgical partner, Dr. Frank Davis, trained at Tulane University in New Orleans, and the neurologist, Dr. Bryan Robinson, was a product of Emory University in Atlanta. Dr. Robinson was the oldest of the three of us, and was an exceptionally bright, well-accomplished researcher who had published a substantial number of laboratory research papers when at the NIH, Stanford University, and the Yerkes Primate Center in Atlanta. Furthermore, he was a man with a vision for the future, something from which the entire community would derive benefit in the years to follow.

We all shared limited office space in the basement of a building owned by a dentist directly across the street from the hospital. Frank and I shared one of two small office suites, and because we had only one desk could not both see patients the same day. For the most part it worked out fine because there was always surgery to be done, and an emergency room needing constant coverage. Our office manager and secretary, Nancy, was an attractive, pleasant and very efficient lady, who incidentally years before had been the fill-in swimmer for "Jane" in the old Johnny Weissmuller Tarzan movies— filmed 15 miles to the south of town at Wakulla Springs.

Although we had a small office set up, it was well conceived and efficient in the way it was run. Little was ever lost where the patient was concerned. Adequate time was always allotted for the initial consultation, and our findings were meticulously typed and recorded in the chart for future reference. While each of us had his own method regarding the neurological examination, I found my background at the University of Iowa indispensable. Something I found of great value was having learned how to quantify such functions as strength and reflexes. This enabled me to discern any changes in the patient's neurological status either pre-or post-operatively over a period of time. It was like having a reference gauge in following the course of his illness. Frank had his own method which worked equally well for him.

Also essential was a small double-tiered, box-shelf on the corner of our desk into the top of which all laboratory, x-ray and pathology reports were placed by the office personnel. Those reports could only be filed in the patient's chart after we had personally read the report and relegated it to the bottom tier. This provided a safety net to obviate overlooking any important patient data.

~~~

Our first house was rather small for a family of five, but it was new and only a short drive to the hospital. There is no greater feeling in the world than to have finished such a long educational process, begun a wonderful family, and settled into our own home within such a fine, gracious community.

After having allotted a few days to move in and find out where to get gas and groceries, I was ready to begin work; thereafter, I left Robbie at home to tend to the children. It didn't take long at all to change my self-identity. For years I had always been a dependent student who was low on the academic totem pole, seldom having any spare change in my pocket. Now, to the contrary, Frank and I as neurosurgeons were to assume positions of strong responsibility— professionals upon whom the rest of the medical community could depend.

My partner and I, because we were the only two neurosurgeons in the extensive referral area, made it clear to everyone that we would be available 24 hours a day throughout the year. And make no mistake— it was by no means an eight-to-five job, whether we were on-all or not. We were guided by our conscience, and driven by virtue of both our difficult training, and what was expected of a neurosurgeon in those days. After deciding early-on that one of us would always be closely available, we forever kept our promise to the community. As a point of emphasis, I can recall a weekend when the phone was out of order at my house because of a storm (that happened frequently in those days), and because Frank was off and out of town, he let me move into his home with my family for the entire weekend in order to have phone service while on-call.

Not all partnerships such as ours are lasting, and it behooves me to emphasize that point at this juncture. The key words are respect and consideration for each other plus a firm commitment to one another's patients. If one of us happened to be off call, whether it was a night, weekend or vacation, before leaving we tried not to burden our partner with undone work or loose ends, even if it might have necessitated working late. It was also understood that when covering on a night when a postoperative complication (such as a hemorrhage) occurred in the
~~~

absent partner's patient, the man on-call approached the problem with the same expediency and dedication as if it were his own patient. Thus, both the patient and his family had the peace of mind knowing that a doctor familiar with their case was but a phone call away.

From the onset, it was prudent to arrange our weekday schedules such that the man in the office on any particular day would take all consultations, whether they were in-house or impending from miles away. He would also cover the ER, and take night call as well. That scheme generally allowed the other surgeon to work unencumbered in the operating room. However, there remained days when the surgeon in the operating room still carried the sometimes heavy burden of the emergency room (for instance on a Friday when his partner was off for the weekend). At times this became quite problematic, as I will point out later.

~~~

It didn't take long to start filling up my surgical log with patients seen in the office. Most of them were spinal disc cases, and it appeared from the onset that they were closely divided between the neck and lower back. Since most readers do not know what comprises a "herniated disc", I shall now take this time to introduce the subject.

The disc is a wafer-shaped piece of cartilage that exists between any two adjacent vertebrae and normally acts as a cushioning material. When its outermost fibers of cartilage break down, the softer interior portion begins to bulge, protrude, or even extrude out as a fragment. This may cause pressure on an adjacent nerve root, resulting in symptoms such as numbness, tingling, pain or partial paresis in the extremities.

My lumbar disc operations were done with the patient in the prone position while draped over a curved, padded frame to allow chest expansion during respiratory movement. The spinal operations in those days were done without using magnification, and the light source left much to be desired. The incisions were relatively lengthy, and after dissecting away and retracting the massive paraverteral muscles, we removed minimal bone from the lamina. We then carefully packed off the epidural veins with small cottonoid pledgets, and while carefully retracting the nerve root, the ligament over the herniated disc cartilage was then incised and the fragment removed. Although this sounds very straightforward, neurosurgeons are a compulsive, finicky group, who
~~~

deplore blood in the surgical field or the careless handling of any tissue. Peripheral nerve tissue is manipulated with the utmost, delicate care and sometimes not at all. While not all disc operations that we performed in those days would receive an "A" grade today, the majority of them did well. In 2008, I ran into a medical colleague from whom I had removed a ruptured lumbar disc in 1972, and Ben was proud to inform me that he had never had another problem with his back since.

Our cervical (neck) cases were done a bit differently. In contradistinction to the lumbar disc ruptures where only nerve roots stand as delicate obstacles to the surgeon, those in the neck are fraught with danger by virtue of their close proximity to the spinal cord. This magnificent structure cannot be disturbed in any manner whatsoever. We could approach the disc from either the front or back of the neck, depending upon the circumstances peculiar to the case. When utilizing the posterior approach, we positioned the patient in the sitting position. This was quite effective in cases of a small disk fragment situated beneath the nerve root axilla adjacent to the side of the spinal cord.

For those cases with large or unusually displaced disc fragments and/or arthritic spurs impinging upon nerve root or spinal cord, we would ordinarily operate through the front of the neck. This is readily done with special instruments specifically designed for that purpose. The anterior approach, of course, necessitated some removal of the adjacent vertebral bodies embracing the disc, but replacement was executed with a bone graft harvested from the patient's ilium by an assistant. Solid bony fusion would then transpire over several months. The advantage of the anterior approach is the wide access to the entire disk space and any bone spurs. The re-stated risk is the ever present close proximity to the fragile spinal cord.

~~~

Concerning the emergency room, I was soon called over from the office early on my first day of work. It was to see a nurse's brother who had been struck by a car while crossing the street. While not a life-threatening injury, he did ultimately prove to have sustained some permanent brain damage. This case served to introduce me to the doctors, nurses and the procedural protocol of the ER. The emergency department, incidentally, is a necessary component of being a community physician, and, before proceeding further, it merits a brief
~~~

comment. Although some cases are interesting; most are not. While often causing a disruption during the middle of a busy day, or interrupting a critical night's sleep, it usually represents the cry of someone in need— and the doctor alone must answer that cry. Emergencies never take a holiday, and can be anticipated on Sundays and Christmas as well. They come in singles or multiples, and vary from the trivial to the complex, sometimes even dehumanizing in nature. But one factor stands consistently above the rest: the anticipatory stress that hangs over the wary physician like a dark cloud; namely, the uncertainty of not knowing what problem lurks ahead, and whether or not he possesses the wherewithal to handle it. In the case of a neurosurgeon, 70% of major automobile accident victims will have sustained head / spinal injury; hence, he must maintain a mental fortitude to accept the responsibility at any given moment. Since many of these major accident victims would have associated multi-system trauma (e.g., chest, abdominal and orthopedic injuries), often with significant blood loss, we were usually the admitting trauma surgeons "in charge" in those early days. This type of activity is not suited for those who are timid. I have always tried to teach others that when faced with a stressful situation, it is best to step up and engage it head-on. On the other hand, if one is not of the proper temperament— it might, indeed, be best to choose another line of work.

While speaking of the ER, I believe I had only been in town for a few weeks when my partner, who had been working alone and very hard for several years, went on a well-deserved two-week vacation. That was my true introduction into the total neurosurgical package. Not only was I occupied with a full office and operating room schedule, but I felt overwhelmed in the emergency room as well.

One afternoon they brought in my first severe cervical spine fracture, one which needed stabilization by cervical traction. In those days our initial treatment was to insert what were known as Crutchfield tongs into the skull. This was a mini-operation performed in the emergency department. After injecting a local anesthetic into the scalp and making bilateral paramedial stab incisions, two twist drill holes were made into the cranium with a small hand drill. The tongs, a miniature version of the old ice tongs, were inserted and held securely by a strong cord ultimately tied to weights draped over a pulley. The patient was carefully placed supine on a narrow, rotating (Stryker) frame with the weights suspended over the head end. Because people with spinal injuries are often paralyzed and unable to turn or shift their body weight, they are prone to skin breakdown and the development of large open wounds (decubitus ulcers), which may often become very deep, infected and ultimately exude pus. The Stryker frame enables the nursing staff to rotate the patient 180° every two hours to prevent these "pressure" bedsores.

Another emergency room case of interest occurred late one evening, when they brought in a man in deep coma, who was not moving the left side of his body. A large bruise on the right side of his scalp was the telltale sign of a blunt force to the head. The history, as given by a witness, indicated a fight in which the patient was struck and fell backwards, striking his head on a concrete floor. I suspected a right-sided brain hemorrhage, but needed x-ray confirmation. After taking the man to the x-ray department, I injected contrast material into his right carotid artery for an angiogram, the latter verifying a deep brain hemorrhage. The clot was indirectly indicated on the film by a displacement of the neighboring blood vessels. Meanwhile, the patient further deteriorated into a moribund state, as evidenced by deepening of his coma and the appearance of labored, irregular breathing. While fully cognizant of the apparent hopelessness of the situation, I felt his only possible chance of survival was surgical evacuation of the hematoma. Despite an uneventful craniotomy, and removal of the entire clot, he lived but a few hours. The nature of this death demanded an autopsy which, as expected, showed extensive traumatic brain injury from the forces to the head. The state's attorney and sheriff's deputy stood by with me, as the pathologist proceeded with his work. Subsequently, the perpetrator was apprehended and prosecuted. This unfortunate case clearly typifies the responsibility of any surgeon when providing service to a county hospital. Injuries and deaths from careless behavior and assaults accounted for a large part our weekend and nighttime practice.

~~~

That first year in Tallahassee seemed to fly by rapidly, perhaps because things were so busy in our small community. On my nights on-call, it seemed that I burned a constant track between my house and the hospital. On my nights off, Robbie and I would frequently sit on our small front porch, enjoying the warm summer nights, which echoed nature's chorus of sounds — the owls, frogs, and crickets. I would ventilate to her listening ear the challenges of work that day; she in turn
~~~

would update me on the children and the domestic home-front. How different this was from the days in Chicago!

~~~

Roughly 30% of my time, when not in the office, was spent in the radiology department. Dr. Raimondi always emphasized at Northwestern that, "neurosurgery is neuroradiology." To the layman, the neurosurgeon must have a firm grasp of radiographic anatomy, for unlike many other fields of surgery where body compartments or regions can be explored, he must know precisely where the problem lies within the skull or spinal canal before entertaining an incision.

As indicated earlier, when discussing the diagnosis of spinal disease, a myelogram was performed by instilling an oily contrast material through a lumbar puncture needle. This provided contrasting of soft tissue shadows enabling visualization of normal and pathological anatomy.

When evaluating the brain, we had basically three diagnostic modalities. The first, angiography, has already been discussed. The second consisted of a nuclear brain scan in which a radioactive material was injected into the bloodstream, and after placing a detector over the head, abnormal masses containing the accumulation of such material could then be seen on a film. Although imprecise, it did provide a vague estimation as to the location of some abnormalities. The third diagnostic radiologic procedure which has been touched upon briefly, entails the installation of air into the ventricles of the brain (discovered by Dr. Walter Dandy in 1918), after removing equal increments of CSF. If a mass such as a tumor is suspected, it is imperative that the air be introduced from above through a burr hole bored into the skull (ventriculography), whereas, if no mass is suspected the air may be safely instilled through a lumbar puncture (pneumoencephalography or PEG). The latter might be used in cases such as suspected hydrocephalus or brain atrophy. Once the bolus of air has been introduced into the intracranial cavity, the patient is then strapped into an elaborate, motorized chair that can be rotated in any number of positions to allow for movement of the air bubble. This air/tissue contrast interface then allows for the indirect visualization of the intracranial anatomy. Injecting air into a patient's head was a dreadfully painful procedure, much likened to a medieval torture. I have seen grown men crying in
~~~

agony, describing it as if the head were being "squeezed in a vise." Though a painful, cumbersome, and very time-consuming examination, it was an indispensable diagnostic tool in those early days. The value of contrasting intracranial air in establishing a diagnosis is well illustrated in the following case encountered soon after my arrival in Tallahassee.

One night while stepping onto the elevator during late rounds, I bumped into a colleague who was a general practitioner. I asked Bob what he was doing up so late that evening, when he replied that he was on his way up to perform a spinal puncture on a young man with a severe headache and fever. He felt in all likelihood the man's symptoms represented spinal meningitis. Having seen me by chance in the meantime, he asked if I would mind taking a look at the patient first. After concluding my examination, I was very suspicious that this delirious man had an increase in intracranial pressure, and for the reasons previously alluded to; I felt that we should rule out a brain mass before entertaining a spinal puncture. The first and most expedient thing to do was a simple x-ray of the skull, looking for any signs of bone erosion or brain shift as indicated by a displacement of a calcified pineal body. When the x-ray rolled out of the dryer, I was dumbfounded to immediately see the diagnosis. With the x-ray having been taken with the patient lying on his back, there was an air bubble with a fluid level within it in the right frontal lobe of his brain. It was the diagnostic sign of a brain abscess! The patient, whom I later got to know very well, and his wife standing nearby, both agreed to emergent treatment. All things being considered at that time, I thought it best to simply drain the purulent material to effect an immediate decompression of the swollen, tense brain. We thus transported him to the operating room, and, after preparation of the scalp, made the trepanation under local anesthesia. A large trocar was then passed into the abscess cavity with the immediate release of putrid gas, followed by the egression of thick, yellow, foul-smelling pus — together representing the products of anaerobic bacterial metabolism. The trocar was replaced with a small red rubber catheter. Because the organism proved to be a Streptococcus on the Gram stain, penicillin was used both in irrigating the abscess cavity through the catheter and was given intravenously for several weeks. Jordan's initial recovery was uneventful, but he did have a grand mal seizure several weeks later for which he was placed on medication. An elective craniotomy was then undertaken six months later to excise the contracted, then sterile, abscess capsule which was the nidus for his seizures. At the time of his craniotomy, evidence of an old unrecognized head injury and fracture of the skull base, containing herniated brain tissue into the frontal sinus, was discovered and repaired. Dr. Robert Snyder, one of our otolaryngologists, in a later trans-facial operation obliterated the frontal sinus. The latter, thereby, consummated final closure of the portal of entry which had led to the onset of the original infection. Jordan has subsequently done well, has remained seizure-free, and has since been taken off his anticonvulsant medications. Later, as a fish and wildlife officer for the state of Florida, he introduced me to fishing in the bayous of the St. Mark's Wild Life Refuge.

Injuries about the face and paranasal sinuses not infrequently lead to brain infections. Another closely related and interesting case comes to mind that presented to me during that first year. My neurologist partner, Dr. Robinson, while treating a 20-year-old man in the hospital with meningitis, found out that he had experienced four previous attacks of this life-threatening disorder dating back to early childhood. Dr. Robinson learned through a careful history that, when the patient was a small child, he was running with a pencil in hand, and had stumbled and fallen only to drive the instrument far up into his nose. Not only did he develop subsequent attacks of meningitis through the years, but also noticed profuse dripping of clear fluid out of his nose, especially after arising in the mornings, and bending over to put on his shoes. Astutely, Dr. Robinson suspected CSF leakage from a perforation of the skull base, and asked me to consult on the case. We were able to document an old injury in the floor of the skull by introducing a radionuclide into the spinal fluid through a lumbar puncture. Cotton pledgets were then inserted high into the nasal cavity by an ENT specialist. A Geiger counter then proved that the fluid circulating up and around the brain carrying the isotope was leaking into the nasal cavity onto the pledgets. A frontal craniotomy later exposed the defect in the skull base, which was repaired with a pedicle flap graft of soft tissue (pericranium). This was the first of several such cases of frontal CSF rhinorrhea I was to see and treat during the years to follow. The majority of them were the result of motor vehicle accidents with craniofacial injury from secondary collisions with the dashboard and steering wheel.

~~~

In 1972 our small neurological group moved into our own, newly constructed, office building located three miles from the hospital.
~~~

Although not quite as convenient where the hospital was concerned, we had modestly increased our space to eventually accommodate four doctors and an EEG lab. Later that summer another neurologist, Dr. George Slade, joined us. Dr. Slade, also a product of Emory University, had special expertise in the electromyographic diagnostic techniques (EMG) of neuromuscular disorders, expanding our group's diagnostic capabilities.

My own office and examining room were spacious and elegant indeed, enhanced by pictures of my family adorning the bookshelves and by those hard-earned licenses and diplomas hanging on the walls. Always conservative after having been raised in a modest childhood home, I initially felt out of place sitting behind a beautiful walnut desk atop a thick, deep-red, carpet; nonetheless, it certainly made the office work more pleasant.

During the weekdays in the operating room, Frank and I assisted one another on all major cases. Sometimes that meant the assistant's mere presence in the operating room and availability in case of a surgical question, whereas, at other times another pair of hands might have been needed. Weekends were an entirely different matter because the man who was "off" was out of touch, and not infrequently out of the city altogether. If a surgical assistant was needed on a weekend, we had to scurry around to find one— usually a general surgeon or often times an orthopedist. The following story illustrates very dramatically how a weekend "on-call" might unfold.

At 8 A.M. one Friday morning, Frank, who was scheduled to be off for the weekend, began operating upon a rather complex arteriovenous malformation (AVM) of the brain with me as his assistant. What was initially thought to be a straightforward case became a very lengthy procedure. Meticulously, he dissected out and clipped the arterial vessels feeding this entangled mass of veins. Under these circumstances, the surgeon must exercise care not to interrupt the blood supply to normal brain tissue. The operation went very well, but demanded many hours of careful work. Success arrived at about 11 o'clock that night as he delivered the mass from the brain, and, I might add, the patient did very well. Tired myself, I drove home at midnight, hurriedly ate a late supper, and immediately collapsed into a deep sleep. At 1 A.M. I was awakened by my bedside phone, and an excited emergency room physician, in a town 35 miles away, related to me the following horrific, inconceivable story.

It seemed that a 10-year-old boy was spending the night with a friend, and, as curious pre-adolescent boys have been known to do, was playing with a loaded shotgun. The gun tragically discharged into the child's head. To the horror of all concerned, he was transported to the local hospital where, because of the seemingly hopeless nature of the injury, he was treated expectantly. The child, deeply comatose and bleeding, was totally covered up with a sheet, and the cart upon which he was lying pushed against a wall in the hallway. Several minutes later, someone happening by noticed movement of one of the boy's toes sticking out from beneath the sheet. In total disbelief, the ER personnel suddenly realized that the child might survive after all, hence, the phone call requesting my assistance.

The very nature of this disaster and the mere anticipation of what I was to encounter and deal with in the emergency room triggered such a "fight or flight" response, I gave no thought, whatsoever, to either the tedious prior day's work or the fatigue incurred.

As they wheeled Jerry into the emergency room, the staff was aghast at the sight of the wound, sparking great urgency to the situation in order to save this boy's life. Hours before, when first hearing about this tragedy, I had alerted the operating room personnel to prepare for immediate surgery. Urgently, we first needed to draw the patient's blood for the necessary laboratory studies, and had to begin an immediate blood transfusion. Portable radiographs were taken to demonstrate in-driven bone fragments, while the head was rapidly being shaved.

When in the operating room, we inspected the wound which, as one might well surmise, was both untidy and extensive, consisting of massive tissue destruction involving virtually the entire right posterior quadrant of the child's head. Once he was on the operating table, the anesthetic having been administered and blood having been rapidly infused, his condition stabilized such that we could proceed. Inspection of this grotesque wound revealed a major loss of scalp and skull with the underlying brain being unrecognizable as such. The entire right occipital and parietal lobes were pulped from the blast, and large inferiorly depressed shards of bone were seen to have imploded into the brain, and were also obstructing the major transverse venous sinus. I could only surmise that was the reason he survived the long ambulance trip, for the bone was serving as a tamponade of the lacerated venous sinus, thereby preventing exsanguination. Dr. Luther Parraro, a general surgeon, was my assistant that night as we struggled to save little Jerry.

The operation was straightforward, and consisted of standard surgical debridement of all devitalized tissue. In essence, the procedure was a total right parieto-occipital lobectomy of nonviable brain. The blood loss was extensive, and I can vividly recall Dr. Parraro having said, "Oh my— I've never seen so much bleeding." Once this gaping wound was tidy, and the bleeding totally controlled, we spent the rest of the early morning hours trying to obtain a watertight wound closure with fascial tissue taken from his leg.

Later as he was being wheeled over to the intensive care unit, I gazed at the small, childish, angelic face beneath the large head dressing, and was in awe that such a fragile human being could have withstood such a devastating war-like wound. Jerry remained neurologically stable, although deeply obtunded, over the next 24 hours— his overall prognosis remaining guarded.

Thinking ahead to the next 24 hours, I knew it to be imperative, because of the short window of time to avert an infection, that we proceed with scalp reconstruction in order to cover this large defect. We had only one plastic surgeon in Tallahassee at the time, and C.W., an avid sailor, was somewhere out in the Gulf of Mexico on his sailboat. I had little choice but to proceed with the operation myself, giving full credit to my brief experience in plastic surgery both in Chicago and the Air Force for enabling me to do so. We were able to rotate a frontal full-thickness pedicle scalp graft (hinged on its own blood supply) posteriorly to cover the entire defect. Then, following standard time-honored procedure, we covered the defect over the frontal bone of the skull vacated by the pedicle graft with a large split thickness skin graft harvested from the thigh. Within days all appeared well, and it seemed that we would escape from this without an infection after all. Fortunately, the luxuriant blood supply to the scalp tends to preclude infection, providing any necessary surgery is promptly done.

During the extensive course of recovery, we were ecstatic over the fact that the child failed to show any signs of paralysis of either extremity on the left body side contralateral to the blast. Even more remarkable was the fact that his sensorium slowly, yet steadily improved, eventually resulting in normal speech and cognition. Years later, in retrospect, our head neurological intensive care nurse, Teddy McQuat, reminded me how Jerry would, "cry like a cat" for hours on-end during those early weeks after the operation.

Six weeks after hospital discharge, the little guy walked into the office with his dad. He was fully alert, spoke fluently, and exhibited minimal blunting of his affect. As expected, he was left with a complete left visual field defect being devoid of the right occipital lobe. His strength in the left arm and leg were absolutely normal. However, because of the absence of the right parietal lobe, he lacked any awareness of the left side of his body. Expressing great concern, his father told me that the entire family had to constantly be on the look-out that Jerry would not hurt himself; for instance, on several occasions he came close to shutting his ignored left arm in a car door. It is important, however, to point out that if Jerry visibly looked at his left arm and leg, he could direct them in any desired motor activity with reasonable coordination and good strength.

Six months later we readmitted him to the hospital, and successfully constructed an artificial skull plate out of acrylic. No further surgery was ever necessary. Of interest during the next decade, Jerry was followed by Dr. Sam Moorer, Director of the Children's Medical Services for the State of Florida, who presented him to other medical personnel as an illustrative case of a pure "parietal lobe neglect" syndrome — an extremely rare, yet fascinating neurological abnormality.

Ten years later in 1982, a young man briskly walked into my office, and politely reintroduced himself to me as Jerry McWhorter. His ambition was to join the Army, but because he had just been rejected for his disability, he asked that I write President Reagan on his behalf. Instead, I did ask a friend of mine, who was chief of neurosurgery at Walter Reed Army Medical Center at the time, to see what he could do to help Jerry; it was to no avail. The last I learned of the young man's whereabouts was in an article written in our local newspaper, reflecting that Jerry McWhorter had ridden his bicycle all the way from Tallahassee to Washington, D.C. He wanted to prove to the president that, despite his brain injury, he was fit for the Army. Although most can appreciate the Army's reluctance to accept someone with such a severe disability, they can equally appreciate this young man's courage, self-confidence and determination to succeed and move forward in life.

Several other non-trauma-related pediatric entities were encountered during my first year in practice. One such condition immediately coming to mind was the sudden development of an inexplicable increase in intracranial pressure occurring in babies during the early months of life. Several such alarming cases presented to us. These babies initially presented with an unexplained febrile illness which then rapidly progressed into a state of deepening coma. Based upon the signs of dangerous increased intracranial pressure, we were reluctant to initially perform a lumbar puncture to necessarily exclude meningitis or encephalitis, and needed first to rule out a space-occupying mass. I can recall a number of instances in which the attending pediatrician and I wrestled with these desperately ill babies on the x-ray table in an effort to obtain a diagnostic arteriogram. After excluding a tumor or other mass lesion, we were left with an unusual type of encephalitis to which the infant almost invariably succumbed, despite our best medical efforts. This was a terrifying disease for parents and physicians alike. Years later, this condition of unexplained malignant brain swelling, known as "Reye's syndrome," was ascribed in large part to aspirin, and its incidence was greatly reduced with the discontinued use of that drug in newborns and infants.

Another pediatric condition frequently referred to the neurosurgeon is termed craniosynostosis. Normally, the multiple bones which form the skull are not united at birth and are displaced centripetally as the underlying, unconstrained brain grows. By age three most of the brain growth has occurred, whereupon the edges of the individual bones fuse along what are termed "suture lines." In a small group of babies this fusion process occurs prematurely (shortly after birth), setting the stage for a permanent misshaping of the head. A prominent cosmetic deformity may ensue which, later in school, may become a focus of ridicule by other children. Such an extreme example was the man previously alluded to at Iowa City who had the tower skull. When presented with such an infant during the first two years of life, the neurosurgeon can redirect the head shape by creating artificial sutures, and, by so doing, can induce a cosmetically pleasing head conformation.

Shortly after my arrival in Tallahassee, I attended a medical staff meeting at the hospital in Perry, Florida, enabling me to meet the local doctors for the first time. Out of that contact, a little baby girl was sent to me as my first case of craniosynostosis in private practice. After surgical repair, there was a satisfying normal reconfiguration of her skull. Years later, the proud parents sent me pictures corroborating the good result. We were destined to operate upon several similar cases during the ensuing years, and, while not a life-threatening condition, the parents were invariably grateful for our preventing conspicuous permanent cranial deformities in their children.

The dynamics of hydrocephalus have already been discussed, but a patient seen within months of my opening my practice merits description. I was presented with an infant boy, not more than three months old, with a very rapidly enlarging head. A bedside test commonly used in those days entailed holding a large flashlight against the baby's skull while in a pitch-dark room. In this child's particular case, the entire head trans-illuminated, as if shining the light through a water-filled balloon, indirectly inferring an absence of brain tissue. An ensuing air encephalogram, at first glance, seemed to corroborate the absence of a cerebral cortex. However, upon very close scrutiny we thought we could discern a brain mantle no more than 3 mm. in thickness. Based upon this miniscule evidence of probable cortical tissue being present (as opposed to the developmental absence of the cerebral hemispheres altogether, a condition known as hydranencephaly), we elected to install a ventriculoperitoneal (VP) shunt. One year later the infant seemed to be developing normally, and a repeat PEG remarkably demonstrated the unequivocal presence of a thickening cerebral mantle.

During the ensuing years, little Archer showed continued normal progress in growth and development. After his skull bones eventually fused, he became shunt dependent, meaning that any obstruction to the drainage system would result in a rapid dangerous increase in intracranial pressure. This calls for an immediate shunt revision. At times throughout his childhood, obstruction of the shunt did occasionally recur, but his parents would alertly recognize the symptoms, and whisk him quickly to us, despite their living far away by the Gulf Coast. Because his father later left the area for work in Louisiana, we temporarily lost track of little Archer MacCluster, but we will revisit his case later in the book.

~~~

Things seemed to go pleasingly well for our neurological group. We were quite congenial and freely communicated with one another regarding interesting cases. As a point of emphasis, this becomes one of the great advantages of a small group practice when a perplexing diagnostic problem is encountered. It was considered important that we should not only offer but welcome other opinions under such circumstances. Early on in the practice, we would meet on the south side of town at the old Silver Slipper restaurant for supper once a month, and would discuss pertinent articles which we had recently read in the neurological literature. This "journal club" attested to our desire of
~~~

remaining current on medical issues, and in maintaining high academic standards in our practice.

A unique opportunity presented itself in 1972. For a number of years, Dr. James Lyerly, to whom we referred as having been the first neurosurgeon in Florida, took the train on a monthly basis from Jacksonville through Tallahassee en route to the Florida State Mental Hospital in Chattahoochee. While there, he would examine —and at times operate upon— patients with various maladies of the nervous system. After his retirement he handed the job over to the neurosurgical group in Pensacola, whereupon, after many years of service they asked whether Frank and I would take over. We didn't hesitate in accepting that responsibility, one which we did not relinquish until several years after retirement from our Tallahassee practice. Frank and I alternated on a monthly basis to attend a clinic set up by the attending physician and his head nurse. One can only imagine the array of unusual patients which we encountered at FSH. Routinely, we would examine and order a disposition on between 8 to 16 clients, some requiring surgery, but more often they did not. Most of them were meek and hardly vocal. Others, of a highly unpredictable, vicious or even potentially dangerous nature, were escorted while in restraining devices. It was comforting, indeed, that there always existed several attendants who would promptly hustle away those out of control.

~~~

Back at home our family moved out to the edge of town during the second year. I picked up a scenic eight-acre piece of property upon which a local dentist had previously constructed a rather unusual, old-appearing, stone two-story home. He and his sons had transported the large stones from a long-vacated structure, which he had purchased several miles away. Of interest was the fact that the majority of the stone blocks each weighed 60-80 pounds; consequently, because of their extreme weight, only a single layer could be cemented in at a time to maintain integrity of the interposed concrete. It was a marvelous place in which to raise a family, there being abundant surrounding acreage for future animals and a pool. One of the disadvantages to living out in the country became readily apparent when telephone communication was lost with the hospital during a storm outage. Not infrequently, the hospital had to send the police out to notify me in times of need.
~~~

~~~

The variety of clinical material we encountered in our practice proved intriguing. We saw an abundance of the common neurological conditions, and, when least expected, an unusual disorder would present itself. As an example of the former, during my first two years in practice we had a run of cervical spine fractures involving the odontoid process of the second cervical vertebra. The odontoid is a peg of bone which is an extension of the body of the second cervical vertebra, the axis, around which the skull and uppermost cervical vertebra, the atlas, rotate. A fracture through this peg, because of the instability produced, poses a risk of severe spinal cord injury or possibly even death. A standard operation consisted of wiring together, and fusing the superior three cervical vertebrae with autogenous bone. We did this with the patient under cervical traction and prone on a Stryker frame. I counted 12 such cases of this condition which we had operated upon within the first 24 months I was in practice, certainly enough to write up a series for publication. Some of the larger medical centers do not see that many fractured odontoids over such a short time span; hence, I felt that we were fortunate to gain valuable experience in this type of surgery, while simultaneously providing specialized spine treatment for the community.

Thus far we have not discussed the subject of brain tumors in our clinical practice. To become successful in this type of work necessarily requires the confidence of the entire community. Over the course of time, we were fortunate that our clinic developed a very favorable reputation in the eyes of the referring doctors. Although we performed a significant volume of charity work, the majority of our patients were of the middle class. In due time, we then began to see patients within the upper middle-class as well from our rather large referral area. One such patient was a prominent businessman from a town in Georgia. Mr. Chad Sewell was a visible figure in both the timber and real estate businesses. He was an intelligent, fluent man who, out of the blue one day, experienced a grand mal convulsion. Bryan first admitted Chad to the hospital, and performed the diagnostic angiogram himself. This study showed an enlarged artery leading to a tumor- blush located high up in the cranium near the middle of the head, and straddled by the cerebral hemispheres. This tumor, known as a parasagittal meningioma, abutted against the great major draining venous sinus of the brain, the superior
~~~

sagittal sinus. Pathologically, a meningioma is ordinarily a perfectly benign tumor if it can be totally removed. However, they may on occasion be quite intimidating to the surgeon, for they can be very large and extremely vascular; furthermore, they may be imminently associated with important venous sinus structures. In Chad's particular case, I felt postoperatively that I had been able to remove the entire neoplasm, including that portion very closely applied to the wall of the superior sagittal sinus. Chad recovered uneventfully from his operation, and had no neurological sequelae at the time of his discharge. He was treated with medication for his seizures. This affable man even wrote (and later published) a clever poem, which amused us all, about his total hospital experience. Although he was not to be seen again for several years — this was not to be the end of his story.

~~~
~~~

FIVE

The Dawn of Mr. Hounsfield's Revolutionary Machine

~~~

In 1973 Godfrey N. Hounsfield first described what was to become a major innovation in medicine — the development of computed axial tomography or CAT (18). This was destined to revolutionize our diagnostic approach to diseases of the brain and spinal cord. By looking at a programmed series of two-dimensional, axial-cut x-ray plates, we could gain a three-dimensional perspective as to the location of lesions within the intracranial cavity and spinal canal.

In its simplest form this may be described as a collimated planar series of 160 x-ray beams with a detector on the opposite side of the patient's head, the entire ensemble rotating 180 times through an arc. The 28,800 transmitted x-ray measurements (160x180) — the latter based upon the x-ray absorption coefficients of the disparate tissues— are analyzed numerically by a computer and displayed as a visible brain slice. By repeating the process at multiple, pre-designated brain levels, the entire organ can be pictorially represented. The first generation of this scanner was made by the EMI Corporation in England; hence, they were first known as EMI scanners.

My partner, Bryan Robinson, a man of vision, flew to England soon after hearing of this device. After viewing, firsthand, the scanner's great potential, he returned to Tallahassee while envisioning a neurological foundation which could finance an EMI machine for our hospital. He wasted no time in setting up such a foundation whose board members consisted of some of Tallahassee's most prominent and influential citizens. Soon the generous contributions from our community enabled the purchase of the machine. The expediency with which this project was completed might best be illustrated by the fact that, when the Tallahassee
~~~

scanner was placed on order, there were but two EMI machines in place in the entire United States — at the Mayo Clinic in Rochester and the Massachusetts General Hospital.

Until such time as this space-age diagnostic tool could be installed in Tallahassee, we continued to rely solely on the neurological examination, clinical judgment, and the time-honored radiographic procedures of cerebral angiography and pneumoencephalography (PEG) for the diagnosis of intracranial pathology. This serial method in logic was often problematic, and in some instances was fraught with a potentially dangerous delay in treatment as illustrated below.

One day in Tallahassee while on her way home from school with a friend, an eight-year-old girl was amusing herself, as kids often do, by tandem-walking on top of a wooden rail fence. Upon losing her balance she fell to the ground, striking the back of her head on the cement sidewalk. Reportedly there was no loss of consciousness, and, although complaining of a headache, she was able to walk home. Because of the nature of the injury, her mother took her to the hospital emergency room. After an examination and brief period of observation, the child was dismissed home. Several hours passed, whereupon, the concerned mother, sensing things were not right, returned the child to the hospital. A different physician evaluated her, and he too sent the child on her way home. In the meantime the mother was given instructions as to any warning signs or symptoms that might subsequently occur. After several more hours of anguish over the little girl's headache and overall appearance, mom headed to the hospital for a third emergency room visit. Still another physician unfamiliar with the case examined little Jill. Even though a linear occipital skull fracture was visualized on a radiograph, the child remained perfectly alert, had no vomiting, had not lost consciousness after the fall, and was neurologically intact. In view of her stable condition at that point, now several hours after the injury, the emergency room staff again began making preparation to release the child under further observation by the responsible parents. One of the hospital staff pediatricians, Dr. Sam Moorer, happened to be standing nearby in the emergency department at the time and overheard the dialogue between the mother and the staff. Concerned about what he was hearing, he stepped forth and suggested to the emergency physician that the little girl be seen by a neurosurgeon. Shortly thereafter I was summoned to evaluate the case.

Although my neurological examination was unequivocally normal at the time, I did admit the child to the intensive care unit with half-hourly evaluations. My focus of concern was the occipital skull fracture, and the fact that it crossed over the large transverse venous sinus draining blood from the posterior aspect of the brain. This sets the stage for a potential, posterior fossa epidural hemorrhage. Such an event may occur because the traumatic force fracturing the very thick occipital bone can also tear the dural wall of the venous sinus, whereby it is stripped away from the interior of the skull. The potentially grave nature of a clot in this location is attested to by the dearth of symptoms, other than headache, as the hematoma expands in size to a critical life-threatening mass. At that point the brain stem may be compressed at the medulla oblongata, which can result in sudden death. These concerns notwithstanding, the child remained perfectly stable for an additional 24 hours. When making evening rounds on the second hospital day, I told the parents that if, by the next morning, the child were still asymptomatic, I would discharge her home. At that point it was beginning to look like the initial three ER physicians had been correct in their assessments after all.

Late that same night I received an alarming phone call from the intensive-care nurse stating that Jill's headaches had abruptly intensified, and that she was now vomiting—clearly a significant change in her status. I requested the nurse to immediately notify both the x-ray department to prepare for an emergency angiogram, and the operating room to prepare for an emergency craniotomy.

There were two distinct possibilities which could have accounted for the child's deterioration. The first, and most likely, was a posterior fossa epidural hematoma as already discussed. In that case, we would operate through the back of the head with the patient in the prone position. A second possibility was the development of a contrecoup frontal subdural hematoma, mandating a frontal craniotomy with the patient supine. Time permitting, an arteriogram would provide critical information to help answer this diagnostic question.

Close analysis of my right brachial angiogram revealed the study to be entirely normal, thereby excluding a frontal lesion with a brain shift. Without further delay we transported her from the radiology department to the operating room, and prepared the child for a suboccipital craniectomy. An element of uncertainty still persisted in my mind regarding the diagnosis; yet, I drilled with conviction the exploratory burr hole through the occipital squama to exclude a life-threatening clot.

Upon emerging through the inner bone table of the skull, that burden of uncertainty was lifted— solid dark-red (classically described as "currant-jelly-like" in the textbooks) blood clot was encountered. A large window of bone (craniectomy) was then fashioned to ensure total clot evacuation. Finally, in recalling the technique shown to us years previously in Chicago by Dr. Ed Sequeira during that frightful operating room hemorrhage, the rent in the venous sinus wall was obliterated, obviating any further bleeding.

I would have a hard time ever recalling a more gratifying moment in my medical career than when I stepped into the waiting room and told the anxious parents that their little girl was going to be okay. The child subsequently proceeded to make a full recovery. When last seen in the office several weeks later, the mother graciously handed to me a gift-wrapped box. It contained a stone statue of a small girl with braids, sitting down while holding a little doll; a brass engraved plate at the statue's base read—"Thanks for Jill's Future."

~~~

Until now, I have not addressed pain management. Prior to 1980, many cases of severe peripheral body pain due to debilitating diseases, such as cancer, were treated by an operation called a cordotomy. This procedure entailed the creation of a precise destructive lesion within the tract of the spinal cord conveying pain sensation to the higher pain centers of the brain. Initially, we used the percutaneous radiofrequency approach discussed when I was a resident at the Evanston Hospital. Understandably, the advantage to the patient was the absence of a deep, painful incision and the necessary convalescent period for healing. The primary disadvantage, in my mind, concerned the fact that the electrode placement was not done under direct vision, but rather by x-ray control. As a result there was always some element of uncertainty as to the exact location of the electrode tip; for example, it might have merely displaced rather than penetrated the spinal cord, even though on the x-ray film things might have looked optimal. The results were mixed, but it was a laudable procedure, indeed, when successful.

During the ensuing years, we began performing more of our cordotomies with the patient draped over the curved padded frame while awake and using local anesthesia. Under these circumstances, there is certainty as to where the spinal cord lesion is being made, but the
~~~

lengthy duration of the operation often led to a restless, complaining patient, already in pain from his underlying disease. After the extended period of time required for the exposure of the spinal cord, it always seemed that about the time I was ready to make the delicate pain-relieving incision into it, the patient would shout out from beneath the surgical drapes, "I can't stand this position any longer — I have to move"; whereupon, at times he did!

Two interesting cases immediately come to mind regarding cordotomies. The first was a morbidly obese, middle-aged lady who, because of her excessive weight, had destroyed her right hip joint. There was no such thing as a total hip replacement in those days, and she was non-ambulatory because of incessant, deep, agonizing pain. A cordotomy was undertaken, whereby she experienced immediate and permanent pain relief. Subsequently, she became totally mobile and was able to go on with her normal daily activities. Several years later, however, because she lacked any pain sensibility on the right side of her body, she developed an acutely (initially unrecognized) fulminant gallbladder attack—devoid of pain— from which she nearly died. Our operation had been such a success that this vulnerable lady almost perished as the direct result of the loss of the normal protective pain response to injury.

The second intractable pain case concerned a man who had previously managed to get his arm caught in a conveyor belt while at work, having it horrifically avulsed at the shoulder joint. He later not only experienced the phantom-limb phenomena, a condition in which (unless directly observing its absence) he thought his arm was still attached, but also experienced continuous excruciating pain in the phantom. Although the probability for a complete and lasting ablation of his phantom-limb pain after a high cervical cordotomy was low, we proceeded in hopes of sparing this man further misery. The immediate result of the operation was that of total pain relief, and upon his last follow-up office visit many months later, he remained pain free.

~~~

In the summer of 1973, my partner and his wife embarked upon a four-week vacation to China. After counting the days until he returned, I then planned to take the entire month of September off. Incidentally, those extended vacations were so punishing to the man left covering the
~~~

practice that we never did that again. My time off, however, was consumed with preparation for my final examination in neurological surgery. I had previously taken and passed the written part of the board examination; now after two years in clinical practice I was eligible to sit for the oral exam. I had heard unpleasant stories of fully trained, very competent neurosurgeons taking the test as many as three times, yet, still failing. That alone was enough motivation to spur me into a comprehensive review. When October arrived, I flew up to Rochester, Minnesota, the day before I was to be given the examination at the old Mayo Brothers' house. I'll never forget the morning of the exam, when 20 candidate neurosurgeons climbed aboard and sat on the chartered bus outside of the hotel, anticipating the drive up to the Mayo house. There was utter silence, and one could have cut the tension with a knife. I personally felt like an animal being led to slaughter. Once there, and despite the pressure of the three-hour oral examination before world eminent neurosurgeons and neurologists, I felt it an honor to sit for the examination in that historic building which resonated with both charm and mystique. Each candidate would independently spend the first of three hours in a nicely decorated, old room while being questioned by two senior examiners. The latter were free to ask any questions varying from the minutest, such as a nerve-tract connection in the brain, to the more practical, like the description of an entire operation. If they saw for a moment that the candidate knew the answer to any given question, they would promptly change to another subject in an effort to canvass his total fund of knowledge. At hour's end, each candidate would then advance to another room to engage with another duo of examiners. I think the stress of anticipating our fate leading up to the examination was far greater than the examination process itself. No one would argue, though, that we were all relieved when it was over.

Because of far advanced scheduling from my office, later that afternoon following the examination I met with the chief neuroradiologist at the Mayo Clinic, who was going to give me a personal tour through the EMI scanner department. I was curious to see the physical workings of this revolutionary machine and the images which it produced. That experience rivaled the board examination in excitement (albeit more pleasant), especially, since we had ordered our own device for Tallahassee Memorial Hospital.

This entire story concludes with my later receiving written notification that I had passed the examination, and was now certified by the American Board of Neurological Surgery. Of historical interest is the fact that the secretary of the board at the time, Dr. Kemp Clark, was the man who had escorted us through the Mayo house that day, and who had later signed my letter of accreditation. He was also the physician who had pronounced President John F. Kennedy deceased after the assassination in Dallas 10 years previously, nearly to the day.

~~~

A leading sequela of traumatic brain injury causing death in those days was an acute subdural hematoma. Even in modern times, the mortality rate from this devastating entity remains at 60 to 80%, the reason being not only the pressure from the clot itself but also the associated brain injury and swelling. Despite clot removal and drugs that would reduce brain swelling, the treatment often fell short. As a result, neurosurgeons were forced to become more aggressive in their attempt to improve survival. As generally recommended at the time, we therefore began performing hemicraniectomies on the side of the hematoma, and would discard the large bone flap —in essence, half of the skull — after removal of the clot itself. This allowed the brain to swell unconstrained until the fury had subsided.

One such case involved the teenage sister of one of our intensive-care nurses. The young girl was brought in deeply comatose after having been struck by a car. An emergency arteriogram revealed a massive, subdural hemorrhage with a prominent brain shift. The clot was evacuated, and a hemicraniectomy was performed. She remained in dire straits for days-on-end, and I felt the outcome could have gone either way. However, after finally stabilizing, she then slowly began to improve. Over the course of many weeks, the patient made a remarkable recovery without any lasting neurological deficit. Six months later we covered her large skull defect by constructing a stainless steel wire-reinforced acrylic plate. Gertrude subsequently continued her education, pursuing the challenging x-ray technologist curriculum. She has not only supported herself since then, but has also provided a needed service to the community as a very competent x-ray technician. After 35 years, I have yet to fail receiving an annual Christmas card from this grateful patient. Unfortunately, not all similar head injury cases had the same favorable outcome that Gertrude did.

~~~

In 1973 it was our pleasure to welcome the first two anesthesiologists to the hospital staff. One of them was Dr. Charles Deal, whose professionalism I could not have done without throughout these many years. Among his many contributions, he was indispensable in working closely with us relative to the overall care of small infants during surgery, including vital blood replacement. In addition, I appreciated his tireless presence during long tedious tumor and aneurysm cases, and his help on multiple weekend emergencies. It gives the surgeon great peace of mind knowing that the anesthetized patient is physiologically and pharmacologically in good hands, allowing him to concentrate on his demanding work.

~~~

When neurosurgeons discuss brain tumors, there is no greater challenge than a particular one which exclusively resides in the daunting posterior intracranial fossa —the acoustic neurinoma. While neurosurgeons have referred to intracranial aneurysms as the "king" of intracranial operations; the acoustic neurinoma has been dubbed the "queen."

This tumor derives its origin from the sheath of the VIIIth (auditory) cranial nerve; predictably, the patient usually presents himself to the doctor with a history of unilateral hearing loss. Most commonly, the tumor springs from that portion of the nerve within the bony internal auditory canal, a point well lateral to its exit from the brainstem. Because the VIIIth nerve is accompanied by the VIIth (facial) cranial nerve throughout its intracranial course, the expanding tumor encroaches upon the latter as it grows medially out of the canal back toward the brainstem. With further unconstrained growth, the tumor may attain a critical size, not only thinning out both cranial nerves to the point of transparency, but also becoming draped with important arteries as it begins to invaginate into the vital brainstem. The latter brain structure represents a conglomerate of nerve tracts and clusters of neurons, many of which control such critical functions as respiration. With the pathological anatomy having been described, it doesn't take much imagination to appreciate the challenging task involved in both diagnosing and removing these neoplasms. However, there is a positive side: these are histologically benign tumors, and when totally removed—the patient is usually cured.
~~~

With regard to the diagnosis itself, in years past we relied foremost on the otologist to confirm the patient's hearing loss as being secondary to VIIIth nerve damage; i.e., in contradistinction to a bony or infectious malady of the middle ear. If we were fortunate, plain x-ray films of the internal meatus of the internal auditory canal might have revealed tell-tale erosion of bone. If the tumor were larger, the PEG or angiogram might have assisted us with the diagnosis; and in the case of a very large tumor, one of the old nuclear brain scans might have proven of value. Because often the patient's signs and symptoms were either meager or absent, and the radiologic studies equivocal, these tumors would attain an enormous size before they could be diagnosed. Under these circumstances it was indeed a challenging task to affect a safe total removal — to say nothing of sparing the nerve to the face. The radiological studies noted above were at times not only difficult to perform, but often did not clearly depict the problem.

Parenthetically, the complexities of radiological diagnoses of the nervous system were later to fall within the province of a new breed of specialist— the neuroradiologist. We soon began actively looking for such an individual to join us in Tallahassee.

Once unequivocally diagnosed as an acoustic neurinoma, the individual was prepared for surgery which, in those days, was done with the patient in the sitting position. This position is best demonstrated on the cover of the book in which the author is removing another type of tumor from the skull base (foramen magnum). This approach provides the neurosurgeon a clear visual advantage, unobscured by the welling up of fluid and blood. With direct access to the neoplasm, both arms are free to manipulate the instruments. Brain retractors were very carefully, yet monotonously held by the assistant, and poor overhead illumination was supplemented with the old, standard, reflective-headlamp used by the otolaryngologists.

It isn't difficult to recall my first encounter with this imposing tumor. As mentioned previously, we had to begin setting up the operating room at 4 P.M., well after the senior surgeons had finished their day's work. Because of the inordinately long preparation time, it was 6:30 P.M. before we even made the skin incision. After the mass was exposed, we first removed a tiny portion of the internal auditory canal's bony posterior wall; this enabled us to dissect around the far lateral extent of the tumor, a prelude to separating it from the facial nerve. Once done, we then entered the middle of the tumor mass and carefully de-bulked it. All of this took several hours of work. By midnight we were ready for the most delicate and dangerous phase of the procedure, namely, dissecting the tumor capsule and the blood vessels away from the brainstem. Hours later, it was indeed gratifying to, at last, deliver the remnants of the tumor capsule from the surgical wound, thus affecting a total cure. Although giving it my best effort, I was unable to preserve the patient's facial nerve — a difficult sacrifice to accept. Despite the paralysis of one side of her face and the obligatory ipsilateral loss of hearing, she was free of this large brain tumor, which likely would have otherwise threatened her life.

In subsequent cases of large acoustic neurinomas in which I had to sacrifice the facial nerve, I was able to employ a procedure universally used by neurosurgeons to transpose another cranial nerve in a grafting procedure. My preference was to first expose the distal (the proximal segment having already been effaced intracranially by the tumor) portion of the facial nerve as it exited from the skull base, and then anastomose it directly to the XIIth cranial nerve (the nerve normally innervating one side of the tongue). Those nerves fibers from the latter would then eventually grow into the peripheral VIIth nerve fiber-sheaths in the face. Ultimately this would serve to preserve facial muscle tone, and even restore some degree of facial movement. Despite the necessity of another operation, this was cosmetically preferable to a total facial paralysis.

These acoustic nerve tumors were among the most challenging operations of our entire careers. They demanded the utmost of our intellect, skill and endurance, as attested by my own record case of 12 hours duration; but even that was far exceeded by my partner, who once labored for 22 hours to totally extirpate one of these difficult neoplasms.

~~~

In 1974 we encouraged a highly recommended neuroradiologist, Dr. Donald Beeckler, to join the neurological community in Tallahassee. He became a partner in the radiology group rather than our clinic, but we always considered him one of us. Don, as expected, brought in a fresh set of ideas regarding the radiologic diagnostic approach to any number of neurological disorders. Furthermore, he assumed full responsibility for the daily technical work in neurodiagnosis. This lifted a tremendous time-consuming burden from us. It used to be said that neurosurgical procedures would come in groups of two or three in any particular patient's case. I can recall instances in which Frank and I would have to
~~~

perform bilateral cerebral angiograms and ventriculography preceding a given craniotomy, and, not infrequently, these were done on an urgent basis. With Dr. Beeckler now here to assist, he could execute the diagnostic workup while we were freed up to examine patients and work in the operating room.

As previously stated, our neurological group maintained a strong sense of academia, and Dr. Beeckler was a welcome addition in that regard. Citing an example, the hospital procured a large, high-capacity, revolving, x-ray viewing machine onto which all of the prior day's neurological imaging studies were mounted. Each and every morning at 7:30 A.M. our neurological group would gather around with the neuroradiologist to discuss the previous day's radiographs. Routinely, there followed a rather erudite exchange of information much as one might expect to see in a university setting. The primary beneficiaries of these conferences were ultimately the patients themselves.

~~~

The much-anticipated day finally arrived when the hospital engineer began revamping the radiology department to house the magnificent EMI machine ready to be shipped from England. Months later, we watched with great enthusiasm as the scanner was eventually bolted to the floor and heavily wired into the hospital circuitry in preparation to accept its first patient. While again acknowledging with a strong sense of gratitude the efforts of Bryan Robinson and the generous contributions from his newly formed neurological foundation, that day finally arrived. What a wonderful device was this Mr. Hounsfield's scanner! No longer did I have to scramble around in the middle of the night, preparing to puncture and inject contrast material into the restless (if not combative) head injury patient's carotid artery in anticipation of a craniotomy— recall the homicide victim who had struck his head on the concrete. Nor did I have to deal with the infrequent occasion of failing altogether to obtain an acceptable diagnostic study, always a possibility in the thrashing, semiconscious patient. Here now was a machine into which we could simply transfer the supine patient from his emergency room cart, and inflate the water bag encompassing his head; we could then sit down and let the scanner do its work. Time and again, while I sat there with a late-night cup of coffee in-hand waiting for the computer to analyze and churn out the brain slice images, I would actually feel out
~~~

of place and lazy. After all, for so many years— dating far back into my residency training— I had been engaged in the rigors of performing emergency angiography under the direst of patient circumstances.

~~~

At home we were a closely knit family, but everyone's time was largely occupied, particularly during the week when the children were busy with school and their many extracurricular activities. Most of our time spent together was on weekends, and much of it centered on sporting activities. There was ample space in the paved driveway area behind the house, where there were many basketball games played (and plenty of skinned knees to show for it). The large front lawn was a splendid location not only to play touch football, but the family was large enough that we even enjoyed an occasional game of softball "workup." The spirit of competition was engendered in my children at an early age and has never ceased.

The front yard was also contiguous with a field where my son Jeffrey first developed his interest in baseball. When he was a small boy I taught him the basics in fielding, pitching and hitting. I remember the little kid holding up a mitt twice the size of his head as he stood far down by the fence, catching a fly ball hit well over 200 feet. He never shied back from the ball, and soon became skilled at the sport. Jeff later grew up to be quite a baseball player, starring in high school. I have always been very proud of all of my children's many accomplishments.

Our swimming pool also provided a great source of family fun during the warm season. As a carryover from my own childhood, I taught my children how to swim, perform life-saving maneuvers, and to dive off of our one-meter board. Because we didn't have cell phones in those days, I ran a sixty-foot telephone line out of the living room and up by poolside, always anticipating a call from either the physician in the emergency room or one from some distant town. Although frequently interrupted from our fun in the pool, we always cherished those moments that we did enjoy together.

The traditional American holidays were never lost to my family, and best demonstrated by our quality time spent together. Years later as adults my children often fondly recall those events, and have perpetuated the spirits of Halloween, Easter and Christmas within their own families.
~~~

Worthy of emphasis was another characteristic of the "Lucky Few" generation, where the mother generally remained at home and assumed both the household responsibilities and those regarding the children. Robbie and I considered that important in our own family structure, especially in view of the demands placed upon me at the hospital.

Because I had spent most of my life up to that point in the study and practice of medicine, I felt that I very much needed another outlet from my work in addition to the family. Even Osler recommended that the physician have some hobby or outlet away from the daily grind of medicine as a means of keeping both the body and the mind in good health.

Heretofore, I had always enjoyed the great game of golf, but had little to show for it. Granted, I had achieved low scores during any number of good rounds, but honestly, there were many bad ones that I would like to have forgotten. It seemed that I had arrived at a point in the game where I could not consistently improve any further. I seriously needed to give thought to an alternative hobby. In retrospect, golf was a major consideration in my originally moving to Florida, yet I never chose to pursue it after arriving here. Eventually, I gave my clubs to Jeff.

At some point it finally dawned on me that I finally had the opportunity for a hobby in which I could creatively account for my spare time. Why not build furniture for all to enjoy? Now, as a source of relaxation, those well-honed skills used in the operating room could be applied directly in the shop at home. How satisfying it would be to learn the techniques of complex joinery leading to the construction of beautiful pieces of furniture without any metal fasteners. Ever since those memorable days when I was a little child taking in the sights of those robust, magnificent power tools and the pleasant odor of lumber in my grandfather's high school workshop, I had aspired to have a similar shop of my own someday. When that day finally arrived, the cornerstone tool of my garage workshop was a floor-model Craftsman table saw with a 12-inch blade. Soon thereafter I acquired in succession: a bandsaw, drill press, lathe and an assortment of hand tools as well. I felt a strong incentive to expertly learn to use these tools, even though my surgical friends around the country were appalled that I would even think of subjecting my hands to such risk, merely for a hobby. I was very much aware that I needn't necessarily lose a hand nor even an entire finger— but simply the mere tip of a finger— to eliminate me from a neurosurgical career. As a relevant point of emphasis: In our field we must necessarily discern tactile sensation as it is transmitted from the remote distal ends of delicate instruments through our fingertips as we engage in our work.

My first few years in the shop were spent in a self-teaching mode, both finding my own way in the use and maintenance of the tools, and also learning basic woodworking techniques. With regard to the latter, most of the acquired information was gleaned from reading past material written by the old master-craftsmen and from sparsely published woodworking periodicals. Shop time was initially spent making various and sundry simple cabinets, book / file cases and table stands, which I took pride in designing myself. These projects were generally constructed from the inexpensive soft woods of pine and fir. In the years to follow I planned on purchasing and gaining expertise in additional tools, designing and building more complex items, and utilizing more expensive, often figured- hardwoods in doing so. I envisioned it as providing me with countless future hours of challenging activity, pleasure and self-fulfillment away from the arduous task of the demanding, yet interesting practice of neurological surgery.

~~~

One morning I received a phone call from a physician across town at the Florida State University clinic. The doctor related to me that he was currently confronted with a freshman football linebacker who complained that each time he would engage in a hard tackle, he would experience pain in his neck and "shock-like" sensations in his arms. The doctor was deeply concerned about a perplexing x-ray film of the young man's neck. I immediately had the physician send the athlete directly to my office with radiographs in hand.

Upon entering my office I found him to be a tall, strapping, muscular chap as one might expect of a college football player. He was in no visible pain at the time, and a thorough neurological examination was entirely normal. I was astounded, however, when I flipped the x-ray film onto my viewbox in the examining room. The reader will recall my previously having discussed the odontoid process as a site of cervical fracture, rendering the neck unstable and risking spinal cord injury. In this particular football player's case the odontoid process, as such, was congenitally absent, there being only scant evidence of a rudimentary ossicle present, an anomaly known as *os odontoideum.* To everyone's bewilderment, this young athlete had transcended his entire early life of
~~~

growth and development while playing contact sports without the bony support of an odontoid process. Only the supporting ligaments of his spine had served to prevent his neck from dislocating during forceful motion— a potentially disastrous scenario. It was difficult for both the student athlete and his family to comprehend such a state of affairs in view of his muscular development, strength and athleticism all through high school. Nonetheless, it became imperative that he no longer participate in football. Moreover, in order to prevent a future spinal cord injury from an automobile accident or even a minor fall, we recommended a surgical operation to permanently stabilize his cervical spine. After realizing the potential gravity of the situation, the entire family consented to the surgery, and he was admitted to TMH. Because he lacked a functional odontoid process altogether, we had to go one step beyond the operation previously described for a simple odontoid fracture. It was necessary that we wire and fuse with bone the upper three cervical vertebrae to the base of the skull. Despite minimal limitation of neck motion after the operation, he did fine, later becoming gainfully employed and eventually raising a family. When seen in the office 25 years later for an unrelated problem, the bone fusion was found to have remained solid, and the neck stable as demonstrated by a series of dynamic radiographs.

Thus far several representative neurosurgical cases, as encountered both in the office and the hospital, have been cited. The following case history presents a very unusual set of circumstances, but requires some basic background knowledge.

I have previously discussed the lethal threat of acute subdural hemorrhage accompanying serious head injuries. Usually these space-occupying clots are the result of venous hemorrhage from torn bridging veins between the brain and the venous collecting systems within the fibrous membrane (dura mater) overlying the organ. Under ordinary circumstances there is a time frame after the injury allowing for prompt diagnosis and treatment. There exists yet another entity which may result from a substantial blow to the head— generally to the side of the skull— also resulting in an intracranial hemorrhage, but the pathology is different. Parenthetically, many people have been warned at one time or another early in life, that if struck on the side of the head —"they might well die." Indeed, there is an element of truth to that statement. In point of fact, the temporal bone of the skull in front of the ear is one of the thinnest bones of the calvarium, and closely applied to its inner-surface is an artery. If the skull is fractured in that location, the artery may well be torn, resulting in a very brisk, sustained hemorrhage. Given a sizeable clot in that region, the temporal lobe of the brain may be displaced medially by the clot and may herniate, impacting the brain stem and rapidly causing death. An injury such as this demands immediate diagnosis and emergent treatment to avert such a catastrophic result. In contradistinction to relatively slow venous bleeding, it bears emphasis that arterial hemorrhage is rapid and pulsates with each beat of the heart. One of my professors in Chicago once told me, "When you are summoned to the hospital from home to treat a subdural hematoma you must hurry, but may have time to put on your shoes and socks while dressing. If an epidural hematoma is suspected, there is no time for the socks."

And now for the story: Late one weekend afternoon, I received a concerned call from an Air Force physician at Tyndall Air Force Base, well over 100 miles from Tallahassee. The partially trained young general surgeon related to me that he was in the process of evaluating a 12-year-old boy whom they had just brought in after a fall in which he struck the side of his head on a hard surface. He continued... and while the boy had not initially lost consciousness, he was left with a headache, had a bruise over his temple, and had x-ray evidence of an underlying linear temporal skull fracture. Also, it was noted that the pupil of the boy's eye was slightly larger on the side of the fracture. Of utmost concern was the fact that, as we spoke, the child's headache was steadily worsening.

Upon hearing this alarming history and learning of the findings, I felt reasonably certain that the child was developing an epidural hematoma. What's more, there wasn't enough time, even by air, to transport him to Tallahassee for emergency surgery. As we were conversing, I briefly reflected back on my own training as a first-year general surgical resident. I was lucky to have just observed a burr hole being made, to say nothing of having trephined one myself. Nonetheless, I asked the young surgeon if he had ever participated in such an operation. With some hesitation, he replied that several years before he had had… "very limited experience." The doctor fully concurred with my feeling: That in order to save this child's life, he alone must step up and trephine the child's skull. As he quickly wrote things down, I listed in order the steps to be taken: exactly where the incision was to be made, the instruments to be used, and how the operation was to proceed from there. If the exploratory burr hole revealed the anticipated clot, he was advised to increase the size of the bony opening by creating a silver-dollar-size craniectomy, enabling him to both remove the entire hematoma and ligate the suspected bleeding artery. After repeating things back to me, clear in his own mind what he was supposed to do, he hastened the child to the operating room. A couple of hours later I received another phone call from Tyndall AFB— the surgeon proudly informed me that he had successfully removed the suspected clot and had staunched the bleeding. After having unquestionably saved this boy's life, he then agreed to aerovac him to Tallahassee, where I would tidy up the wound in our operating room, and later follow the patient up in the office. Needless to say, when the little guy arrived at TMH, the pertinent work had very competently been done, and there was very little left for me to do. Upon dismissal from the office in six weeks the child appeared perfectly normal, despite his ordeal.

I don't believe that I have ever been prouder of a colleague during my career than I was of that Air Force captain that Saturday afternoon. After all, it hadn't been that many years since I had been in those shoes as a partially trained general surgeon responsible for an Air Force base emergency room. It was easy, indeed, for me to empathize with his plight. Regrettably, I never had the privilege of meeting him; nonetheless, I wrote to his commanding officer, commending the captain for his courageous venture outside of his field of expertise in saving a child's life.

~~~
~~~

SIX

Entering the World of Microsurgery

~~~

1975 was a very interesting year in my life from several different standpoints. The first one to be mentioned had a major impact as to how operative neurosurgery would be practiced in the future.

In 1957, as background information, Dr. Theodore Kurze at the University of Southern California (one of the author's oral board examiners in 1973) was the first to use the operative microscope in a human craniotomy. Over the succeeding 15 years there were many pioneers in the further development of microneurosurgery as we see it today (47).

Dr. Albert Rhoton, Jr., professor and chairman of the Department of Neurosurgery at the University of Florida in Gainesville, later began writing the book on the microscopic vascular anatomy of the human brain. Through meticulous cadaver dissections under the surgical microscope, Dr. Rhoton and his staff were able to methodically dissect and pictorially demonstrate the microvasculature of many important brain regions. While many of the larger parent vessels depicted had been recognized for years, the true extent of their perfusion had remained unknown; moreover, a multitude of much smaller perforating arteries and their respective areas of circulation were demonstrated for the first time. Over a period of several years, integral segments of this monumental work were subsequently published, collectively exhibiting clear, artistically accentuated photographs of the dissected vessels. In the years to follow much of this material became indispensable to most neurosurgeons for any number of reasons. I personally found it most useful both during the dissection and clipping of intracranial aneurysms, and also in approaching tumors at the base of the brain. But to fully appreciate this atlas-like compilation of anatomy, one had to first not
~~~

only become proficient in the use of the surgical microscope, but also in microsurgical techniques as well. Dr. Rhoton was to offer this opportunity to any neurosurgeon desirous of following this innovative path. Accordingly, he envisioned, organized and implemented a splendid course in microneurosurgery at the University of Florida.

Frank and I were two of the surgeons among the early groups taking Al Rhoton's informative course. Frank went first for his five-day rather intensive session, and after his return to watch over our practice I then drove to Gainesville for my participation.

The setting provided was a clean, well-illuminated, small, yet very comfortable teaching laboratory with roughly six to eight neurosurgeons participating in the course. Most of those in my group were from Florida. We sat at a long centralized bench, each individual having his own desk-top space with a surgical microscope and the necessary instruments. While Dr. Rhoton was the primary instructor, there customarily was a second microvascular surgeon of national prominence assisting — in my group it was Dr. Robert Crowell from Boston.

I have very pleasant memories of that entire experience from the onset of the first day. Interestingly, there was some pressure to learn under duress, for most of us had basically had very little previous experience with the surgical microscope, and virtually none with the tiny structures with which we were about to deal. One doesn't relish the thought of making a mess out of a new and difficult surgical exercise in front of his peers. But we were all quite congenial, had strong senses of both empathy and humor, and all possessed similar degrees of surgical skill. Any difficulties that anyone might have encountered were appreciated by all, and were assuaged by Dr. Rhoton, an excellent and tolerant teacher, indeed. The atmosphere in my mind was pleasantly conducive to learning; the information gleaned, indispensable; and the friendships, everlasting.

As expected, the early part of the first day was used to introduce us to the surgical microscope and its intricacies. I immediately recalled the day back at the Evanston Hospital when Joe Tarkington shouted at me, as a surgical resident, for not attaching the correct lens to the scope. To the contrary, our instruction now began with a basic, thorough discussion of the optics of this complex device, including the indications for lenses of variable focal lengths. This knowledge would enable us to work either deep within the brain, or on more superficial areas, depending upon the geometric plane of interest. We also learned that the visual beam could be split into a second ocular pathway utilized by an assistant/observer, television monitor or camera, depending upon the circumstances. Heretofore, I had no conception of the numerous applications of the surgical microscope. After further instruction in the use of the various microsurgical instruments, we were then ready for our first hands-on experience.

Vivid in my mind was that first exercise in which we performed a tracheotomy upon a large, anesthetized white rat. The trachea in this animal was perhaps one half the diameter of a pencil, a good starting point in getting the feel for microsurgical technique while navigating within a field of magnification. We were all soon able to appreciate the tactile sensation of working with jeweler's forceps and fine dissecting/cutting instruments under superb illumination and magnification without roughing up the rats or causing their demise.

The second exercise entailed the dissection of the structures within the carotid sheath of the animal's neck, followed by the performance of a side-to-side vascular anastomosis between the carotid artery and the jugular vein— namely, the creation of an arteriovenous shunt.

The final challenge consisted of constructing an arterial bypass by dividing the 3mm. carotid artery on one side, and re-routing it behind the esophagus to suture its cleanly incised stoma (end) to the side of the contralateral carotid artery. The surgical goal, of course, was to create and maintain a patent, water-tight, functioning arterial bypass. Once completed, I can recall how satisfied we all were as we observed our individual bypasses through our microscopes, the efferent vascular loop rhythmically pulsating with each beat of the animal's heart as it competently diverted blood to the contralateral side of the rat's brain. We had just entered a new and exciting chapter concerning our neurosurgical armamentarium.

At the end of the vascular session, several questions were raised by the group. One of mine concerned the possibility of an aneurysm rupture during its dissection under magnification. It seemed to me that with blood suddenly flooding the magnified field and obscuring the anatomy, it would be a very treacherous problem with which to deal. Dr. Rhoton assured us that once the blood was evacuated from the operative field of vision, it was in fact easier under magnification to secure the aneurysm without an errant clip placement.

The remainder of the week was occupied with a variety of micro-neurosurgical exercises, including cadaver microvascular anastomoses such as we might encounter when treating a patient in the operating room. Also under magnification, we performed bone dissections with a small high-speed drill of the type used both in the transsphenoidal approach to the pituitary gland and in the unroofing of the internal auditory canal during the surgery of acoustic neurinomas. These bone dissection specimens from the microsurgery course remain in my display case some 34 years later, having since been used upon occasion for teaching purposes.

~~~

A second experience highlighting1975 also bears mentioning. There are a number of milestones one hopes to achieve during the course of one's professional development as a surgeon. For instance, the importance of board certification cannot be over-emphasized. This is not merely a question of self-fulfillment, but reflects a level of achievement which may be important to the prospective patient in choosing a specialist. Yet another level of relevant achievement was my induction into the American College of Surgeons. This prestigious organization is the largest collective group of surgeons in the United States, representing virtually all of the surgical specialties. Among its primary goals are the continuing education of all surgeons, and, in the public's best interest, the setting of sound policies and standards for the practice of surgery. To gain membership into this organization one must have been trained at a well-recognized university center, met certain stringent educational requirements, and been certified by his/her own specialty board. In addition, records of all surgical procedures (including those performed in the radiology department) done by the candidate during the two years preceding application had to be submitted for scrutiny. Finally, the applicant had to be recommended by two standing members of the ACS as personal references. After my acceptance in the fall of 1975, my wife and I flew to San Francisco where I joined my class for that year in a formal cap-and -gown induction ceremony.

Of added significance on that honorable occasion was listening to the keynote guest speaker. This prominent man, Dr. D. Carleton Gadjusek, was later to share the 1976 Nobel Prize in medicine for his work on what were then called, "the slow viruses." The distinguished group of several hundred surgeons listened spellbound as Dr. Gadjusek spoke of what was a recently discovered killer of mankind.
~~~

He began by describing a disease in sheep long known as Scrapie, which was manifested by a rapid deterioration of the nervous system. His point in discussing Scrapie was the fact that the disease had been recognized for many years in the veterinary literature, but because of poor cross-referencing it was never compared with similar diseases in humans. The next related illness Dr.Gadjusek alluded to was named "Kuru", a CNS disease attacking the brains of a primitive tribe in the highlands of New Guinea. The infectious agent in the case of Kuru was spread among family members during the ritualistic practice of cannibalism. The modern, human proto-type of the slow virus group of diseases, Creutzfelt-Jakob Disease (CJD), was finally discussed. This terrifying illness had long been recognized in the neuropathological literature as "diffuse spongioform encephalopathy" —a disease universally fatal in one to two years after onset. It causes widespread destruction of the central nervous system, often presenting as a rapidly progressive presenile dementia. These disorders all had common features among which are a very long incubation period often as long as 12 to 15 years after exposure (hence, the reason for calling them "slow viruses"); a constellation of characteristic neurological abnormalities at the time of presentation; and a relatively rapid, downhill course ending in death. Postmortem examination of the brains revealed widespread loss of neuronal tissue, and a spongiform appearance under the microscope. Conspicuous by its absence was a lack of a cellular inflammatory response contrary to what is normally seen in cases of encephalitis. Of paramount concern was the fact that these diseases, a variant being the modern day mad cow disease, were all caused by a transmissible agent—one very difficult to inactivate or destroy by conventional means. Several cases had been reported in the surgical literature which had clearly been traced to the ineffective sterilization of instruments, for example during corneal transplantation. Instruments exposed to the tissues containing the "slow virus" could not be sterilized by boiling, autoclaving, ultraviolet light, antiseptics such as iodine or even formaldehyde. Soaking them in Clorox was the only effective method of disinfection.

Upon returning to Tallahassee, I expeditiously delivered a hospital lecture to the general medical staff and our pathologists on this alarming group of "slow virus" diseases. Not only were cases springing up in the current medical literature after organ transplantation, but we suspected one or two cases in our own institution for which we added Clorox to our sterilization routine.

Only in more recent years have we come to learn that the transmissible agent in these diseases is not a virus after all, but rather a misfolded (abnormal) copy of a normal brain protein called a prion protein (PrP). In 1997 Stanley B. Prusiner won the Nobel Prize in medicine for his discovery of the prion. While current research has not yet uncovered the origin of the abnormal prion, once present it alarmingly and uncontrollably induces normal PrP to misfold, resulting in the relentless destruction of the brain leading to death.

In closing on a personal note, it is only fitting that both my interest in this group of transmissible diseases and my deep admiration of Drs. Gadjusek and Prusiner reflect back to my original interest in medicine as a child, which was spurred by reading De Kruif's, *"Microbe Hunters."*

~~~

While the acoustic neurinomas are now familiar to the reader as occurring exclusively in the posterior fossa as one of the most seriously challenging tumors to the neurosurgeon, we are now reminded that there are other tumors located in that region. The majority of primary brain tumors in children also occur in the posterior fossa; more specifically, most are found within the cerebellum— an important brain mass modulating balance and coordination. Of the primary neoplasms occurring within the cerebellum of children, there are two predominant types, each usually presenting in children under 12 years of age and manifesting similar symptoms. That, however, is where the similarity ends. One tumor, the astrocytoma, is benign; the other, the medulloblastoma, is extremely malignant.

The reader will recall my 1970 experience in Atlantic City, when I presented a clinical research paper, co-authored with Dr. Bucy. That paper was entitled, "Astrocytomas of The Cerebellum in Children — Long-Term Study" (10). The case material in that paper entailed contacting and examining a series of adult patients operated upon many years before as children. The essence of that clinical research was to emphasize the fact that with a timely diagnosis and total surgical removal, long-term survival could be achieved. We had several patients living 20 to 30 years after extirpation of their primary brain tumors. As made evident by that paper: The alarming discovery of a primary brain tumor does not necessarily predispose one to an early death.
~~~

During my years of private practice in Tallahassee, I have had the opportunity to evaluate and operate upon several similar cases. As a point of emphasis, these children most often present to the primary care physician in serious condition, and when seen by the neurosurgeon they frequently have signs of increased intracranial pressure secondary to obstructive hydrocephalus. If not immediately relieved of this pressure, a fatal issue is certain to follow. Given such a child in dire straits with headaches and vomiting from pressure, the opportunity of being able to affect a cure by totally removing the tumor is a very rewarding operation for the neurosurgeon. I shall reflect on my last such experience with this lesion.

As so often the case it was an evening phone call, this time from a family physician whom I had helped to train many years previously in Tallahassee. Having been sent to us from Panama City, the child, a seriously ill boy with headaches of mounting intensity and vomiting, arrived later that night. After admission, he was expeditiously worked up with laboratory and imaging studies in preparation for early morning surgery; by late the next afternoon, we had totally enucleated his tumor. In spite of the fact that the child entered the hospital with dangerously elevated pressure on his brain from hydrocephalus, he was discharged totally asymptomatic just a few days later— in all likelihood permanently cured of his brain tumor.

The malignant counterpart childhood tumor within the cerebellum, the medulloblastoma, carries an entirely different prognosis, with the initial presentation of headaches and vomiting being the same as the previous patient. We had the opportunity to treat several of these patients as well. As shown below, the age spread was significant.

My first encounter was caring for a cute, thirty-month-old toddler, whom my partner had operated upon when the child was one year of age. I happened to be on call the weekend that she came in at the end-stage of her disease and quietly passed away. I'll never forget those totally devastated, grieving parents as they choked and sobbed over the loss of their angelic, little, blue-eyed, blonde girl. Maintaining my own composure has never been tested to a greater extent than it was that sad day while attempting to comfort them. I strongly empathized with their grief, for I also had a little blonde, two-year-old girl of my own at the time.

The second patient with a medulloblastoma fell near the other end of the age spectrum. It was an 8-year-old boy upon whom I had operated. His tumor mushroomed inferiorly out of the cerebellum while encroaching upon the roof of the vital brainstem, and was visibly plugging the Sylvian aqueduct. With the aid of the microscope I was able to remove all visible tumor within the surgical field, as later confirmed by enhanced, high- resolution CT scanning. Despite what appeared to have been a total gross removal, we all knew that the natural history of this lethal tumor would eventually prove us wrong. Realizing that tumor cells had probably seeded out in the spinal fluid, the child was given a full course of irradiation therapy to the entire craniospinal axis. After he had fully convalesced, I referred him to a pediatric neuro-oncologist at the University of Florida in Gainesville, who administered an extensive course of chemotherapy.

Years went by, and everyone was jubilant over what appeared to be a cure. This bright, affable, handsome, lad grew up, and graduated from high school as one of the most popular students in his class. But sadly, and despite the valiant efforts of a host of medical personnel, his tumor relentlessly recurred, sweeping this young man's life away from his loving family and friends.

Neuropathologists for years have informed us of the predictable nature of the medulloblastoma. Because the primitive germ cells from which the tumor is derived are present at the initial time of brain development, the predictive length of the patient's survival seems to be double the chronological age at the time of surgery plus nine months—even with aggressive treatment. This rule certainly seems to have held true in these two illustrative case histories, but someday we will hopefully defy that rule, and find a solution to this relentless neoplasm so lethal to youngsters.

~~~

The reader might well ask, at this point, what my experience has been concerning the often discussed topic of medical malpractice. In my case, this subject dates back to a conversation I had with Dr. Joe Tarkington during my first day as a neurosurgical resident, when we were discussing a patient while studying his x-ray on the view-box. The doctor was trying to make a point to me when, in a very serious tone, he said, "Jim, here at this institution, we look upon every patient as a potential threat for a lawsuit." Obviously very naïve at the time, I had difficulty comprehending what the man was talking about. At that time the definition of medical malpractice, as I had been taught by a law
~~~

professor in a medical jurisprudence course at the Northwestern medical school, was basically defined as: "A deviation from the prevailing standard of practice of medicine in the community at the time of the incident, thereby directly resulting in the bodily injury or death of the patient." I would not have even considered deviating from the standard of medical practice, but to the contrary, expected to practice with the highest standards and to the best of my ability. In my own mind I had studied far too hard and been too conscientious to stray off of the high road of medical virtue by cutting corners or exhibiting carelessness.

Nonetheless, I was in for a rude awakening, for I hadn't been in Tallahassee a year before an incident occurred. Keeping in mind that definition of malpractice, I shall describe the case, and allow others to judge.

Several months into my practice, a middle-aged fellow presented to me in agony, having sustained the sudden onset of severe pain from a ruptured disc in his back. His low back pain radiating down his leg was of such intensity that he could barely stand. We put him at total bed rest in the hospital and on pain medication for a week, as was both customary and affordable in the early 1970s. He showed no improvement and continued to manifest both pain and a compromise of nerve function in his leg from the pressure of the disc. We recommended surgery on his back to remove the offending disc fragment from beneath the nerve root, and, without hesitation, he requested that I proceed. It was standard procedure for me to give him what we called "informed consent," concerning the risks of surgery. I then recited an extensive list of potential side effects which, although very unlikely, could possibly occur in association with the operation. Among many possibilities these included: infection, blood transfusion, loss of bowel, bladder or sexual function; paralysis of his legs or even unexpected death. In view of his disabling pain, he clearly accepted these risks and requested that we proceed with the operation.

In the operating room, the surgery was carried out with the patient positioned prone on the padded frame. The outstretched arms were carefully flexed at the elbow, generously padded with protective blankets and rolled towels, and supported on arm boards. The operation progressed uneventfully, the nerve root having been released from its compression by the disc fragment. The man awakened from the anesthetic free of leg pain. The next morning when I made rounds, he reported that his back and leg were fine except for the pain in his incision. However, he was experiencing numbness over the inside of his hand, and had difficulty spreading his fingers sideways. In short, he had an ulnar nerve palsy in his arm, probably the result of pressure on the nerve at the elbow, albeit, remote from the site of surgery in his back. We simply don't know how or when this occurred. It could well have been during the operation, but the entire operating room staff attested to my obsession with positioning and protecting the patient in preparation for surgery, including the thorough padding of all pressure points in the arms. The palsy could have also possibly occurred in the recovery room or even in his hospital bed while still under some late influence of the anesthetic, his body position having remained largely unchanged throughout the night.

Because during the ensuing weeks the patient failed to show any significant improvement of his hand despite physical therapy, another operation was carried out to release the ulnar nerve at the elbow. Meanwhile, he made a full recovery from his disc operation with no evidence of nerve damage and no further pain in either his back or leg.

Several months later I was disheartened to receive word from his attorney that he was filing a lawsuit against me, alleging negligence. His lawyer conceded that I given the patient and his wife informed consent, including the possibility of paralysis in the legs or death, but I failed to mention the possibility of a potential nerve problem in either his arm or hand. Realistically, I hadn't mentioned it, simply because it was totally unexpected, remote as it was from the operative site. When I appeared before the judge on this case, he looked at me, and openly admitted that I had done nothing negligently wrong. However, at the same time he invoked the Latin phrase, "*res ipsa loquitur*" or "the thing speaks for itself." In elaborating, he found me responsible for this man's injury, simply because I was "the captain of the ship"—declaring that anything adversely happening to this patient under my watch was my fault.

There is more to come in the book respecting medical malpractice. For the moment, however, there are certain facts to be addressed in this case. First, the patient did sustain a permanent injury, whether it was in some way indirectly related to the operation or not. Second, it was not due to negligence as a result of my having deviated from the accepted standard practice of surgery, if we use that time-honored definition. Third, doctors of the future coming under scrutiny by similar judicial decisions, even though they are totally innocent of misconduct, risk losing their reputations or even their licenses to practice medicine. Finally, most will agree that patients in some way need to be compensated. Several options have been suggested in that regard, including some type of state managed patient compensation fund. Suffice it to say, at that point very early in my professional career during a relatively straightforward operation, an event not directly related to the operation itself did occur; and despite the fact that I had attempted to do everything correctly, I was held liable.

Medical malpractice claims escalated throughout the United States in the 1970s, and Florida was not exempt. Physicians' insurance premiums in high-risk specialties, such as ours, skyrocketed, and both the increasing incidence of malpractice claims and the high jury awards became nearly intolerable. In 1975 professional liability carriers began pulling out of Florida, and many doctors were left without any insurance at all. There was a three-month period in which Frank and I could not obtain a malpractice policy, forcing us to "go bare" for that period of time. It defies the imagination to think of practicing neurosurgery without protective insurance in an environment where adverse things beyond our control may happen at any time. We initially agreed to send off the high-risk cases to the University of Florida, because the university center is considered the "last bastion" of treatment, and probably somewhat less susceptible to a law suit should an injury occur. But consider for a moment: Everything we do within the province of brain and spinal cord surgery is high-risk. I can recall vividly one such patient whom I absolutely could not bring myself to accept; perhaps I was unfair in judging him. He was a huge, bullish man in severe pain with a ruptured disc in his neck. His case called for an approach through the front side, a potentially dangerous operation, simply because of his thick, short neck. His anatomy dictated a deep narrow surgical wound in close proximity to the spinal cord. Although I had performed a substantial number of these anterior cervical operations, and had never personally experienced an adverse incident, I saw this man as a serious risk. Despite his languishing in pain and his sincerity in asking me to perform the procedure, I felt compelled (while practicing defensive medicine) to send him to the university for treatment. Frankly, I had a bad intuitive feeling about that particular patient.

With an ever-increasing strong distaste concerning the negative and always threatening subject of medical malpractice, I became active on the legislative committee of our Capital Medical Society. We lobbied legislators, attended numerous political dinner functions, and even audited committee meetings at the State Capitol building. Eventually, by winning the major support of the state legislature, the Florida Medical Association was able to help draft and implement passage of a bill supporting the concept of a "state mediation panel" to aid in alleviating the crisis. The panel was to consist of a doctor, lawyer, and a judge who would provide a forum to hear the grievance. The mediation panel would listen to the merits of the case, if any, and then make a recommendation. The panel's decision was in no way legally binding, and the plaintiff, irrespective of the recommendation, was still free to take his case to court. We felt confident that such a mediation panel would go a long way in reducing frivolous lawsuits and high insurance premiums, thereby encouraging the companies back into the insurance pool in Florida. But the doctors of our state were shocked when the Supreme Court of Florida ruled that: "a mediation panel was unconstitutional."

At the request of some of the officers of our county medical society, I then wrote a rather lengthy, comprehensive article describing the problem and our enigma in solving this malpractice conundrum. In trying to deliver our message to the public in order to enlist its understanding and support, the officers of the medical society enthusiastically hand-carried the article to the local newspaper for publication. The paper refused to publish it! They retorted that the lawyers insisted that they be given equal space for a rebuttal article. For some reason, that was never done. Interestingly, some of the contents of the article leaked out of Tallahassee; for soon thereafter, I caught a glimpse of fragments of it— copied verbatim— in a newspaper down in the southern part of the state.

The long hours of work concerning all of these measures were merely exercises of futility; it was perfectly clear that the cards were heavily stacked against the medical profession. The future impact on society regarding increasing medical costs and physician availability will be discussed later.

~~~

An important snapshot into my personal life occurred on October 18, 1976, when our second son, Roger, was born; and because the other children were growing up, it was an exciting day for everyone! I kept the other three kids out of school that day so that they could be with me to celebrate the birth of their little brother. That day for brunch I took them to Burger King for hamburgers and teased them that the "truant officer" might be looking to catch them out of school. It was the first
~~~

time that they had ever heard of such a character, and they all anxiously looked around the booths for him, wondering what he might look like as they ate their hamburgers. While we have since laughed about it as adults, when they were little they told me they had been fearful that he would throw them in jail. Later that morning the baby was born, and since my wife and I had always planned on four children, we couldn't have been happier now with two of each sex. I have always enjoyed them immensely, our relationships changing with each passing year. As adults, I look upon them more as companions in life; nonetheless, I never seem to quit worrying about their welfare.

Speaking of children, a dramatic chain of events occurred on Father's Day of that same bicentennial year. I was deeply engaged in my workshop trying to cut some tapered legs for a television cabinet on my table saw when I received an emergency call from the hospital. The operator informed me that Dr. Carey Farmer's son had sustained a head injury, and was en route to the hospital. It seems that the little nine-year-old boy was standing on a 3-meter diving board at the local country club pool when he slipped off, striking his head on the cement deck nearly 10 feet below. Immediately after the fall there was a complete and sustained loss of consciousness, which persisted when I intercepted him as the ambulance pulled up to the hospital unloading dock. His father, Carey, was, ironically, one of our emergency room doctors at Tallahassee Memorial, and an excellent one indeed. Although I had known him for some time, we were about to become much closer. His child was deeply comatose from the severe closed head injury (today commonly referred to as "traumatic brain injury" or TBI), hence, we promptly maneuvered him into the EMI scanner. Carey, understandably, was beside himself with worry, having personally tended to so many head injuries himself. As the pictorial brain slices slowly emerged from the machine, we were relieved that there was no major intracranial hemorrhage or brain shift. However, there were indications of diffuse contusions, namely, bruising of the brain tissue. We took the child to the operating room, and inserted an intracranial pressure monitor to help us better manage the brain swelling commensurate with such an injury. For days, the boy remained comatose but otherwise stable. Carey, persistently agonizing over his son's serious injury, and I spent literally hours together discussing potential outcome scenarios for the child. At that early stage after the injury, we could not rule out significant lasting brain damage. Then one day, the little guy began to spontaneously move his extremities and later opened his eyes. The prognosis, which is often better in children than adults with comparable degrees of injury, suddenly became more favorable. Once having turned the corner he continued on to make a complete neurological recovery. What a joy for all of us it was to see this little boy begin to smile and run again. Carey Farmer, whom I had come to know as a close friend, was a man of many talents. He was not only a physician and a lawyer, but several years previously, had also been elected to the Florida House of Representatives from a congressional district in the southern part of the state. Because of that broad experience, he was invaluable during that period of time in which we were involved in trying to solve the medical malpractice crisis. But events in that family were to later take another tragic turn. At 42 years of age Cary, also a pilot, and his wife were flying a small plane 150 miles east of Tallahassee on their way home from a trip to Orlando, when they encountered a violent thunderstorm. The news of the inescapable crash killing them both shocked the entire community. I will always remember Carey as a truly good man with a very positive attitude, and one who was often at my side in dealing with serious trauma cases in the emergency room. I have sorely missed him both as a colleague and as a friend.

~~~

One of the advantages of my having trained in Chicago, and my partner in New Orleans, is the fact that we were each able to learn unfamiliar surgical techniques from one other. While I had performed any number of disk operations through the front of the neck, I had no prior experience in the surgical treatment of burst fractures of the cervical vertebrae. Reference has already been made to the rather high incidence of spinal fractures brought into our emergency department, both from the nearby highways as well as far distant towns. The burst fracture presents a unique set of problems, not only where cervical spinal instability is concerned, but also because of the loss of spinal height. Frank taught me the technique of vertebral body replacement, which interestingly bears a strong resemblance to the mortise and tenon woodworking joint. While the patient is maintained in skeletal traction, the shattered vertebral body is totally removed through the front of the neck, and is replaced by a solid rectangular block of bone fabricated from the patient's ilium. The graft is snugly fitted into mortises cut with a high speed air instrument into the normal intact vertebrae above and
~~~

below the burst. A metal plate with pre-drilled holes is then fastened with screws to the graft (now functioning as a vertebral body) and the two adjacent vertebrae, thereby holding it in place until the fusion is complete in three months. Several months later, after healing was complete and the spine radiographically stable, we usually re-operated to remove the hardware. This minor procedure was done to prevent future backing out of the screws, and their migration into the soft tissues. With cervical fractures of such magnitude, the patient invariably sustains an immediate severe and irreversible spinal cord injury resulting in quadriplegia, but that doesn't obviate the need for spinal stabilization. The latter becomes particularly important if it is a low cervical fracture, and the patient left with some residual functional use of his upper extremities requiring rehabilitation.

~~~

Thus far we have described a variety of cases, most of them having ended favorably. It would be a gross misrepresentation, however, to leave the reader with the impression that everything in neurosurgery turns out perfectly well every time; unfortunately, that is by no means the case, as illustrated below.

Soon after having taken the microsurgical course, I had an opportunity to utilize what I had learned down at Gainesville. A young family man in his early twenties was brought in one day by ambulance after having sustained the sudden onset of a severe headache. His initial evaluation showed a man in distress with severe pain, but other than having a stiff neck, his examination was completely intact. A lumbar puncture revealed bloody spinal fluid, leading us to perform arteriography of the brain. While suspecting a ruptured aneurysm as a cause of his intracranial hemorrhage, we were surprised to find much more than just an aneurysm. The left internal carotid artery was perhaps 30% larger than normal as it coursed up the neck and through the skull. Indeed, an aneurysm of the circle of Willis was found at the base of the brain. However, distal branches of the carotid artery coursing posteriorly from the aneurysm remained distended as they fed into a large arteriovenous malformation (AVM) of the posterior temporal region. The reader will recall that we experimentally created an AV shunt in the rat during the microsurgery course, when we sutured the side of the carotid artery to the side of the internal jugular vein. What
~~~

we saw in this patient was much the same; namely, in an AVM there are no intervening capillaries, and the blood flows directly and unimpeded from the feeding arteries into the veins. Because there is little resistance, the vessels become enlarged, and the AVM takes on the appearance of a cluster of grapes. As the walls of the enlarged veins gradually thin out, they also have a propensity to rupture, and, like an aneurysm, may cause a subarachnoid hemorrhage. In short, the patient under discussion had tandem lesions, each posing the threat of bleeding and therefore requiring treatment.

We planned our operation utilizing a large craniotomy flap, hoping to remove both vascular maladies from the brain circulation in a single sitting. The aneurysm took priority in treatment for, based upon the angiogram, it was the source of his current hemorrhage, and remained a substantial risk at re-bleeding within days. Once secured with a metal spring clip, it was then our intent to move distally to deal with the AVM. We had to constantly bear in mind the increased pressure-head of blood rapidly coursing through the artery in close proximity to the aneurysm, dangerously enhancing the likelihood of the rupture of its thin dome during the dissection.

Under high magnification with the microscope, we carefully approached and dissected the neck of the aneurysm. After perhaps two hours of work, the brain was finally relaxed, the field cleared of blood, and the neck of the aneurysm clearly delineated. Just as I was applying the clip, the fundus of the aneurysm literally exploded, savagely unleashing a torrential hemorrhage. Within an instant the entire brain wound was overflowing with blood. As expected, the profuse bleeding was greatly augmented by the low resistance of the distal AVM, which commanded an inordinately rapid blood flow. We used two large bore suction devices over protective cottonoids to effectively clear away the blood. While carefully protecting the brain, I was able to reestablish excellent visibility with the microscope (as Dr. Rhoton had indicated in his course) in order to again delineate the aneurysm neck and apply the clip. Meanwhile, the anesthesiologist kept the patient stabilized with immediate blood replacement. All of this disconcerting activity took several minutes of intensive work and quite graphically demonstrates how quickly a bad turn of events can occur in the operating theater. In this particular instance, being both aware of the time that it took in bringing things under control and also fearing the consequences of vascular spasm and brain hypoxia—we forewent any attempts to deal with the AVM at that time. We were just relieved to have gotten out of this complicating hemorrhage with a live patient.

When I entered the intensive care unit before coming home late that night, it was very discouraging —but not unexpected—to find the young man unable to voluntarily move the extremities on the right side of his body. The following morning after the entire anesthetic had dissipated, I found him unable to speak as well; in short, he was totally aphasic and hemiplegic. We transported him to the radiology department where I performed a postoperative angiogram, needing reassurance that I had not inadvertently occluded a major vessel within the aneurysm clip. The clip placement was satisfactory, but as greatly feared, the patient had sustained severe, diffuse arterial spasm. Many of the run-off arteries looked like small, used pipe-stem cleaners, being both irregular and markedly reduced in diameter. There was no evidence of a postoperative blood clot. We could now only hope that by supporting his blood pressure at a reasonable level (mindful of a potential hemorrhage from the AVM), and controlling brain swelling and hypoxia, that we could carry him through this rough postoperative period. I tried to remain optimistic of seeing some recovery —no matter how slight—from his devastating loss of neurological function. But as the days passed, he regrettably failed to show any substantial improvement. A part of me died each day when I made rounds on Don, his loving wife always at his side, and often holding his hand while his little children sat nearby. I would try to encourage him to speak, but although he looked at me alertly, he could only respond with guttural, unintelligible sounds. We followed up with months of extensive speech and physical therapy, but Don remained an invalid and unable to ever work again to support his family. It was a crushing experience!

This was my first serious therapeutic failure, and by no means my last. My wife, when seeing me distraught that night, tried to re-assure me that I had done my best. Frank and I both felt that we had given all that neurosurgery could offer at the time. The aneurysm was well clipped, and all major vessels were patent — little consolation, however, when looking at this decimated young man and his family. For the first time I now fully appreciated Dr. Tarkington's having been discouraged with his results in treating aneurysms back at the Evanston Hospital.

Having discussed this tragic case, I find it timely to again bring to the reader's attention one of the important teachings of Sir William Osler — *aequanimitas*— a word I have referred to in a previous chapter. The term pertains to the physician's imperturbability or physical and mental self-control and "cheerful" equanimity at times of both success and failure. Furthermore, the physician must maintain a "calm" under all circumstances in order to both foster clear judgment on his part, and continue to engender confidence in the patient and family as well. Dr. Osler (1849-1919), one of medicine's most distinguished figures, was the physician's teacher of medical ethics and important facets of the doctor-patient relationship; he also illuminated for us a "medical way of life." Dr. Osler spoke of this subject in his graduation address to the students at the University of Pennsylvania Medical School in 1889 (15).

As a word of advice to any prospective young surgeon: One must not allow an adverse outcome such as this to affect him personally, for he must remain composed and effective when confronted with the next difficult case. If one reads of Cushing or any of the other of our great surgical forbears, he will find that they were all confronted by circumstances virtually beyond their control. We can only try to learn from each experience, anticipate adversity, and be forearmed as we do our absolute best in moving forward. By far, the majority of the most difficult and challenging cases do well. I often recall those early days back in my surgical residency when it seemed like many of the very tough cases in neurosurgery did not do well at all. I hoped that perhaps someday I could make a difference.

~~~

In attempting to maintain a balance in the book by frequently citing personal experiences aside from my professional life, I shall now turn to a much lighter subject. One cannot begin to write about Tallahassee, Florida, without mentioning the Florida State University Seminole football team. Before even having made a commitment to come to Tallahassee, I had been intrigued with the college football program there. On Chicago television, my wife and I had enjoyed seeing the wide-open, pro-style offense of FSU with its ability to put quick points on the scoreboard. This was in marked contrast to the image of "three yards and a cloud of dust," conjured up by coach Woody Hayes at Ohio State, and generally true of the Big 10 conference in those days. The reader will recall that I had spent many years at Northwestern watching Big 10 football, the stands often being sparsely filled on a cold Saturday afternoon. To the contrary, the 1971-72 Seminole team was fun to watch. I can recall the excitement of the final game that year, despite a losing
~~~

effort, against Arizona State in the inaugural Fiesta Bowl. Thereafter, things seemed to steadily deteriorate despite changes in the coaching staff. Years later, the alumni became disenchanted, and began looking for a good new head coach to turn things around. There were rumors of such a man by the name of Bobby Bowden up at the University of West Virginia, and general interest in him soon gained widespread attention. After having read about him, I can recall telling my wife at the dinner table one night that I hoped the university could entice this man down to Tallahassee. In 1976, to everyone's delight, FSU was indeed able to talk coach Bowden into leading the Seminoles forward in their future football program.

In those days Doak Campbell Stadium was a relatively small structure, not much more than a large city high school stadium. Before coach Bowden came on the scene, I would frequently take the family out on a muggy, Tallahassee Saturday night to see FSU defeated in a low-scoring affair by, at best, a very mediocre college team. And usually while out there, if on-duty, I would get summoned to the hospital emergency room. No—there were no cell phones in those early days. The announcer in his unmistakable drawl would call, "Doctor—number—1-5-2" over the public address system right in the middle of the slow-moving game, instructing me to call "Talla— hass—ee Memorial emer— gency room." For years the same man, with the same deep inflections in his voice, would frequently break the silence of the game while calling a doctor's number. Promptly I would get up, digging in my pocket for a quarter, and then searching around under the bleachers for a pay telephone to call the hospital. We soon learned to drive two cars to the games. In the event that I should have to leave, I could bid farewell to my wife and kids before heading off to TMH. Little did I realize during those dark, hot, Saturday nights, while driving en route to see some accident victim at the hospital that things would eventually change. With a new coach and perhaps a new team on the horizon, coupled with innovative cellular phone technology, the future became brighter for this Seminole fan and his football family.

~~~

After several years of practice and innumerable frustrations, it became clearly evident that if Frank and I were ever going to move forward in our desire for excellence in neurosurgery, we were going to
~~~

have to make some major changes. A recurring and very frustrating problem concerned any surgical case running late into the evening hours, whether it was a scheduled lengthy elective case or a late-night emergency. A hospital- employed instrument technician would often appear on the scene who either didn't know the names of our instruments or the order in which we would need them. I recall specifically late one afternoon when such an individual showed up at my side as I was about to install an emergency VP shunt in a newborn with hydrocephalus. When I began asking for instruments with an outstretched hand, my full attention remaining focused on the operative field, she would invariably hand me the incorrect instrument. Two things resulted from that frustrating incident. First, I angrily summoned the operating room supervisor, and, in making a long overdue point, asked her to please fetch for me someone who knew the instruments — at least for the sake of the baby! In addition, I later conferred with my partner who was also frustrated with some of the surgical technicians who weren't interested enough to invest the time in learning neurosurgical procedure. This was no longer acceptable. We had come to highly depend upon those few, interested, competent assistants employed by the hospital who were, in fact, very efficient. But unfortunately, those technicians were not always available to us. We agreed that we would immediately begin searching for our own private instrument nurse. In a short time, we found an energetic, efficient woman to help us. With Martha's assistance, appropriate instruments were always at hand for the forthcoming surgical case; furthermore, we had a nurse always present to assist us who was knowledgeable of both the instruments and the operative procedures as well. In addition, we taught Martha all about the floor-model surgical microscope which the Robinson Neurological Foundation had recently purchased for TMH.

What's more, things began to improve in other respects as well. The hospital administration was beginning to realize that the two brain surgeons, relatively recent additions to the hospital staff, not only seemed proficient in their field of expertise, but were also engaging in many surgical procedures ordinarily performed only in the university centers. Not only were we able to bring to the community hospital an assortment of the more common adult and pediatric neurosurgical cases, but also many of the unusual and highly technical operative procedures as well. As a result, the hospital, under the direction of its administrator, Mr. M. T. Mustian, began to assist us in our endeavors. For example, the administration saw to it that we were provided with the latest state-of-the-art neurosurgical instrumentation. Heretofore, we had to "apply" for our instrument needs to a select, antiquated "committee" of surgeons who would begrudgingly ration any expenditure to us. Specifically, I recall that it almost "took an act of Congress" to acquire a new cordless drill for craniotomies or the frame used for our laminectomies. M.T. later saw to it that we got what we needed. In addition, we were given an equal opportunity to compete with the now fading "old guard" of elder surgeons for reasonable early operating room starting times, particularly for lengthy complicated cases. Furthermore, by virtue of the Robinson Neurological Foundation having supported the hospital by both procuring the first EMI scanner and the most advanced model of the surgical microscope, we were forging a strong and lasting alliance with Tallahassee Memorial Hospital.

After roughly one year Martha and her husband moved away, and we began searching for her replacement. We had our eyes on a very bright, efficient, operating room circulating nurse who not only was an RN, but also possessed a BA college degree as well. When offered the job Jenny was happy to accept it, admitting upfront that she had never had any experience as an instrument nurse in the operating room. It certainly didn't take her long to develop that expertise and proficiency which, in the years to follow, she passed on to others. Our clinic nurses in the future not only assisted in surgery on week-days, but were sometimes available for complex emergency procedures on weekends as well.

~~~

Having taken the microsurgery course at Gainesville, we wanted to prepare ourselves for an emergency arterial bypass procedure, should the occasion arise. There were several indications for that operation, the details of which are beyond the scope of this book. Suffice it to say, that at that time there were a number of recognized clinical conditions in which the brain might be deficient in blood/oxygen perfusion, such as a symptomatic patient with an inoperable occlusion of the internal carotid artery at the skull base, and poor contralateral cross-circulation through the circle of Willis. Such a patient was considered ideal for the bypass procedure. In an effort to increase the flow of blood to the deficient side of the brain, a bypass graft could be constructed; specifically, a vessel from the scalp is anastomosed directly to an arterial counterpart on the brain surface.
~~~

By way of introduction, the operation began by dissecting out and preparing the scalp artery (usually the superficial temporal artery), which was then led through a small craniectomy, and sutured to the side of a branch of the middle cerebral artery on the surface of the brain. While easily stated, it was a very demanding and lengthy procedure done under high magnification with the surgical microscope. The vessels used were 3 mm. in diameter, and the suture material was 1/6th as thick as a human hair. It is hard to imagine that the circumference of the mouth of the completed anastomosis contained 12-15 interrupted sutures, and was the size of the "o" on a penny in the phrase, "in God we trust." The obvious question asked is... How can something that small possibly deliver enough blood to the brain to improve oxygen supply? More aptly stated, an anastomosis 1mm. in diameter delivers a meager 20 ml. of blood per minute to the brain. We know, however, that an artery will expand with increased demand, which is the reason for augmenting collateral blood flow to the heart in time of need by medically recommended aerobic exercise. Citing yet another example of the applicability of high school physics, the interested student will recall that the flow of a liquid through a tube is a function of the fourth power of the diameter. Therefore, out of demand, if our anastomosis doubles in size over a few weeks or even months in enlarging from 1 mm. to 2 mm. it will carry 16 times as much blood; i.e., $2^4=16$. In turn this translates into a delivery of 320 ml. (16x20) of blood per minute to the brain, certainly a reasonable volume in supplying a zone starved of oxygen.

In anticipation of a future bypass candidate, we needed to be ready well in advance for performing this operation. I thus prepared a list of all conceivable necessary instruments, suture material, clamps, irrigation devices for the tiny vessels being manipulated, etc. This list was given to Jenny, and within days, she had assembled, organized and sterilized a complete surgical pack. Then one evening after the operating room had shut down for the day, we performed a "mock" anastomosis, using some tiny cadaver arteries which I had obtained from the pathologist. That exercise gave each of us a feel for passing the instruments and fine suture material, and provided me with valuable practice in the technique. It is much like an athlete preparing for an event, namely, to re-train the brain and the eye-to-hand coordination for the job ahead. These mock sessions were subsequently done prior to each future elective (non-emergent) bypass procedure. The theory behind such miniscule work is: "The hand can do what the eye can see." It is a learned process which simply takes practice. Of added significance, man, by nature, has a fine hand tremor which coincides with each heartbeat. Under high magnification that tremor is visually amplified in the hand, the surgeon obviously being unable to eliminate it. Instead, he must simply learn to work with it. When passing a tiny needle through a mere translucent "veil" of tissue, such as comprises the arterial wall, the surgeon must coordinate each clean needle pass with his heartbeat and breathing, lest he irreparably tear the delicate artery. Tying down and cutting each interrupted suture must also be coordinated in the same manner, constantly remaining intently focused for each and every independent precise move.

Without any advanced warning on a Sunday afternoon several months later, I received a call from a neurologist, claiming that he had a potential candidate for a bypass operation. An angiogram had to be done first to demonstrate suitable scalp and brain arteries for the arterial anastomosis. Meanwhile, the patient was in the precarious, "stroke-in-progress" mode. We recommended the bypass procedure to the man and his family as the only remaining chance of helping him to avert a major completed stroke. We were also very cautious in predicting a favorable outcome, emphasizing that there was only a short time-frame in which to accomplish this.

I immediately notified Jenny at her home, asking her to begin setting up as quickly as possible. Within 2-3 hours we had the patient in the operating room, anesthetized, and prepared for surgery. The operation, being my first of this kind, took no less than six hours; and it culminated in our wheeling him into the recovery-room early Monday morning. The procedure itself, aside from the anticipated long duration, went surprisingly well. A postoperative angiogram the next day gratifyingly demonstrated a small, yet patent anastomosis with a trickle of blood perfusing the patient's brain. We were all satisfied with our technical achievement, but ultimately disappointed that the patient failed to show any substantial neurological improvement from his cerebrovascular accident.

~~~

From a manpower standpoint our clinic continued to grow with the addition of two well-recommended neurologists, both of whom having previously been on the faculty at the University of Florida. Dr. Fred Vroom had special interests in epilepsy and stroke management, and Dr.
~~~

Bill Kohler was a board-certified pediatric neurologist. It is pertinent to mention that with the passage of time the future need for additional neurologists became apparent, being commensurate with the increasing population in Tallahassee and the surrounding referral area. Dr. True Martin, who had become interested in neurology as a college student while making rounds with Bryan in the early 1970s, later matriculated through Vanderbilt University as an outstanding student in medicine and neurology, ultimately joining our group. Finally in 1984 Dr. Gerry Maitland, a Hopkins trained neuro-ophthalmologist, served to round out our clinic.

Equally important, the radiology group added to their rapidly growing roster a second neuroradiologist, Dr. Frank Melichar. We were extremely fortunate in Tallahassee to have two neuroradiologists on the hospital staff. There were university medical centers, throughout the country at the time, that were not fortunate enough to have even one such specialist on their faculty. Not only were these men very helpful to us in performing daily interventional work, and providing expert interpretations of brain and spinal cord imaging but were also invaluable in their recommendations relevant to the purchase of future innovative equipment of a highly technical nature.

~~~

In 1977 I ventured further into the hobby of woodworking. Until that time I had been reluctant to invest in expensive hardwoods, merely to have them end up as sawdust and scraps thrust into the garbage bin. I had a physician friend relate to me that one time he had managed to latch on to a rather substantial quantity of expensive, beautiful hardwood while living far out west during completion of his medical training. He paid handsomely to have it hauled about with him over the course of several subsequent moves and countless miles during the remainder of his residency training. He was forever anticipating that someday he would build a masterpiece out of it. Years later when time finally permitted, he attempted to construct a table; I believe it was the first (and quite possibly the last) decent thing that he had ever planned to build. After finishing the project, the proportions in his design apparently didn't suit him, and he admits to having torn it apart in order to try again. After a second attempt, he still wasn't happy with the table's appearance. With a dwindling supply of his coveted wood, he timidly started over for the
~~~

third time. Ultimately, with mounting dissatisfaction and exasperation, he trashed what little of the elegant wood remained. This proved to have lasting negative consequences for him. My friend's experience should serve as an important lesson for all of us: In order to build confidence in excelling at something, one should probably begin with learning the basics. As painful as it might be, one's best interests are served by patiently building up one's talent level over a period of time, and not initially going for a home run.

I was basically self-taught in first learning how to use and maintain all of my tools, both hand and power-driven. The next step led me into studying the fundamentals of design and joinery. Thereafter, there was no limit. The medium itself also has to be studied, for each type of wood is unique in its grain pattern, machining characteristics, and movement during extremes of temperature and humidity. For those seriously interested in this subject, I highly recommend Hoadley's classic book, "*Understanding Wood.*" I have found that this book also makes for a nice Christmas gift for woodworker friends and relatives (16).

Over a period of time in building straightforward projects, I became satisfied with my skill level to the point that I wanted to reach for something more elegant, yet practical as well. As a young boy, I had developed a keen interest in guns and had become a junior member of the NRA. As an adult I had ventured into hunting, but my gun collection was overtaking the space in the corner of my closet. Upon reaching for a tie, the barrel of a gun would often start to fall sideways. It seemed to me that an ideal project would be to build a nice gun cabinet. To begin formulating ideas on design and proportions, I wandered into every sporting goods store in town and many out-of-town establishments as well, especially when on trips to medical meetings in large cities. To my dismay, I failed to come even close to seeing one that I would consider having in my home. The store-bought cabinets were fraught with negative features of size, design or eye appeal, and not one was constructed up to my standards. They were usually built of inexpensive wood and synthetic wood products, and were poorly assembled, often being laden with cheap metal fasteners. Furthermore, they frequently had very unappealing surface finishes. It was clearly evident that the profit margin was probably too slim for most manufacturers to invest the time and expense in producing a quality cabinet. This was in marked contrast to the pre-World War II years when quality pieces of furniture were the rule.

In designing mine, I began with a size estimate based on future guns and supplies. I envisioned all of the wood as consisting of mahogany, including the back. Also proposed was having two large rectangular doors, the rails and styles of which would be jointed around permanent glass panels. The two bottom shelf cabinets were to be enclosed with jointed panel doors. Ornate trimmings would be fashioned with the router. There were other features such as full-mortised locks and hinges plus interior holders preventing the guns from shifting when opening a door or removing a gun. Many days were spent in design, and re-drawing the case before the table-saw was first switched on. By virtue of only working nights and weekends the cabinet took me months to build and apply the final finish. It was my first quality piece and indeed a confidence-builder, which, to this day, stands in my office as I write this manuscript. Through the years, a few visitors have wanted to commission me to build one of these attractive, dark red, glass-fronted cabinets for them. But in defense of the gun cabinet manufacturers — I wouldn't be able to sell such a quality cabinet for a price sufficient to compensate me for my time and materials.

~~~

On a personal note, in 1977 a most damaging event occurred regarding my family of origin, when a ghost arose out of the past. Very early in this book, brief mention was made of my father as a lawyer with an outwardly aggressive, contentious personality. This often resulted in verbal and physical abuse within our family, and regrettably there developed some far-reaching consequences. After I left home for college, my mother finally divorced the man. In the years to follow both parents remarried, and having been raised to respect them I had carried no lasting animosity. As mentioned, I always gave my father full credit as having been the primary driving force in encouraging me forward in my education, especially when things got tough. Certainly he never let me down when it came to financing tuition and books. But despite the passage of time, there was always a lingering tension between us.

During that summer of 1977, it was finally time for our family vacation out to Colorado to see the grandparents. With all four children aboard, we filled up our new Volvo station wagon for a much anticipated venture out west. We hadn't seen my parents for years, and had visions of a wonderful time visiting, fishing and hiking. After spending a few
~~~

hours visiting with my ailing mother in Denver, we were then off into the beautiful Rocky Mountains to Central City, Colorado, an old mining town which had prospered during the Gold-Rush days. My father and stepmother owned a 19th-century, frame house built on the side of a hill in the middle of town. As we drove up in front of the rustic, old place late one afternoon, the kids joyously waving out of the windows of the car, my dad strolled out of the house to greet us. At first glance, rather than seeing the face of a man displaying happiness at the sight of his family, I perceived in him the appearance of one with an underlying hostility, reminiscent of the days when I was a little child growing up. It was the facial expression of a man right on the edge— ready to explode with the least provocation. His negative appearance was perplexing in view of the long time interval since we had last seen him. Nonetheless, I promptly dismissed that perception as an unreasonable thought on my part at this early time in the family's reunion. Happily, things that evening seemed to go all right; after all, we hadn't seen the folks for a couple of years. The conversation that cool summer evening was light and relatively pleasant, for we had a great deal to catch up on.

The next morning after breakfast, I inexplicably seemed to sense in my father even more tension than at the time of our arrival the prior afternoon. The hostile facies he was displaying, subliminal to others in the room, was all too familiar to me— I had grown to fear it as a little kid. Who can possibly surmise what the psychodynamics were? Perhaps he was merely feeling the tension of having all of the grandchildren in the house. A few minutes later we gravitated to the unpleasant subject of medical errors and medical malpractice. Respecting him both as my father and an attorney, I ventured further into the subject, fully expecting to gain his paternal support and advice. It was, indeed, a serious miscalculation on my part. I described to him our plight in 1975 when the liability crisis peaked in Florida, and the insurance companies pulled out of the state. Continuing further, I proceeded to describe how Frank and I had to practice neurosurgery for three months without any malpractice insurance whatsoever; consequently, if sued, we ran the inconceivable risk of losing our homes and all of our assets. Finally, I concluded by saying, "But dad, we were extremely careful in everything we did, so that we could avoid any potential lawsuits." With that said, I inadvertently triggered him. I had unleashed his pent up wrath and all the anxiety and aggression that I had sensed upon our arrival. With his face becoming increasingly bright red, his teeth tightly clenched and with the glazed eyes of a predator, he shouted— "I could find something to sue you over!" Needless to say, I was absolutely dumbfounded. Before us stood a man who was angrily posturing himself as a trial lawyer against his own flesh and blood — imagine, his own son and family! In this moment of blind rage, he seemed to forget the many years of study that I had endured to become a successful neurosurgeon, now the provider of both the healthcare of our community and the security for his grandchildren. This enraged, malevolent man placed his own ego and the mind-set of the trial lawyer above all else. My ire reached proportions never previously realized, as all of those threatening childhood experiences flashed before me in an instant. Never before have I had to exercise more restraint than when I turned and said to my wife, "Gather up the children and prepare to leave, before I do something I might later regret." The crazed man taunted me further saying, "Just try it." Without a further word, we did indeed leave — never to return. We drove 150 miles south to Pueblo to spend the remainder of the vacation with my aging aunt and uncle, who had been such a stable force for me during the war.

I would like to think that over the succeeding years he was remorseful over this incident, but the harm was irreparable. Just as differing ideologies turned brother against brother during the Civil War, the bitterness between lawyers and doctors roiled the emotions of my own family.

~~~

In returning to the subject of neurosurgery, let me bring to the reader's attention two rather unusual cases of penetrating head injuries as seen in a civilian practice.

Most careful adults are familiar with the potential dangers posed by projectiles being hurled by rotating power lawnmower blades, and usually avoid exposing others to injury. Such was the case of a South Georgia man, who began mowing his front yard one fall Saturday afternoon. Fully aware of the hazards associated with his power mower, he instructed his eight-year-old daughter to remain up on the front porch at a safe distance well away from the lawn. Several minutes into his task, he happened to look up only to find the child lying on her back, sprawled out on the front porch floor. He rushed to her side to find her whimpering and writhing in pain, clutching the sides of her head. In a state of disbelief and terror, he gazed down upon a large gauge wire
~~~

(perhaps 4 mm. in diameter) protruding 3 inches from her forehead. Being very careful not to allow either her or anyone else to touch the offending missile, she was rushed to the local hospital. A Life Flight helicopter then flew her to Tallahassee 50 miles away.

When I first saw the patient, she was an understandably frightened, yet well composed, little girl who remained alert and coherent. Skull radiographs revealed a one and a half inch intracranial penetration of this dirty piece of farm wire. Appropriate antibiotic and tetanus protection were given prior to her departure to the surgical suite. Special care was then taken not to alter the position of the projectile during the operation, for to do so, could both run the risk of hemorrhage and obscure sight of the entry wound, vital for appropriate wound cleansing. To this end, we left a small attached cantilever of bone to secure the wire until full exposure of the brain wound could be achieved. Upon finally withdrawing the wire from the cerebrum, pulped semi-liquid brain tissue and clotted blood exuded from the track left by the wire. Fortunately for the child, this was a “silent” brain area of no recognized functional significance, such as visual, speech or motor control. The wound was thoroughly purged with irrigating fluid and closed in the usual manner. Her recovery was complete and free of infection, seizures or any other recognized neurological complication.

Comment: Despite the father’s serious attempt to protect his daughter from an injury, it occurred anyway. Fortunately for the child, the missile did not penetrate her eye or heart with lasting dire or even fatal consequences. Cited below is another, even more unusual case.

One day in the local newspaper I read that the renowned Harlem Globetrotters were going to play an exhibition basketball game in Tallahassee. At that point in time, Tallahassee didn't have an indoor sports arena of any kind. The FSU basketball team, then a member of the old Metro Conference, would play their home games in Tully gymnasium. Tully gym (much like the old football stadium) was relatively small indeed, and the temporary bleachers were necessarily of low seating-capacity. Of course there was an advantage: A spectator, even with bad seats, was very close to the action, the players and their often nationally prominent coaches.

Having previously told my children for years about the antics of the Globetrotters, we now finally had the opportunity to see them in person. The family looked forward to the event for weeks on-end, and even though my partner was off-call and out-of-town that Saturday afternoon, I piled the family into the car and we were off to Tully for some long anticipated amusement. It was exciting as we took our near floor-level seats, watching the team go through its pre-game stunts and entertaining warm-up drills. Just as the game was about to tip off, and the excitement pitch was at a high level, my pager went off with that formidable beep! After so many years, I finally at least had the luxury of a pager, rather than having to be called over the public address system, but I still had to thread my way through the loud, excited crowd to find a pay telephone. Once on the phone to the hospital, the ER nurse tersely said, "Dr. Geissinger… Hold for Dr. T. J. Billingham." T.J. was a general surgeon and longtime friend, who related to me that one of his wife's sorority sisters from college had just learned that her husband had been shot through the head, and had just arrived in the emergency room. T.J., after having been asked to first see the man himself, told me that the patient was still alive, and that I needed to get over there right away!

After arriving in the ER, I was given the full, incredible story about what happened to this fellow during the previous 18 hours. Apparently he had become deeply despondent and had checked himself into a local motel room the night before. Planning to end it all right there, he held a 22-caliber pistol against his right temple and fired. Surprisingly, aside from the noise, nothing seemed to happen! Again he repeated this attempt at his own life, but apparently with the same negative result. As a third and final effort, he firmly squeezed the revolver's trigger, this time slightly angling the gun against his temple. With the gun's discharge, he did notice a sudden loss of vision in his right eye, but nothing more. Discouraged by the futility of it all, he decided to abort his suicidal attempt; instead, he bedded down for the night. The next day, upon awakening, he was startled to find blood on his pillow, and promptly drove straight home. Upon confronting his wife when entering the house, she was horrified to see blood streaming down his face and neck from his macerated eye and scalp.

Upon my examination I found a man who was fully awake, and who gave a full lucid account of the series of events just described. His only physical complaints were those of headache and loss of vision in his right eye. Indeed, I found his right ocular globe to have been decimated and still oozing blood. Upon further examination, and to everyone's astonishment, this man did in fact have multiple gunshot wounds of his head. In the right temporal region there were three distinct points of entry, each consistent with a 22-caliber bullet, and each associated with tattooing of the scalp by powder burns, thus corroborating an attempted suicide by the close proximity of the barrel. The most astonishing aspect of the examination, however, was the demonstration of two exit wounds in the left fronto-temporal area of the scalp and skull. In summary: This man had sustained two independent, frontal through-and-through gunshot wounds of the brain, and a third which had exited through the right orbit, destroying his right eye. And, to the wonderment of all, he had both driven home and had lived to tell about it!

In the operating room we shaved, prepared and draped the entire front of the head for surgery in the standard fashion. Bilateral craniectomies were performed for purposes of debridement, removal of in-driven bone fragments and cleansing of the missile tracks with irrigation. An assisting ophthalmologic surgeon enucleated what was left remaining of the right eye. Antibiotics and tetanus prophylaxis were given, and his post-operative course was uneventful. Leonard subsequently made a full recovery without any evidence of paralysis, speech disturbance or cognitive deficits. Follow-up psychiatric counseling was successfully administered, deterring any further attempts at suicide. Six months later, we returned him to the operating room in order to cover the skull defects with bilateral acrylic cranioplasty plates, and the ophthalmologist fitted him with a prosthetic eye. To later see this amazing fellow on the street would belie any previous cranial trauma. As a matter of fact, several years later there was an article in the local newspaper relevant to him as a successful local businessman. I always thought this case was one for Mr. Ripley!

~~~

If I may turn to another interesting but quite unrelated subject, the neurological surgeon is frequently called upon to relieve facial pain. In a previous section we have discussed the treatment of peripheral body pain; let me now address the treatment of a well-recognized condition causing facial pain.

The subject of interest is an affliction of the face which is called trigeminal neuralgia, also known as tic douloureux. This condition of unbearable, facial pain was recognized by early civilizations as depicted on figures and statues. According to Stookey and Ransohoff, it was John Locke who gave the first well-documented account of the malady, when he was called to treat the wife of the English Ambassador to France on December 4, 1677 (42).
~~~

According to Locke:

> "On Thursday night last, I was sent for to my Lady Ambassadrice, whom I found in a fit of such violent and exquisite torment, that... it forced her to such cries and shrieks as you would expect from one upon the rack, to which I believe hers was an equal torment, which extended itself all over the right side of her face and mouth. When the fit came, there was, to use my Lady's own expression of it, as it were a flash of fire all of a suddaine shot into all those parts, and at every one of those twitches, which made her shreeke out, her mouth was constantly drawn on the right side towards the right eare by repeated convulsive motions...."

Throughout the years, I have personally borne witness to this condition in a number of my own patients. The first, and perhaps the most graphic, case involved a humble, graying, elderly man who presented himself in my office during a period in which he was having a cluster of these spells. When attempting to speak, he would suddenly seize up as if paralyzed while clutching at his face and groaning in agony; and with his eyes watering, a look of despair descended over him like a veil. Within seconds, this shock-like, lancinating pain vanished as rapidly as it had appeared, whereupon he would then continue briefly with his medical history until another such attack struck him. Fearful of triggering further episodes, he became literally petrified to speak. Being sensitive to his intolerable agony, I then formulated my questions such that he could shake his head, or merely utter yes or no.

For the last 250 years tic douloureux has been recognized by its well-known constellation of symptoms. As a brief anatomical background: The main sensory nerve to the face (trigeminal or Vth cranial nerve) has its origin, like the other cranial nerves previously discussed, within the brainstem in the posterior fossa. Traveling forward to exit the skull, it divides into three major divisions, each ultimately destined to innervate roughly one third of the side of the face. There are two primary hallmarks of the affliction: a trigger mechanism such as touch, shaving, talking, cold air, etc., followed by the ensuing pain itself. A trigger point over one of those primary nerve divisions will cause a flash of pain over that same division. For example, touching the cheek (middle division) will cause radiating pain not only in the cheek but over the entire area innervated by the middle division of the nerve (central ⅓ of the face). The intolerable pain, which is of sudden onset, is often best described as having an "electric-shock-like" quality. It lasts moments to many seconds and then completely disappears. Clusters of these attacks may occur, followed by up to months of pain-free intervals. The patient has no associated evidence of nerve damage, such as facial numbness or paralysis. For many years medical science had absolutely no idea as to what might cause this dreadful disorder, and treatment was therefore purely symptomatic. It was not uncommon for a patient to come into the neurologist's office having had numerous dental extractions after prior attempts to relieve the pain. Over the years we were asked to treat a number of these patients; generally they were referred to us by the clinical neurologists who had already tried various medications. Tegretol has, for the most part, been an effective drug and probably the drug of choice, but it does carry potential undesirable side effects. Dilantin, while it has fewer side effects, is generally less effective in treatment. If either the patient had experienced some adverse reaction to drug therapy, or had become refractory to the medications, the neurosurgeon might then be called upon to offer surgical relief of the pain.

Throughout the years, the neurosurgical armamentarium for treating trigeminal neuralgia has been substantial, but often not of lasting benefit. Factors such as the patient's age, severity and frequency of attacks, and whether or not they had previously had surgery would determine our approach in any given case. In the early 1970s, we usually followed the protocol described below.

The simplest and safest procedure was the injection of 95% alcohol into a facial branch of one of the nerve's major divisions innervating the trigger zone in question. Often this would cause subsidence of the pain attacks for as long as a year, after which they would usually recur. If the patient again returned with symptoms, the next step was ordinarily to incise the small nerve branch, and remove it as it emerged from its bony foramen in the face. This also was usually only temporary in relieving the pain. If the pain continued to recur, we could then offer the patient a more radical operation such as a radiofrequency (RF) thermo-coagulation procedure.

We have previously alluded to this procedure when treating severe pain syndromes in the trunk or limbs requiring a percutaneous cordotomy. The reader will recall that we passed an electrode into the appropriate area of the spinal cord where the heat lesion was to be made. In the early 1970s this technique was adapted to treating trigeminal neuralgia as well. Parenthetically, it should be mentioned that this operation may also be used for alleviating severe, intractable facial pain from other causes. Immediately coming to mind was a man with a grotesque, extensive, cancerous destruction of one side of his face, the pain from which having been totally abolished with an RF lesion..

Just as we did in the case of the spinal cord, an insulated wire electrode was passed within a large bore needle through a foramen in the skull base under x-ray control, directing it intracranially in such a manner that the tip of the electrode entered the Vth nerve precisely at its junction into the three major divisions. Once the appropriate location was confirmed by both x-ray and electrical stimulation, that portion of the nerve incriminated as causing the pain was partially interrupted with a thermal lesion. We seemed to have immediate and very good pain relief with this procedure. The elderly man, whom I initially described with tic, was treated by this method, and his results were quite gratifying. I have used his exemplary case in lecturing medical students about tic douloureux, as photographs of him before and after the surgery are dramatically telling. Graphically, I have pictures of him rubbing his face and smiling during the immediate postoperative period, motor acts which he could not have even begun to contemplate just hours before when entering the hospital. Because there was no surgical incision, and the patient was out of the hospital in one day, it was an excellent therapeutic modality in the frail or elderly patient. The primary disadvantage was its failure to address a recently discovered actual cause of the condition.

For several years, when treating the facial pain by directly interrupting the Trigeminal nerve after its emergence from the brain stem, surgeons noticed in approximately 50% of the cases that there was encroachment on the trigeminal nerve by a small blood vessel. Usually, this proved to be a branch artery supplying the cerebellum. Initially, not much thought was given to this variation in anatomy as an actual cause for the facial pain. However, many years later when using the microscope, surgeons discovered that by dissecting these offending vessels off of the nerve, and interposing between the vessel and nerve a piece of muscle used as cushioning material, the majority of these patients were then permanently relieved of their attacks of pain. In the mid-1970s, this became accepted in the neurosurgical community as a well documented and treatable cause of this devilish condition. After attending a number of national neurosurgical meetings in which this was discussed in detail, my partner and I began routinely performing this microsurgical procedure. We subsequently felt, like many other neurosurgeons throughout the world, that it was probably the procedure of choice in the relatively young and otherwise healthy patient who had responded poorly to medications. In those cases where I found a compressing vessel (not always an artery but sometimes a vein), it was cleanly dissected off of the nerve and a synthetic sponge material was interposed. The results from the surgery were gratifying, indeed. We did have a few cases, however, in which upon exploration no compressing vessel was found. In those we carefully coagulated and divided only the inferior two thirds of the trigeminal root resulting in good pain relief as well. This latter ablative operation, used as our last resort in treatment, was originally advocated as a routine approach to trigeminal neuralgia in 1932 by the skilled neurosurgeon, Walter Dandy, at Johns Hopkins. Of major importance, Dr. Dandy found that his operation was not only successful in relieving the unbearable pain, but also preserved facial sensation (touch), particularly critical to the cornea of the eye.

At this juncture I would like to bring to the reader's attention a point worthy of emphasis. Years ago, when one used to think of neurosurgery, he could only envision any number of complicated, somewhat mysterious and often futile operations deep within the brain to treat life-threatening tumors or aneurysms. Contrary to that thinking, we have just discussed a perfectly benign, non-life-threatening condition— tic douloureux— which if successfully treated results in an eternally grateful patient. Although some of these operative procedures for tic are delicate and fraught with risk, they nonetheless offer a bright ray of hope to someone totally incapacitated with this dreadful condition. Recalling again what John Locke described so many years ago, "...it forced her to such cries and shrieks as you would expect from someone upon the rack...."

To pull someone from the jaws of such torture serves to reinforce the feeling of fulfillment that comes with being a physician.

~~~
~~~

SEVEN

Academic Opportunity and Advancements in Surgery

~~~

It was mentioned earlier that the members of our Tallahassee Neurological Clinic had always tried to maintain high academic standards. We agreed from the onset that we would all obtain board certification, and any new members of our group would also need to receive such recognition in order to become full partners.

Our journal club and early morning x-ray conferences have already been mentioned. In addition, each member of our group alternated in presenting monthly neurological conferences for the medical staff in the hospital auditorium. This was often of the grand-rounds format in which an interesting or illustrative case was presented, and the subject matter of that particular disease or topic then discussed in detail. These conferences were designed with several objectives in mind, foremost being educational. By alerting the doctors to certain neurological / neurosurgical disorders, we hoped that the “front line” physician encountering a patient with a particular malady would recognize it. Secondly, they serve to educate the staff on conditions that we could treat locally in our own hospital, thereby obviating the need for referring the patient to some far-off center for therapy. It is pertinent to cite at this point a good example which illustrates the importance of disseminating such information by using conferences as a vehicle.

Late one afternoon, I received an urgent call from a nurse in an ophthalmologist’s office in a small town several miles away. She expressed great concern in relating to me that they had a man in his twenties whom they had just seen because of the sudden onset of severe headache and blindness in both eyes. With a great sense of urgency, I instructed her to immediately send him to us by ambulance. When I
~~~

examined this acutely ill young fellow, he could only questionably perceive even a very bright light shined into either eye, and by no means could he detect any hand motion presented close to the eyes. An emergency CT scan clearly demonstrated a hemorrhage into a large tumor within the pituitary gland (at the base of the brain), the entire hemorrhagic mass distorting the optic nerves. Without any delay we took him to the operating room that night, and removed the tumor through a frontal craniotomy. Although we successfully decompressed the nerves to the eyes, regrettably, it was too late! The patient remained permanently blind from this condition, known for many years as "pituitary apoplexy."

To his misfortune, this patient had been complaining for a long time of progressive visual loss, but he had simply been fitted with new glasses from time to time. A timely diagnosis as to just why he was losing visual acuity was unfortunately never made. It is very likely that had the tumor been recognized as recently as 24 hours prior to his hemorrhage, this tragic outcome could have probably been averted by a surgical decompression. The optic nerves, in contradistinction to the peripheral nerves of the body, are unique in that they are a true extension of the brain. As a result they are extremely sensitive to external stresses, and once injured the damage to the cells is usually irreversible. Through the years we had the occasion to see a number of cases of very large pituitary tumors, which we successfully treated with gross tumor removal followed by irradiation therapy. Left untreated, these tumors may enlarge to that point at which they outgrow their blood supply, necrose, and hemorrhage; moreover, this may culminate in a sudden critical increase in tumor volume, creating dangerous tension on the delicate overlying optic nerves.

As a result of this tragic case of potentially preventable visual loss, we planned a hospital neurology conference on pituitary brain tumors. We proposed to discuss their various presenting symptoms with special emphasis on the visual system in general and the topic of pituitary apoplexy in particular. I requested that my nurse specifically notify all of the ophthalmologists not only in Tallahassee but in other neighboring communities as well, informing them of the important subject matter of the hospital conference. The purpose, of course, was to heighten their vigilance as to the early recognition and treatment of large pituitary tumors in preventing blindness and to inform the medical community that surgical treatment was readily available locally.

These monthly lectures were not only informative with regard to any number of neurological disorders and their various treatment modalities but also were formatted to be of general medical interest to the entire staff including the nurses, medical technicians and various therapists as well. These noon conferences were to continue for nearly three decades.

Another aspect of our ties with academia was related to scientific writing for publication of our experience with unusual or instructional case material. Every member of our clinic participated. My partner and I enjoyed a close and lasting relationship with the neurosurgeons at the University of Florida, and I can recall two such articles that we published in association with them. In 1976, Dr. Al Rhoton had discussed with the editors of the *Journal of the Florida Medical Association* the feasibility of dedicating one edition of that journal specifically to neurosurgical disorders which might confront the general practitioner. He asked whether we would contribute to that issue by writing an article on cervical disc disease and other causes of upper extremity pain. We were pleased to comply with his request, and our article was published in November 1976 (11).

In Tallahassee we were fortunate to have at our disposal one of the initial first-generation computed-tomography scanners in the country. With the further advance of CAT technology, the hospital subsequently acquired later-generation scanners as well. We were not only afforded an opportunity to make timely, noninvasive diagnoses of many of the more common neurological disorders, but were also privileged to gain an early insight into some of the more unusual conditions, theretofore poorly delineated. Below I will illustrate such an example.

In 1976 we were presented with a six-month-old baby girl who had been followed by her pediatrician since early infancy, carrying the diagnosis of a seizure disorder. While the seizures had been well controlled with medication, there had been a 3cm. increase in her head circumference during the month prior to our seeing her. This placed her well above the upper limit on the head growth curve for an infant of her age. An earlier CT scan done 10 weeks prior to admission (as part of her initial seizure workup) had shown only a slight decrease in brain density on the left side. Of dynamic importance, a repeat scan done at the time of our hospital admission surprisingly showed the rapid development of a huge, cystic structure occupying a major portion of the left side of the intracranial cavity, and which was simultaneously shifting the brain to the right. We operated upon the child through a craniotomy and encountered an enormous fluid-filled cyst compressing the convolutions of the brain, displacing the latter into the right hemicranium. No neoplasm was found. We installed a shunt (similar to those used in the treatment of hydrocephalus) to drain the cystic fluid into the abdominal cavity. A follow-up scan showed a remarkable disappearance of the cyst, with full re-expansion and return of the brain to its normal position. In June 1977 she became irritable and began protracted vomiting, whereupon the shunt was found to be obstructed and nonfunctioning. After the system was revised, her symptoms of increased intracranial pressure promptly abated, and she eventually went on to develop normally.

Without the CT scan, the fluid dynamics concerning those abrupt changes within the cyst could not have been detected either as timely or thoroughly as they were. If allowed to continue unchecked, this rapidly expanding lesion could have indeed become life-threatening, and, at the very least, would have caused severe damage to her brain. The benefit of the shunting procedure was clearly demonstrated.

Interestingly, we collected a small series of four of these cases, and after researching the literature on the nature of these particular cysts, published a well received article in one of the neurosurgical journals (12). Based both upon our personal experience, and also upon some of the cases in the literature with poor outcomes, we recommended careful follow-up of these patients. We proposed that both large symptomatic cysts and those in the process of enlarging, as demonstrated by serial computed tomograms, should be shunted. These recommendations were generally endorsed as accepted treatment, and in the months to follow the American College of Surgeons made reference to our work in its self-assessment examination.

~~~

While again departing from the subject of medicine, another important aspect of my life will now be introduced. In reflecting back to those early childhood days during the war when I spent a great deal of time with the farm family in Colorado, I had since longed to have a farm of my own. As I have often told others in later years, my first dream was to become a doctor, and my second was to be the proud owner of a ranch. My wife had also been raised on a farm in northern Illinois, so together we began looking for a piece of agricultural property to purchase.
~~~

In 1978, we came upon three adjoining parcels of land in Monticello, Florida, a small town 20 miles east of Tallahassee. Several years previously, these three tracts together had constituted a small, dairy farm, but they had subsequently been split up after the owner passed away, having been sold off as separate entities through the years. By gaining the assistance of a savvy "old-time" agricultural realtor, Rufus Hodge, a man familiar with the entire area, we were able to purchase all three parcels back, thus reconstituting the original 218-acre tract. Practically speaking, 100 acres were totally cleared and suitable for cropland and grazing, while the remainder was low-land and abundant both in timber and a nice variety of wildlife. The elevated cleared portion was broken up by trees and small, rolling hills into five potential separate fields, each being unique in its configuration and topography, and each lending itself to future fence enclosure. The trees bordering the fields isolated them both from the perimeter road and from each other, yet allowed for the future strategic placement of gates. The fields were contiguous with one another, the entire ensemble curving as a cleared, concentric ring around a small central forest. Within that forest and on a shallow grade were three natural springs giving rise to a small stream that wound its way peacefully down through the property. Early in the game I had the State Bureau of Water Management inform me that it would be an ideal site for a dam and pond. The entire landscape was very picturesque, a perfect site to develop into that ranch of my childhood dreams. While any existing fencing was in poor condition at best, with a great deal of work and modest expense we could envision exciting future possibilities for the place. For the time being, I was just content in obtaining financing and calling the land my own. Meanwhile, the cleared portion of the property was leased to a nearby dairy farmer who raised corn and grain sorghum for his herd. For the next few years, the family simply took pleasure in driving over to the farm site as an escape from the weekly routine, enjoying the wildlife and the fragrance of the foliage as we hiked through the fields and forests, always envisioning its future potential.

~~~

In refocusing attention back to the hospital, there were continued improvements concerning the way neurosurgery was practiced, particularly with regard to the treatment of certain tumors and
~~~

intracranial aneurysms. The value of magnification with the surgical microscope cannot be overstated, and the improved success rate from operating upon aneurysms must be attributed in major part to this device. But there were other contributing innovations which enhanced our ability to deal with these formidable lesions so often the cause of death or severe disability. I shall attempt to highlight a few of the mechanical developments and newer concepts that we found very helpful relevant to aneurysm surgery.

A head-holding device was developed, which provided for a stable three-point fixation of the skull. It is mechanically anchored to the operating table itself, which disallows any head movement during the operative procedure. This allowed reproducible preoperative orientation of the head into a permanent, fixed position such that the brain was always spatially oriented the same way. It provided the surgeon with a consistent pathway to the circle of Willis at the base of the brain where the vast majority of the aneurysms are located. Such consistency becomes vitally important not only for anatomical recognition during successive operations (visualize a familiar landscape to the base of the brain), but in the event of a premature aneurysm rupture during the approach, the surgeon is constantly aware of his precise location at any given point in time.

Also developed was a flexible, two-armed, self-retaining retractor. As opposed to the inconsistent and cumbersome, hand-held retractors of the past, this device when set in position, constantly and gently retracted the brain with very little to no pressure on this delicate structure. At the same time it allowed optimal access through a very small portal of entry.

Instrument makers, upon request from preeminent aneurysm surgeons throughout the world, were consistently providing improved, high-quality products; e.g., scissors, dissectors, bipolar coagulation units and suction apparatus— each with variable lengths and angles. This allowed us to work in very small, awkward spaces during the dissection. In addition they manufactured a wide assortment of aneurysm clips and appliers. While both large and small, they were forged at varying angles to suit most geometrical situations encountered in reference to aneurysm position. Furthermore, these spring-loaded clips were strong, and the jaws designed not to slip. We also had at our disposal an abundance of temporary, "softer" clips, which could be placed, only if necessary, on a parent vessel for a few moments just prior to final aneurysm-neck dissection and permanent clipping. When encountering an aneurysm in a difficult position or projection, the surgeon finds all of these devices indispensable.

There was also increasing emphasis in the world literature on the salutary features of a relatively small fronto-temporal craniotomy flap to access the circle of Willis. Once this small flap was elevated, the arachnoid membrane over the Sylvian fissure was opened, and time was taken to carefully aspirate CSF to relax the brain. Relaxation was further enhanced by the anesthesiologist's control of blood gases. We then carefully removed a slim margin of bone along the interior of the skull base while working medially. Collectively, all of these maneuvers permitted the surgeon to "slide" along the base of the skull in gaining access to the circle of Willis, while maintaining good visibility and yet minimizing retraction on the brain.

Even though there were a number of neurosurgeons worldwide who, through the years, had contributed to the advancement of the microsurgery of intracranial aneurysms; once again, one man's name seemed to stand above all of the rest — Dr. M.G. Yasargil of Zürich, Switzerland. The vast array of instruments, operative approaches (namely, the one cited above) and techniques conceived by him were conveyed to his generation of neurosurgeons through illustrative papers, textbooks and personal presentations at meetings. Largely as a result of his efforts there was a dramatic decrease in the operative morbidity and mortality of intracranial aneurysm surgery. Dr. Yasargil was later the Honored Guest at the 1986 meeting of the Congress of Neurological Surgeons in New Orleans. After one of his fine presentations, several of us ventured forth to the front of the auditorium, humbly shaking the hand and paying our respect to the man who had contributed so very much to neurological surgery during his lifetime.

This detailed discussion is intended to demonstrate how technology and the human experience have immensely improved the safety and efficacy of aneurysm surgery over a relatively short period of time. From a personal point of view, I cannot think of either a more challenging or rewarding facet of neurosurgery then to operate upon, and exclude from the circulation, an intracranial aneurysm. While my partner and I both operated upon aneurysms with regularity, we always remained cautious and humbled by them. Furthermore, nothing can replace sound judgment in knowing what constitutes one's limitations. As will be cited later, it is both prudent and wise to constantly remain cognizant of those limitations, always being prepared to refer away to another institution those lesions with which the surgeon feels uncomfortable. Consistently good results from operating on the more common and readily-accessible aneurysms are well within the capability of most well-trained neurological surgeons, providing that they are inclined to venture into this aspect of neurosurgery. This stands in contrast to the days back in the late 1960s, when the results of the highly skilled Canadian neurosurgeon, Dr. Charles Drake, were very difficult—if not impossible— to duplicate.

~~~

In 1978 we invited Dr. and Mrs. Paul Bucy down to Tallahassee for a visit. Through the years I had grown close to my mentor, as had many of his former residents. As a matter of fact, my wife, children and I had spent an entire day and night with the Bucys at their beautiful retirement home on a mountainside in Tryon, North Carolina, a few years before. It was indeed a privilege and an honor. In turn, when they came down to our small Florida town, they were our guests for a few days. Despite his being a very high profile figure in the field of neurosurgery, he was a warm, affable, and very personal human being as well. Many of us, as his surgical residents, looked upon him as a second father. I can still recall my driving him out to my farm one day, conversing about the days of old in Chicago and our mutual neurosurgical colleagues. He was an extremely sharp man, even in his later years, always seeming to have a firm grasp on everyone's whereabouts and what they were doing. On another day, we and our wives drove down to Wakulla Springs, the filming site of the old Tarzan movies. Even though the four of us were all out on a boat looking at unusual tropical birds, plants and alligators, he and I never ceased discussing neurosurgery. In his retirement he had both originated and edited the new neurosurgical journal, *Surgical Neurology.* After having personally seen and been impressed with our private neurosurgical practice during a brief visit to Tallahassee earlier in the 1970s, Dr. Bucy requested that Frank and I write a special article for that journal. The article, which provided guidelines in establishing a private practice in neurological surgery, was published in 1975, much of that information being applicable to this day (7).

His new journal was one of the many topics he and I discussed, and certainly one of which he could rightfully be proud. He later asked if I would be interested in writing occasional book reviews, concerning newly released neurosurgical textbooks, for publication in *Surgical*
~~~

Neurology. That was something that I subsequently did for many years, thereafter. There is little doubt that having had that opportunity to frequently review current concepts in neurosurgical disorders and advanced operative techniques served to make me a better neurosurgeon.

One evening while he was here, we had him speak at a dinner gathering of neurologists and neurosurgeons both from Tallahassee and some of the remote cities in the Panhandle. He was a dynamic speaker who didn't use notes, and who possessed a gift for totally captivating the audience, as he reflected on his experiences in the early history of neurosurgery. The group was enthralled while listening to his story.

The following day, we initially escorted him on a tour of Tallahassee Memorial Hospital, showing him how medicine was practiced at our institution, thereafter introducing him to both our neurosurgical facilities and a cross section of our case material. He had always said that he had hoped that I would engage in the academic practice of neurosurgery within a university setting as so many of his former residents had done. In that respect I have always felt that I let the man down. However, later during that visit he told me that he was impressed with our hospital and with the challenging variety of neurosurgical cases and quality of our work. By having said that, the professor couldn't have paid us a greater compliment.

At noon that same day he was scheduled to give a lecture to the hospital staff. As we were leaving the house that morning I was concerned that he hadn't mentioned any slides to present to the group. Thinking that I might need to scrape up a projector, I asked him whether he had any slides to show. Dr. Bucy looked at me with that twinkle in his eye and said, “Should I have?” When the time came for his talk, he stepped up to the podium in his usual confident manner and, within seconds, had the audience captivated with his presentation. Speaking strictly from the cuff, he was an impressive orator, who spoke about his youthful learning experiences with the prominent neurologists and surgeons of old, the majority of whom were in Europe at the time, and also of his time spent with Dr. Percival Bailey at the University of Chicago. Finally, he mesmerized the audience when asked to discuss the syndrome bearing his name — the Klüver-Bucy syndrome. Briefly stated, it is an experimental animal model resulting from bilateral temporal lobectomies in subhuman primates. Among other things, it is manifested by striking changes in visual recognition, emotional and sexual behavior in these animals. While this syndrome had never been reported in humans, I once had a patient who had sustained a violent rotational head injury resulting in severe bilateral temporal lobe contusions; he later bore a very strong behavioral resemblance to the bilaterally temporal lobectomized monkeys.

Dr. Bucy's extensive research work at three of Chicago's great universities has contributed very significantly to our knowledge concerning the function of the brain and spinal cord in humans in both health and disease. It was a pleasure and an inspiration to hear him recount his vast experiences.

While I would later visit my professor again in Tryon, I shall never forget that memorable experience with him in Tallahassee. In closing the chapter on this preeminent neurosurgeon, I would like to add the following afterthought: Throughout my career he had encouraged me to write an assortment of reviews and articles for publication, always reiterating that I should do more writing. Perhaps this was a subliminal motivation in my undertaking this book so many years after his death.

~~~

Neurosurgery differs from other subspecialties in a number of different respects, notably, during nights and weekends. Conditions which we are called upon to deal with during "off-hours" are often urgent, if not emergent. A fractured cervical spine must be immediately stabilized, if only by traction; a cranial gunshot wound must immediately be taken to the operating room; compound depressed skull fractures must be urgently cleaned and elevated; and intracranial blood clots, in any number of locations, must often be promptly evacuated.

Another such emergency confronting the neurosurgeon is the older child with hydrocephalus, who has entered into a state which we call, "shunt dependency." I shall attempt to shed some light upon this interesting, yet potentially dangerous condition. Earlier we discussed the infant with hydrocephalus in whom, under conditions of either obstruction to the flow of CSF or its malabsorption, the ventricular chambers of the brain enlarge. If unchecked, the brain mantle thins out as the ventricles expand, causing the entire head to enlarge as well. This can only occur because the multiple, individual, unfused bones of the baby's skull are displaced both apart and centripetally by the expanding intracranial contents. Years ago when visiting a state facility in Illinois, I shall never forget the disturbing sight of several severely advanced hydrocephalic children existing in a vegetative state with basketball-
~~~

sized heads, yet tiny faces, as they lay quietly in large bassinets. While this sometimes grotesque head-enlargement occurs at the expense of brain destruction, it also acts as a means of dissipating the pressure within the intracranial cavity. But today's early therapy of installing a shunt during infancy not only prevents that abnormal expansion of the head, but also maintains a normal pressure within the chambers of the developing brain. As normal brain growth later decreases, the individual skull bones begin to fuse together into a sturdy, solid, cranial vault, much of that fusion having taken place by age 3. After that point, any obstruction to the shunt system will cause a sustained pressure buildup within the cerebral ventricles, the head no longer capable of enlargement as a pressure-relief mechanism. Again, if we may refer back to a basic concept learned in high school physics — liquids are non-compressible. This, of course, is the basis for the immense forces generated by hydraulic cylinders. When at Iowa City, Dr. Sahs drove home that important concept to the residents and students with the following analogy: If one should have a large steel vessel completely full of a liquid, and if by some means he could force just one more drop of liquid into that vessel through the tiniest and strongest of valves— the vessel would explode! Imagine the pressure building up in a shunt-dependent child's head to that point in which something must give, necessarily causing the brain to shift. If unchecked, this will result in a fatal issue. Let me share a dramatic such case with the reader.

One Saturday afternoon I was at home playing with my children in the swimming pool, when my answering service called instructing me to immediately call the emergency room. Once on the line, a distraught nurse informed me that a 10-year-old child's parents had appeared, totally unannounced, with their little girl crying with an intense headache and violently ill with projectile vomiting. It seems that when born with hydrocephalus in another remote town far away, she had a valve-regulated shunt placed shortly after birth. There had been no subsequent problems, whatsoever, until that Saturday morning when she awakened complaining of headaches. Realizing that the child was getting into trouble with an ever intensifying headache and subsequent vomiting, the parents hastily drove her to Tallahassee. While unaware of the particular shunting device that her doctors might have had installed 10 years previously, I suspected that there had to be a small, residual opening in the bony skull beneath a shunt reservoir. In an effort to save valuable time while en route to the hospital, I asked the nurse to palpate the scalp, and to shave the hair over any discernable flushing apparatus beneath it.

I also asked that she procure from the operating room supervisor a large bore ventricular needle with a stylet. Mindful of the fact that this little shunt-dependent child could stop breathing at any moment, I believe I well exceeded the speed limit in driving to the hospital. After parking my car in front of the emergency department door, I hastened into the holding room. By now, I found the child unresponsive and breathing with a barely perceptible, shallow, irregular effort. After quickly swabbing the scalp with iodine, the ventricular needle was directed through the silicone shunt reservoir beneath the scalp and into the ventricular chamber of the brain. Upon removing the stylet there was an explosive ejection of ventricular fluid, projecting perhaps 3 feet out onto the floor. Within mere seconds, what had been an apneic, moribund child suddenly began to wake up, and exhibit purposive movement. While I had witnessed similar phenomena at the Children's Hospital in Chicago many years previously, I don't ever recall anything more dramatic than this. At one moment this little girl was so very close to death, but once the pressure was relieved, it was as if she were awakening from a nap. By reducing that pressure, we not only temporarily prevented brain herniation, but also allowed normal perfusion of the brain with blood and oxygen. Her suddenly regaining consciousness was like turning on a light switch. She was then taken to the operating room, where the entire shunt mechanism was removed and updated. Her recovery was gratifyingly complete and uneventful.

This represents still another example in which the neurosurgeon is called upon to deal with non-cancerous, yet debilitating, life-threatening disease that ended with a favorable outcome.

~~~

By 1979 there had been several changes regarding the neurological practice in our community. One day out of the blue, a neurosurgeon who had just finished his residency walked into my office for a visit. He told me that he liked Tallahassee and had decided to practice here. The doctor proceeded to query me and my partner as to whether or not we could use another neurosurgeon in our clinic. At that point in time other neurosurgeons had set up practices in Panama City to the south; Dothan, Alabama to the west; and Thomasville, Georgia, only 26 miles to the north of Tallahassee. As a result, our referral area had contracted significantly throughout the years. In view of this regional increase in
~~~

neurosurgical manpower, even though our county had grown in population to partially compensate, we considered it unnecessary to take on another man in our clinic at that particular time. Because Renaldo was predetermined to settle in this locale, he was candid in telling us that he would set up a solo practice here anyway. Since we did have an open hospital staff, he was readily credentialed. By joining the staff he was also obligated, in accordance with the hospital bylaws, to share emergency room call until age 55. By his taking call every third night for emergency patients not already established in our clinic, it was of immense help to us after nearly a decade of having shouldered that responsibility ourselves. We were destined to work in harmony with him throughout the years to follow. Upon rare occasions we would reciprocate in cross-covering for one another regarding the emergency room (for instance during times of national meetings), but ordinarily my partner and I continued to remain available every other night and weekend for our own group practice. Meanwhile, Renaldo was a cautious neurosurgeon and, like the rest of us, was well aware of his limitations. Ego aside, he never hesitated in soliciting our advice on difficult problems, and in some conditions such as intracranial aneurysms, he preferred that we handle them exclusively.

~~~

Another most disturbing event occurred in the spring of 1979 which was to change the face of our clinic forever. In regressing for a moment I will begin by bringing to the reader's attention a series of events occurring in 1970, one year before my arrival in Tallahassee to practice. My partner, Bryan Robinson, had been beset with symptoms of dizziness and imbalance, which ironically were found due to a brain tumor in his posterior fossa. He was sent away to a university center in the northeast by Frank in an attempt at a surgical cure. While the surgeon was bold in his approach to the tumor, a good portion of it involved the vital brain stem and had to be left untouched. The histopathology of the lesion was that of a benign blood vessel tumor called a hemangioblastoma. Although non-cancerous in the true sense of the word, it was malignant by virtue of its location, that is to say, that residual portion of the tumor would continue to grow unconstrained within the brainstem. Bryan recovered nicely from that operation and returned, basically
~~~

asymptomatic, to his busy practice of neurology. Thereafter, for years he remained well and was a very visible leader in our community.

Then late in 1978 he developed the inevitable and dreaded recurrence of his symptoms of disequilibrium. None of us can even imagine what went through the mind of this erudite neurologist as he had to face the reality of his self-diagnosis. Only a neurologist could envision those tumor cells, benign as they might be, continuing to multiply and insinuating themselves between the delicate clusters of nerve-cell nuclei and white matter tracts of the hindbrain— considered inviolate by the neurosurgeon. Furthermore, neither irradiation nor chemotherapy would alter that slow, yet protracted, growth of these cells. To the rest of his family, close friends and medical partners, his announcement of the long anticipated recurrence of symptoms was terrifyingly surreal. The immediate question asked — what therapy exists that might help him?

Frank and I deliberated as to what should be done, and where we could possibly send Bryan to give him the best chance of a surgical cure. The neurosurgeon of first choice was Dr. M.G. Yasargill in Zurich, Switzerland. We felt that if there was anyone on the planet that could save our partner, it was this legendary figure in microsurgery (whom I have already extolled) who could accomplish it. To our great dismay, however, Dr. Yasargill was already scheduled far in advance with other equally desperate patients, in all likelihood many of them important figures like Bryan.

Following considerable further thought, we chose another well-respected, important leader in our field, a superb surgical technician in his own right, who practiced at a university hospital in New York City.

After first being thoroughly worked up in New York, Bryan underwent a very long and delicate microsurgical operation, after the conclusion of which the surgeon felt very confident that he had totally removed this relatively uncommon benign tumor. To everyone's relief, Bryan emerged from the anesthetic neurologically intact, and by the next morning expressed a desire to begin writing thank-you notes to his many concerned friends. However, the optimism was short-lived, for he soon began developing the insidious, yet progressive, unmistakable signs of neurological deficit. He was taken to the x-ray department where a CT scan ruled out a postoperative hemorrhage. An arteriogram, however, indicated an alarming degree of arterial spasm with a concomitant, critically compromising, blood-perfusion deficit throughout the brain. Frank was in constant telephone communication with the New York surgeons regarding the gravity of the situation, and he in turn called me daily in Los Angeles where I was attending a national neurosurgical meeting. Day by day, despite the watchful eye of the neurosurgical staff, Bryan's condition deteriorated into a state of deepening coma in the wake of diffuse and multiple areas of brain infarction (strokes). The spasm could not be broken, despite the administration of a multitude of drugs designed to inhibit the tonic contraction of smooth muscle. Several days later I had the opportunity to meet with his surgeon, who by then was also attending the AANS meeting in Los Angeles. He told me that he had never before witnessed such severe spasm in any condition other than that encountered with ruptured intracranial aneurysms. The surgeon emphasized how desperately they had worked to save Bryan's life, expressing their feelings of helplessness and sorrow during his unrelenting deterioration.

If I may interject: Arterial vascular spasm remains a serious complication of aneurysm rupture and is, for the most part, resistant to drug therapy— indeed a frustrating scenario familiar to most neurosurgeons. It was the general feeling that the similarity between Bryan's high degree of spasm and that seen after aneurysm rupture was more than a chance occurrence. After all, his hemangioblastoma was a blood vessel tumor which probably discharged the chemical products of red blood cell breakdown into the subarachnoid space during its removal, analogous to the hemolysis seen after an aneurysmal subarachnoid hemorrhage.

Despite the best therapy that medicine had to offer and countless prayers from us all, Bryan didn't show any signs of recovery. We had him flown back to Tallahassee by ambulance plane and watched over him in our own intensive care unit until his passing at the young age of 49. A very close friend and colleague had left the rest of us to carry forward. His legacy lives on through those grateful patients he has treated, the physicians he has trained, the research he has accomplished, and, not least of all, through the Bryan Robinson Neurological Foundation.

~~~

Thus far little has been written about the subject of head injury. To gain an appreciation as to the magnitude of this subject, it is apropos to quote a few statistics. From 200 to 300 victims per 100,000 of the population at large are admitted annually to hospitals both in Britain and
~~~

the United States for head injuries. In terms of cause distribution, 58% of severe head injury cases and 56% of head injury deaths occur in motor vehicle accidents. It has been reported that in the U.S. there are 24 head injury deaths per one million population per year. These figures were derived from studies in the 1970s, and cited in the classic book by Jennett and Teasdale (19).

Neurosurgeons less than 60 years ago were limited as to what they could do for the patient under the dire circumstances of a serious head injury. In an effort to improve, Dr. Cushing brought the x-ray machine to Hopkins, but this was of limited value, capable of diagnosing skull fractures only. Later his collaborative effort in developing electrocautery aided in the control of hemorrhage during brain surgery. Finally, he developed the concept, and was an ardent proponent, of subtemporal decompression of the brain. This was an operation employed in cases of increased intracranial pressure from any number of causes, such as tumor, abscess or brain swelling. By removing a window of bone in the temporal region of the skull during a craniectomy, the intracranial contents could be allowed to displace laterally beneath the soft tissues of the scalp, thereby dissipating the pressure. Later, this operation was modified to include the removal of the anterior portion of the temporal lobe itself (temporal lobectomy). In addition, the later development of arteriography by the Portuguese neurologist, Egas Moniz, in 1927 greatly aided in the diagnosis of surface hematomas which, once recognized, could then be evacuated from over the compressed underlying brain.

In momentarily reverting to our discussion of shunt-dependent hydrocephalus, and how the fused cranial vault acted as a "closed box" filled with non-compressible liquid; any event resulting in a space-occupying mass (such as an intracranial hematoma or even simply a severe general increase in brain swelling from any number of causes) will cause a rise in the intracranial pressure. If the pressure reaches a critical level, portions of the brain will shift or herniate out of their respective compartments, compressing the vital brain stem. Left untreated, this may cause irreversible and fatal hemorrhage within the latter. Furthermore, in the case of a blow directly to the side of the head, there may be a direct injury to the temporal lobe. The latter, in becoming "pulped" and swollen, may itself encroach medially upon, and compress the brainstem with the same end result. These are instances in which Dr. Cushing's subtemporal decompression would allow lateral displacement of the temporal lobe instead.

To summarize: When first entering the private practice of neurosurgery, we had the arteriogram at our disposal as our primary diagnostic modality for cranial trauma, plus the surgical wherewithal to both evacuate surface hematomas and, if conditions warranted, to perform temporal lobe resection.

But in pausing for a moment of thought: Let us suppose that the brain is massively contused, and, with the limited surgical options above, the pressure continues to rise to dangerous levels — what is the outcome? Or stated another way, we may ask ourselves: What can we do if the severely head injured patient is brought in from the highway, and a CT scan fails to reveal an intracranial mass, but instead displays diffuse brain contusions and rapid swelling. What can possibly be done?

During the 1970s collaborative studies in Europe and the U.S. gave us further perspective into the treatment of traumatic brain injury. While utilizing well-established, interrelated physiologic principles, coupled with innovative devices, new therapies became available. Collectively, these would allow not only survival in many critically injured patients, but would also preserve neurological function not thought possible in the late 1960s. Briefly, some of these concepts will now be highlighted.

The trauma surgeon has long recognized the importance of establishing an airway in the comatose brain-injured patient. In later years the ability to rapidly analyze blood gases and cerebral blood flow in the laboratory animal has demonstrated the interdependence of the two in the trauma victim. Not only is it important for the cellular structure of the brain to be adequately perfused with oxygen, but cerebral blood flow itself may be regulated by controlling the carbon dioxide level of the blood as well. These blood vessels autoregulate and dilate with increasing levels of CO_2. By placing the patient on a ventilator with a controlled ventilation rate and lowering the blood CO_2 level, the volume of blood flowing into an already engorged brain may be reduced. In essence, we are controlling further liquid streaming into the fluid filled "closed box," already under pressure. Recall for a moment, the terrifying case of the young woman encountered early during my residency from whom we attempted to remove the benign dermoid cyst from beneath her occipital lobe, only to have her expire under our very eyes from malignant brain edema. At that time in history, had we known what we do today about controlled hyperventilation, the outcome might have been entirely different. On numerous occasions, I have encountered an extremely tight brain upon opening the dura mater, but with the help of the anesthesiologist, who rendered the structure "relaxed" through physiologic means, we were able to safely proceed with the surgery. Neurosurgery has become much safer for the patient.

A second factor in controlling intracranial pressure concerns chemically monitoring the mineral and protein content of the blood (osmolality) by which we are able to determine a patient's overall state of hydration. The stress of an injury normally causes body fluid retention, which may in turn translate into more brain swelling. By administering drugs and dehydrating agents, we have another effective means of reducing brain water and, hence, pressure.

Finally, through the years several different devices have been developed to directly monitor intracranial pressure, some of them now being of historical interest only. At TMH we finally settled on using a newly designed catheter directly placed into the cerebral ventricle. The hydraulic pressure of liquid within the catheter is fed into a pressure-sensitive transducer, which converts the mechanical pressure within the ventricular chambers of the brain into an electrical signal which can be continuously monitored at the bedside. This not only provided continuous monitoring of the intracranial pressure, but also allowed the direct removal of CSF from the system if necessary.

In summary: we now had a means of not only continuously monitoring the intracranial pressure, but also the ability to control it by either reducing or removing liquid from the various intracranial fluid compartments —blood, extracellular water and ventricular fluid.

Try as we might in the past, we neurosurgeons, when confronted at the onset with a critical closed head injury, could never with any consistency predict the outcome in any individual case. Because of both the information gleaned from the international collaborative study on head injury and the more recently introduced concepts in treatment, there has been a significant improvement in the outcome. We have come to realize that, when confronted with anything less than an obvious brain-dead patient, we are able to give the patient chances for a quality of survival not thought possible when I first entered this field of surgery. Some of my most grateful patients have been severely head-injured victims.

~~~

At the onset, when discussing entering private practice, I spoke of the total environment in which I was about to enter. However, I
~~~

neglected to emphasize the importance of character judgment in choosing a partner. During the early years of my practice I became aware of instances in which practicing physician partners split up for one reason or another. Sometimes the issue was simply a financial one, but often it involved either a personality clash or inconsideration in sharing the workload, especially during off-hours. The time spent in covering the emergency room, as distasteful as that job can be, sometimes ranks very high on the list of causing discord. I had a very close friend in a large subspecialty group of perhaps 20 physicians who, after 25 years of practice, contracted some intermittent, unexplained, severe allergy problem nearly causing his death. He at times struggled to go to work, often carrying on his person a loaded syringe of epinephrine in the event of a dangerous respiratory compromise. Yet at times when he was severely incapacitated during a period of disability, he had great difficulty getting any of his partners to take call at night so that he could recuperate. Rather, he had to swap entire weekends for one weeknight of call or had to actually pay someone a generous fee to cover for him —a sad commentary indeed!

Conversely, I recently learned of a pediatrician whose practice was covered at night for six weeks by three other colleagues, while he tended to his wife who was dying of cancer.

In retrospectively looking at my practice I picked a fine partner. Granted, I had learned to know him distantly over a two-year period, while I was finishing my residency in Chicago. He and I possessed similar lines of thinking, often leading to the same conclusions regarding neurosurgical problems both within and outside of the operating room. We also shared similar feelings on the management of our office. Because our surgical skills were very much in parity, there was no need for any professional jealousy, but rather compassion for one another in times of perplexity and stress. We possessed a mutual empathy for each other's plight whether it entailed "on-call" coverage on a weekend or during an extended vacation. And, I might add, we possessed similar senses of humor, which carried us a long way, indeed. Finally, money was not an issue, for we agreed at the onset that after receiving my board certification, everything would be split evenly. These are all important considerations for any young physician entering into a partnership.

While on the subject it is timely to say a word about money, for that is often a driving force over which many stumble. When I first came to town, Frank was charging what I thought was, if anything, an unreasonably low fee for removing a brain tumor. With all due respect to his conscience, I felt that we deserved more for our efforts. With a bit of levity, I have said to others that patients won't think you are "worth your salt" if you don't charge at least a reasonable fee for operating upon something as important as their brain. Years later, on a more serious note, I removed a chronic subdural hematoma from the 80-year-old father of a prominent local insurance man. I'll never forget when Ike told me that, as he sat in the intensive care unit waiting room for days-on-end while anticipating his father's recovery, he marveled at how busy Frank and I were. He was impressed by the hospital operators constantly calling our names over the public address system. One morning in passing by him, he collared me to say, "Doc, you and your partner really seem to enjoy what you're doing in practicing neurosurgery. You must never worry about money, simply because it would just come naturally with the good job that you both do." I have always considered that as a compliment, indeed.

If I may offer any advice to the young physician entering practice: Avoid being blindsided by considering only the lucrative aspects of a potential practice. Look not only at the professional potential of the referral area but also at the character profile of your future partner(s). I would now like to present two instances of reciprocation, which best illustrate this fraternal-like relationship.

Previously mentioned was the fact that Frank and I always tried to clear the deck of any undone work in anticipation of the other man taking over the helm. Unfortunately, the gods of medical emergencies don't always respect timing and good intentions. I was in a deep sleep late one Friday night in preparation for a week of covering the practice, as Frank was about to leave early on Saturday morning to attend a neurosurgical meeting in some distant city. Frank, of course, was covering the emergency room that Friday night to give me a reprieve before he departed town. At about 4 A.M. my bedside phone rang, and it was my partner. It seemed that a young woman with a very serious head injury had been brought to the hospital and was on the brink of herniating her pulped, non-dominant right temporal lobe. As we spoke the patient was on the operating table being induced by the anesthesiologist, and Frank was about to commence scrubbing his hands. The problem concerned the fact that my partner was scheduled to catch an early morning flight out of Tallahassee, and needed to get home, cleaned up and able to arrive at the airport on time. I could tell that he was bothered to impose upon me, but, being candid, I was glad to help him out of this mess, knowing full well that he would do the same for me. Upon arriving in the operating suite, it was like a changing of the guard. I scrubbed my hands, walked into the operating room, and no words were spoken as the circulating nurse gowned and gloved me. By that time Frank had the patient prepped, draped and the skin incision made. I stepped in as he took off his gloves, and began explaining to me the details of her injury. As he left the room, he thanked me and said that C. H., a general surgeon and friend of ours, knew about the case and was standing by to assist me, if needed. The air drill was passed to me by the nurse, like the baton in a relay race, whereupon I promptly proceeded to open the woman's skull. There was not a moment lost in the transition, as I engaged in the process of exposing her injured brain. The anesthesiologist controlled the intracranial pressure until I was able to resect the badly injured temporal lobe. Collectively we were all able to interrupt the imminent brain herniation evident on Frank's initial neurological assessment. The case went smoothly, and the patient recovered uneventfully from a potentially lethal injury. As I recall, we had her out of the hospital by the time my partner returned from his meeting the ensuing Friday — well rested, I might add.

Sometime later, another incident occurred late one Sunday afternoon during my neurosurgical watch of the emergency room. Incidentally, this occurred before Renaldo had come to Tallahassee to set up his solo neurosurgical practice. Frank, being an accomplished, avid sailor, had been out on his sailboat in the Gulf of Mexico all weekend.

At about 4 P.M. a deranged young man entered a mission home in Tallahassee which, at the time, was housing several middle-aged women. While three of the women were occupied in their individual rooms, the assailant, wielding a handgun, burst through their unlocked doors, and fired upon each, bringing them down in succession within a matter of minutes. There was absolute bedlam as their unharmed cohorts heard the commotion and observed the slaughter. Amid screams and confusion the man fled, leaving the three injured women on the floor of their rooms drenched in blood.

I arrived at the hospital from home, just as the EMTs were carting these poor souls into the emergency department. Since our small city was not accustomed to this kind of carnage, the ER personnel were caught by surprise; nonetheless, they responded in a very professional manner. Soon the place was abound with law enforcement officers, as laboratory and x-ray technicians scurried about, and both nurses and emergency medical technicians were starting IVs and establishing airways in the victims. Upon my arrival, one of the distressed nurses informed me that all three women had been shot in the head. Seldom have I found myself in a direr situation, simply because of the urgency of the matter, and the fact that I was the only neurosurgeon available to treat all three dying women. During times of war, such tragedy is commonplace and expected, but in what should be a civil society, multiples should neither be intentionally shot nor die as a result.

One by one I entered each treatment room, and proceeded to examine the victims. Each was surrounded by an entourage of an assortment of ancillary medical personnel, each dutifully performing his or her job. In the interest of precious time, I can recall having had to be harsh with them, merely to gain access to the patient, amidst their bodies, for the purpose of a much-needed neurological assessment. The first lady had a single bullet deep within the right frontal lobe of the brain, and even though conscious, she was poorly responsive. Of equal concern was the fact that she had sustained an abdominal gunshot wound as well, raising the important question of ongoing internal hemorrhage.

The second woman, already in dire straights, was deeply comatose from massive intracranial injury. She had fixed dilated pupils and agonal respiratory effort.

The third patient was somewhere in between the first two in her status, but her bullet wound was in the left frontotemporal region, the dominant side controlling speech. She was deeply obtunded, not able to speak intelligible words, and was completely paralyzed on the entire right side of her body; yet, she had no signs of increasing intracranial pressure at the time.

This dreadful scenario demanded that I triage the cases much as one would do on the battlefield. The easiest decision was to treat the second patient expectantly, for it was immediately evident that she had sustained a non-survivable brain injury. While the remaining two cases were both going to require craniotomies, I elected to have the nurses prepare case # 1 first. She was the most likely to survive without appreciable neurological deficit, providing we not only treat her brain wound, but simultaneously explore the abdomen for visceral penetration and hemorrhage. Thus, we shaved her head, had blood prepared for transfusion, and summoned the general surgeon on-call to assist me. Case #3, although she had the greatest neurological deficit, was stable at the time and had no associated injury. Things were also set into motion in preparing her for a craniotomy to follow.

Once in the operating theater and with the anesthesiologist in control, I proceeded with the craniotomy; the general surgeon explored her abdomen through a second, isolated, operative field with his own instrument nurse. With regard to the head wound, it took a standard scalp flap and craniotomy to adequately debride the wound. About half way through the procedure, I received a call over the intercom from the emergency room nurse stating that the other salvageable patient was deteriorating with signs of increasing intracranial pressure, predictably the result of further brain hemorrhage and swelling. I glanced up at the clock, which by now registered 8 P.M. My first thought was that Frank had perhaps returned from his voyage, and was at home by that time. "Please call Dr. Davis at home and tell him my situation," was my reply. Within minutes, the nurse called me back to inform me that Dr. Davis was on his way.

It was a long night for all of us, but the outcome was as good as we could have ever expected under the circumstances. Those two victims on whom we operated both survived. My lady with the multiple gunshot wounds left the hospital several days later without any residual neurological deficit or abdominal complications. Frank's case, understandably, was left aphasic and hemiplegic from her disruptive, dominant-side brain wound, but she became fully alert and cognitively sound.

For years afterward when we recounted that horrific night, he always kiddingly told others that I had picked the patient with the best outcome, and I had made him look bad with his poorer end result. But we all know better. He quickly came to my aid and saved the woman's life, well aware from the onset of her precarious neurological state.

~~~

In moving now to a much lighter subject, 1980 was the year that Coach Bobby Bowden really began to turn things around for Florida State football. After a very successful 1979 season, the fourth-ranked Seminoles played against number five Oklahoma in the Orange bowl. While aspirations were high going in, they lost the game and a possible national championship to a squad with two future very prominent Sooners: J.C. Watts, the quarterback, who was later to become a member of the U.S. Congress, and Heisman Trophy winner Billy Sims.

During the fall of that same year (1980), the team traveled to Lincoln, Nebraska, to take on the Cornhuskers who were ranked No. 3 at
~~~

the time. Bowden's outfit beat that perennial football power 18-14 in their own backyard, causing the entire nation to take notice.

Equally exciting was the following Saturday evening when No. 4 Pittsburgh rolled into Tallahassee. Pitt was a high-powered football machine led by Dan Marino at quarterback and 19 other teammates who were destined to later play in the NFL. Bobby Bowden's offensive coordinator, George Henshaw, was to call an ingenious game. He had the offense check off on more than 50% of its plays against Pittsburgh's vaunted defense, completely keeping the Panthers off balance. The Seminole's offense, called the "Mirror Offense", persisted in deliberately remaining out of phase with the opponents defense, resulting in an outstanding 36-22 Florida State victory. I would have to agree with many others who felt that those two successive victories against such high profile opponents were probably as important as any in vaulting FSU football to national prominence. The games were as exciting as I have ever witnessed and the forerunners of a great future for the Seminoles on the gridiron. However, a catastrophic event with neurosurgical implications occurred here in town as a direct consequence of that historic Pittsburgh game.

If I might regress for a moment: Because of the near certainty of getting snatched away from the stadium on Saturday nights, I had years previously given up going to football games when on-call for the emergency room at TMH. Just knowing that I would probably get interrupted from the game caused enough apprehension that it was difficult to enjoy myself. And should I get called, depending upon the stage of the game, I had to worry about traffic while maneuvering out of the parking lot and across town in time to save someone lying on a cart in the emergency room. It just simply wasn't worth the hassle. Those were the games I either watched on television, or, if that was unavailable, listened to them on the time-honored reliable radio. In those days the expectations for an FSU victory against highly ranked opponents were still guarded, and the TV networks were somewhat wary of televising every high profile game. Because the Pittsburgh game was not televised, it became a radio night. The excitement conveyed by the announcers was scintillating as the game swung back and forth, one touchdown being exchanged for another. After our FSU victory and with my heart still racing with excitement as I listened to the final statistics, I began getting ready for bed. No sooner had I switched off the radio than the phone rang — it was the emergency room. The nurse announced to me that the ambulance was on its way to the hospital with a spinal cord injury case.

Upon my arrival I found a clean-cut, middle-aged man lying on a spine board. A rigid supportive plastic collar was encircling his neck, and reflected on his face was a look of total despair — he was quadriplegic! As I began my examination, his eyes were riveted upon me in trying to glean some expression of hope from my intent face. These very serious spinal cases (usually hopeless at first glance) test the neurosurgeon's "imperturbability" as much as any other. The results of my neurological assessment indicated that he was what is termed a "low quad" since he could weakly flex his elbows and wrists, but he was totally devoid of any intrinsic hand muscle function. His total and irreversible spinal disruption below the sixth cervical segmental level did fortunately spare his ability to breathe. Tragically, he was totally paralyzed in both legs, had loss of voluntary bowel and bladder control, and was void of any sensation over his trunk and lower extremities as well. A cervical radiograph confirmed a severe fracture-dislocation at the level of C6-C7.

The first order of business was to reduce the dislocation of the cervical spine. Previously, I had mentioned the need for inserting Crutchfield tongs into the skull after making twist drill holes in the bone under local anesthesia. This old method was cumbersome, required a special surgical pack, and the tongs did not hold well over a long period of time. Those small tongs for years had been the gold standard in maintaining traction and realigning the injured vertebra in the neck. By now, however, we had a newer device which was named after its innovators— the Gardner-Wells tongs. This was a semicircular tong apparatus which grabbed the skull from the sides, and became engaged in the outer bone table simply by turning two knurled screws. These tongs, which also were inserted under a local anesthetic, were spring-loaded as an added safety feature to obviate penetrating too deeply. In this distressed, hapless man, the tongs were first inserted, and he was then transferred to a Stryker frame for frequent turning of the body to prevent breakdown of his skin. He was then transported to the intensive care unit in anticipation of surgical stabilization of his spine.

Now for the sad part of this story —he too had been listening to the exciting Pitt vs. FSU football game on his radio. But to his great misfortune, he was also enjoying the game while drinking beer and sitting adjacent to his swimming pool at the time. In an uncontrolled moment of exultation, devoid of good judgment after the Seminole victory (disinhibition from the alcohol probably a factor), he sprang from his pool-side lounge and dove into the pool, striking his head on the bottom. I was never told how deep the water was, or if he was even at the deep end of the swimming pool at the time; that is all irrelevant. He was a truly good man simply enjoying a good game, but in a split second, his life was to change forever. Oh my— if he could have just had that moment of uncontrolled excitement and obscured judgment back!

Distractions reign everywhere; it is a dangerous physical world in which we all live. There is little room for complacency, and caution must be exercised every step of the way. Accidents are not limited to cars, skis, small airplanes or table saws. Those of us in medicine who constantly see the end results of these tragedies are perhaps more cognizant of them, and therefore more cautious than the lay person. If we could only deliver this message of caution to the public on an ongoing basis, much heartache would be spared. The public has to constantly be reminded of life's hazards, for there will always be those who drive while deeply fatigued or intoxicated, still others who ignore fastening their seatbelts; and I expect there will, forever, be unwary parents who allow their children to ride tricycles, scooters and ATVs on busy streets.

In terms of spinal cord injury, we have made some inroads in Florida. In our spinal cord injury prevention program, a very well contrived movie was professionally produced in an effort to reach the younger citizens of our state. Locally our head neurological intensive care unit nurse, Teddy McQuat, showed the film to every high school group in our area, hoping to reduce the numbers of these often needless, tragic injuries.

~~~

Since this book concerns the professional life of a brain surgeon, it follows that we should devote adequate space to the important topic of brain tumors. In future chapters this will be a recurrent topic in which specific points will be addressed. Also at this juncture, it is important that the reader understand the concept of cerebral hemisphere "dominance." We are referring to that side of the brain which controls the use of the preferred hand and usually speech, the two often coinciding. In the case of the right-handed individual, we are usually
~~~

correct about 95% of the time in ascribing speech dominance to the left cerebral hemisphere. However, in the case of the left-handed individual whose right hemisphere is dominant for handedness, the side for speech origin is much less predictable— often having been cited at 50-50.

In terms of all types of tumors afflicting the brain, we ordinarily think of perhaps 30% as being metastatic from some remote source such as the breast. As a point bearing emphasis, many lung tumors make their presence first known with symptoms of brain pathology such as seizures, paresis, or imbalance to name a few. At this juncture, I find it timely to make an important statement: Just because a solitary tumor from an outside source takes root in the brain, it does not necessarily mean a hopeless prognosis for that particular patient. The first thoracic surgeon in Tallahassee and a good personal friend of mine, Dr. Nelson Kraeft, referred a patient to me many years ago with a solitary tumor in her cerebellum from the lung. I totally extirpated the intracranial neoplasm, and Dr. Kraeft subsequently resected her lung. The lady proceeded to enjoy seven additional years of quality life before succumbing to her disease. This, indeed, should serve as a source of encouragement for those harboring such a disorder. Both Dr. Kraeft and I were always proud of her relatively long survival with what is usually considered a very lethal disease.

An additional 30% of the total number of all brain tumors or 40% of primary brain tumors, that is to say those originating in the brain tissue from the onset, consist of a group classified as astrocytic tumors. For purposes of clarity the astrocyte, as opposed to the neuron, forms the supportive or cellular skeletal framework of the brain. The neuron (the functioning nerve cell unit itself) fortunately is rarely the source of a primary tumor, while, to the contrary, the astrocyte is commonly so. In the 1920s, Dr. Cushing and Dr. Bailey, to whom we have previously referred, classified (on the basis of cell type) the gliomas of which the astrocytic tumors are an important large subgroup. Through the years, neuropathologists have graded the astrocytic tumors on a scale of 1-4 based both upon cellular and nuclear morphology and also on secondary changes such as blood vessel growth, tumor necrosis, and hemorrhage. In the adult, a grade 1 astrocytoma in the cerebral hemispheres may live for many years after the diagnosis is made, while a grade 4 (the highly malignant glioblastoma multiforme) portends a very grim prognosis. On the other hand, a low-grade astrocytoma in the cerebellum of a child, as we have shown, is compatible with a very long term survival— if not a normal life span. Representative examples of adult astrocytic tumors will be discussed with emphasis on treatment, longevity and quality of life issues.

In 1980 a 30-year-old, right-handed farmer was referred to me by one of our neurologists after having sustained a first occurrence, general-motor seizure. A CAT scan demonstrated a non-enhancing neoplasm within the left frontal lobe convexity. There was no mass effect, that is to say, there was no brain shift or ventricular compression. In view of both the tumor appearance on the scan and the normal neurological examination, we suspected that his neoplasm was in all likelihood an asrocytoma. An open brain biopsy was indicated to both confirm the diagnosis and to dictate any future therapy, if any. He was taken to the operating room, where a craniotomy was performed, and well away from the motor and speech areas of the cerebral cortex a representative biopsy was taken. The histopathology of the tumor was that of a grade 1 astrocytoma. We felt comfortable in offering him a reasonably favorable prognosis in predicting several years of a good functional survival. To the contrary, we did not recommend any intervening therapy at that time other than, of course, the control of his seizures. Irradiation therapy is of little to no value in such a low-grade tumor; to the contrary, it could be harmful. Unfortunately, we were surgically constrained from performing a major brain resection because of the eloquent area of the cortex involved with the tumor. In following this patient's clinical course over the ensuing years, Terry and I , because of common outdoor interests, were destined to become very close friends.

The second astrocytic tumor case involved a man in his 40s who owned a very successful, large scale, blue-collar business in Tallahassee. He also presented medically with a first time grand mal convulsion. His neurological examination was entirely normal, including both cognitive function and affective (emotional) tone. This patient's CAT scan, in contradistinction to the first case, revealed a contrast-enhancing tumor in the anterior portion of the non-dominant right frontal lobe. Under these circumstances, we could afford to be more aggressive than in the previous patient. Through a large right frontal craniotomy, a brain biopsy was first performed. Upon examining the frozen tissue section, the pathologist reported the tumor as being a grade 2+ astrocytoma. Upon receiving the report back in the operating room, we proceeded with a major resection of the non-dominant frontal lobe in hopes of curing this man. The surgery itself went uneventfully, and he left the hospital one week later totally asymptomatic. Sam then returned to his shop business where, for several years, he continued to work. I even had him repair a complicated piece of surgical equipment for me one time. He was followed up annually in the office with repeat examinations and CAT scans both of which were normal upon each occasion. After five or six years I began thinking that possibly I had indeed surgically cured him of his borderline malignant tumor, and even entertained the notion that perhaps he was wasting his time with routine annual visits to our clinic. However, it just wasn't to be. Sorrowfully, after roughly seven years, the lesion rather abruptly converted into a grade 4 tumor (glioblastoma multiforme), snuffing out his still young life, and leaving his wife widowed to run the family business.

The final illustrative case appeared in a popular local TV celebrity. He, like the previous two, also presented initially with a major motor seizure. Calvin, however, differed from the others on his initial neurological examination in that he was found to have some speech hesitation (expressive dysphasia). As bad luck would have it, his CAT scan and arteriogram were suggestive of a malignant, dominant temporal lobe glioma. A left temporal craniotomy and limited brain biopsy confirmed a grade 3+ anaplastic astrocytoma. Because his livelihood depended upon his speech, we dared not surgically go further at that point in time. He was treated with a course of palliative whole brain irradiation therapy. Months later our hand was forced by the symptomatic progression of his disease. I operated again, this time resecting as much as I dared of his temporal lobe, the histopathology of the tumor at that time being the dreaded glioblastoma multiforme. After the surgical decompression, I sent him for a medical opinion to a neuro-oncologist at the University of California, San Francisco, considered by many as the Mecca of brain tumor chemotherapy at the time. Despite everything medicine had to offer, Tallahassee lost its beloved TV personality and friend in less than 14 months. The glioblastomas, like Calvin's, are among the most malignant and relentless of all brain tumors by sparing no one, and have afflicted such high-profile personalities as Dick Howser, manager of the world champion Kansas City Royals, and Senator Ted Kennedy of Massachusetts.

~~~

An academic sidelight will now be interjected as we move to the subject of cerebral vascular disease. Because stroke had continued to be the third leading cause of death in the U.S., we felt compelled to bring
~~~

the message home to the doctors of our local medical community. After receiving the endorsement of our influential hospital medical director, Dr. I. B. Harrison, coupled with the full support of the neurological staff, we were able to organize the Capital Medical Society Seminar in the fall of 1980 on the "diagnosis and treatment of stroke." This one-day seminar was sponsored by nine different pharmaceutical companies, and afforded the doctors seven hours of continuing medical education. The subject matter covered most aspects of the diagnosis and medical/surgical treatment of stroke including: neuroradiological imaging, thrombo-embolism, aneurysmal subarachnoid hemorrhage, intracerebral hemorrhage, arterial endarterectomy and cerebral arterial bypass procedures. It proved to be a very informative experience for all members attending, and a strong testimonial to the high academic standards of our medical staff. I have in my possession to this day a letter which I received from one of the medical directors, thanking me for organizing the conference. The letter kindly read: "The medical seminar was a superb educational experience, and of such high caliber that it was worthy of a national audience."

~~~

In a previous chapter, we touched upon the topic of cerebral arteriovenous malformations (AVM) as being an abnormal developmental cluster of arteries and veins. As we advance further in the book, I will be discussing several cases in which we undertook surgery on these lesions, lending support for describing them now in more detail.

In the normal anatomical scheme of things, the arterial blood flows to all organs of the body through a dense capillary network. In doing so there is a succession of decreasing arterial diameters, much like the pipes in a home having first entered through a large conduit from a well or water main. Before the blood enters the capillary bed, where there transpires an exchange of gases and nutrients with the tissues, it first passes through small vascular "arterioles" whose diameters are controlled by the action of smooth muscle fibers within their walls. Much like the faucet of one's sink, which controls the rate of water flow, these regulatory arterioles control the flow and distribution of blood to the capillary bed. Then, as most of us already know, the blood exits the capillary network into the venous system en route back to the heart.
~~~

However, vascular anomalies may arise in the brain during embryological development whereby the intervening small arterioles and capillaries are excluded. Under these conditions, the blood flows, unregulated, directly from the arteries into the veins. These AVM's are not tumors per se, but during the growth of the brain they enlarge commensurately. Because there is no capillary resistance to the flow of blood, several adverse things may happen. First, the low resistance complex supports an enhanced arterial flow rate, leading both to an enlargement of the arterial vessels feeding the AVM and also a distention of the veins exiting the system. The latter may then become grossly enlarged, tortuous and often cluster-like. Secondly, because of the rapid transit of blood, the tissues supplied may be deficient in their supply of oxygen. This zone of ischemia may then serve as a focus for epileptic seizures. Finally, as the veins become distended, their walls become very thin, and may rupture from the high pressure-head of blood pounding into them through the enlarged arteries. Such hemorrhage from arteriovenous malformations is second only to aneurysms as a cause of primary subarachnoid hemorrhage (SAH). There is, however, an important age-distribution difference between the two conditions. The mean age of SAH from aneurysmal rupture is 55, whereas with AVMs, it is 20-30. In several of the cases yet to be described, AVMs were the source of subarachnoid hemorrhage, all occurring either in children or young adults.

The first case was a man in his late twenties who suddenly one day experienced the onset of an excruciating headache. Within a matter of hours, he became drowsy as the headache continued to intensify. When seen by one of the neurologists, he was found to have a stiff neck, leading to the presumptive diagnosis of a subarachnoid hemorrhage. A lumbar puncture demonstrated bloody spinal fluid under considerable pressure by direct measurement. A neurosurgical consultation was then requested. My initial evaluation of the patient revealed a deeply lethargic individual who was paretic on the entire right side of his body. His speech was garbled, and he followed commands very poorly. His findings were compatible with a left hemisphere lesion. We proceeded with cerebral arteriography which revealed an enormous arteriovenous malformation of his left frontal lobe with a coexisting shift of the brain to the right. The primary feeding anterior cerebral artery and its branches were grossly enlarged, and the AVM cluster eventually drained into the superior sagittal sinus carrying blood away from the cerebral hemispheres.

There was little doubt that this man needed surgery in view of the massive hemorrhage, brain shift, major neurological deficit, and the urgent need to prevent a second hemorrhage. After his work-up and preoperative preparation, he was then taken to the surgical suite. A large left frontal craniotomy was necessary for adequate exposure of this sizable abnormality. Upon opening the dura mater, the underlying contents were immediately seen to have been bathed in blood, the brain being angry-red in appearance and very swollen. The enlarged arteries were visualized as they entered the grape-like cluster of thin-walled distended veins. At this juncture, it becomes important to emphasize a basic surgical principle in dealing with such a lesion: The surgeon must first dissect out each of the feeding arteries, and trace it precisely to that point where it enters the mass, thereafter firmly occluding it with a metallic clip. To mistakenly identify a red-draining vein as an artery and clipping it (the vein is red because of its high content of rapidly transported oxygen) often leads to tearing of and hemorrhage from the vessel due to its thin wall. This bleeding may be extremely difficult to control, and is best avoided from the onset. Once all of the feeding arteries are occluded, the venous mass becomes deflated like a tire going flat. At that point it is like the taming of a life-threatening beast, as things then become totally manageable. The veins themselves, now disgorged of blood and collapsed, are coagulated and clipped distally, whereupon, the entire tissue mass is easily dissected away from the brain and removed. What once appeared to be a monster on the arteriogram now becomes an unimpressive, contracted small mass to be sent off to the pathologist. The brain wound is then quenched of any oozing, irrigated and closed.

The patient under consideration made a nice recovery, and, over a period of time, emerged from his ordeal without any neurological deficit whatsoever. He was maintained on medication for several years as seizure prophylaxis, and was followed up in the office on an annual basis. When last seen 5 years after surgery, he was found to be a fluent, clean-cut young man, always dressed in coat and tie, and still working at a local bank. And, what's more, his former golf game of shooting par had returned to normal!

Now a word about the second case: On February 1, 1981, I received a copy of an essay composed by a former little patient of mine. I would like to share it, word-for-word with my readership. At 11 years of age this child suffered from a ruptured AVM, and, aside from our opportunity to help her, we were gratified to receive this extremely well-written documentary of her experience—

My Most Frightening Experience

My name is Annie Hill. I am writing an exclusive account of an actual experience of mine. I live in southern Georgia where we are surrounded by forests and have only one family of neighbors.

On January 5, 1979 in a school restroom, I was opening a door when it fell and hit me on the head because of a loose hinge. This accident is probably what caused me to have the most frightening experience of my life. The following day, on January 6, 1979, I was playing with my brother, my neighbor and his friend. Nobody else was home. I had a terrible headache and so I decided to go in and lie down. Immediately when I lay down on my bed something inside warned me to get back up quickly. As soon as I got up I was appalled to find my left side was paralyzed.

I fell to the floor and although I was terrified, I quickly realized that I needed help so I pulled myself with my right hand and the aid of furniture, doorways, and the carpet to the front door. This seemed impossible and it seemed like hours before I finally reached the front door. After a long struggle, I managed to get the screen door opened and call for help.

Luckily my brother was still playing nearby and he waved to my neighbor who was getting into his truck to go hunting. My neighbor waved back as a friendly gesture, but he was soon made to realize that something was wrong. He came to check on me and then he left to find my mother.

When my mother got there she called the hospital to send an ambulance. I was taken aghast by the whole thing although my mother was at my side. The last thing I remember was riding in my neighbor's truck and my mother telling me to try to stay awake. My mother later informed me that we had met the ambulance halfway between our house and the hospital at a gas station. The ambulance took me to Bosworth Memorial Hospital, but they were unable to handle my case so they rushed me to the Tallahassee Memorial Hospital, a 60 mile trip from my house. Though I didn't realize it then I am very lucky that there were skilled doctors there to help me, especially my doctor, Dr. Geissinger, who to me is the best doctor there could be.

I was in a semi-coma for seven days. I only remember waking for brief periods of time and knowing that my grandparents, mother, father, and their families and friends were there with me. I also remember that I loved the feel of a cold rag on my forehead and face because the room was hot. I was told that I kept repeating "who" wanting to know who was in the room with me. After I came to I constantly called, where is "Mary" for my best friend

Mary Scoglund. She came to see me as soon as she could. I was also told of the critical state I had been in, the long operation I had gone through, and I was very glad I had not been able to know about it.

In the intensive care unit at the hospital, I was fed small chips of ice because the medicine they had given me before the operation had dried up my mouth and they could not give me any water because it would cause swelling in my brain. I tried to make every small ice-chip last as long as possible. I was fed through my veins, being myself too weak and unable to eat or digest solid food.

There was always someone with me at all times for which I was thankful. My family took turns staying with me. During my 11 days in the Intensive Care Unit, I was moved to a different room at least four times. When my grandfather would come to see me he would go to my old room expecting to find me there and he would almost have a heart attack when he didn't. I thought this was funny because I could see his expression from my new room, but he failed to see any humor in the situation.

When I came out of the first operation my left side was still paralyzed. I was told that I had been born with abnormal veins in my head which is very uncommon, and the paralysis occurred because one of the abnormal veins busted and formed a blood clot. The clot was removed in the operation so the pressure inside my head was relieved and thus my brain cells could begin teaching my left side to move again.

After a while I was moved from Intensive Care to a private room. I started on liquid foods such as soups and broth. A physical therapist came to see me every day to exercise my muscles, but I still could not move my entire left side. Then one day I actually moved my big toe on my left foot. I know that that does not sound like a big thing, but it was to me. I had not been able to move it at all!

My father's birthday is on January 20, and all he said that he wanted was for me to walk again and on his birthday, I did, but I had a lot of help. I know I was happy that day. I had done for my father what many people who had been in my condition could never do again in their lifetime–walk! It took a full three months to learn to walk again on my own, but I had determination and I finally did it.

Before and after my operation I had to have a test run called an angiogram. This is what I considered the worst part of the whole experience. This is a test where they make a slit in your skin in which they place a tube and then feed ink into your veins. Since the ink is alien to your body, it tries to fight back against it. You lie down on a table and have x-rays taken of your skull and your brain. The ink helps to make the veins show up. The uncomfortable part about this is while the x-rays are being taken, the ink in the veins causes a terrible burning sensation. My pain was made a bit more bearable because my favorite nurse, Melanie Gilbert, would go and hold my hand each time.

When the x-rays came back my doctor called my mother out into the hall and I knew something was wrong. The x-rays had shown that not all of the abnormal veins had been removed. I was going to have to have another operation.

The second operation took place in August of 1979. This one was worse to me because I knew what was going on and I had months to dread going through it all again. I was prepared for surgery the night before. This included shaving off all my hair! They performed microscopic surgery and the operation was successful. Now I am in the eighth grade. I am in the Junior Honor Society, I am an A-B honor roll student and I can walk and do almost everything I could do before.

As a result of my troubles, I am glad that if this had to happen then it happened in an early stage of my life and that I now have my whole future ahead of me. But I will never forget this frightening experience.

Annie Lynn Hill
Age 13

This is not only a masterful piece of writing from an intelligent, mature, little girl, but is also a very candid, graphic description of a dramatic neurological event as seen from a patient's perspective, and with all the clarity of an innocent child.

~~~

During a week away from Tallahassee, a prominent civic leader was attending a national meeting in Texas. The conference appeared to be going well until one day when his life was about to suddenly change. As he was listening to a speaker in the lecture hall, and without any warning, while diligently taking notes, he suddenly lost the ability to control the fingers of his right hand. He found himself fumbling and struggling to both hold and manipulate his pencil, the movement and strength of his shoulders and elbows appearing unaffected. The first and most disquieting thought immediately entering his mind was that he was having a stroke. Of some comfort was the fact that his mental faculties appeared entirely normal, there being no other disconcerting symptoms except possibly for some neck pain. Dreadfully fearful of something much worse to come, he wasted no time in checking out of his hotel, and catching an early flight back home to Tallahassee.
~~~

When I saw him shortly after his return to town, I found a man understandably anguishing over this sudden event which threatened to change his life. Moreover, his professional duties largely depended upon the use of his dominant right hand. The details of his ensuing examination are both interesting and instructive, especially for those students entertaining a career in the field of neurology.

First and foremost, there was nothing wrong with the patient's brain; he had no headache, speech disturbance, or proximal arm involvement, any of which might have implicated, for example, an embolism lodged in the left middle cerebral artery. On the other hand, he was found to experience pain on passive manipulation of his cervical spine, implicating possibly the neck as a source of his symptoms. Specifically, the neurological abnormalities were limited to the right-hand, where he had lost what we term “intrinsic hand-muscle function.”

As done in previous sections, allow me to provide some essential anatomical background information. During the first two weeks in medical school, while in the gross anatomy laboratory, every student must learn the nerves of the upper extremity. It all begins with the nerve roots themselves which emerge from the cervical spinal cord, and individually exit the spinal canal in a descending, orderly fashion between the vertebrae. Continuing further downstream, they join to form the fascicles of the nerve trunks and branches which we call the “brachial plexus.” The student also learns that the individual nerves emanating from that plexus are destined to innervate specific muscles of the upper extremity and hand. More specifically, those nerve root elements within the plexus that form the familiar ulnar nerve course down the inner side the arm to innervate the intrinsic hand and finger muscles. The ability for one to coordinate fine, hand-finger movement, as in playing the violin, depends upon that particular nerve, often referred to as the “musician’s nerve.” More precisely, the nerve root elements ultimately contributing to the ulnar nerve are the C8 and T1 roots (predominantly C8) after exiting the spinal cord at those respective levels. In our patient's case we could correlate his neurological findings of intrinsic hand muscle paralysis (C8 nerve root) with his sudden onset of neck pain; moreover, we could postulate a provisional diagnosis of an intervertebral disc rupture between the C7 and T1 vertebrae where that susceptible C8 root emerges from the spinal canal. This is a splendid example of what we call correlative neuroanatomy.

With his history and the information from his examination at my disposal, I was able to reassure him that he had not sustained a stroke, but rather had a spinal condition which we could treat. These are diagnostic points, emphasized elsewhere in the book, that I had made at Northwestern when teaching those medical students on my service who were entertaining the neurological field as a specialty. Few areas of medicine allow one to lay out a strong presumptive diagnosis at the bedside, simply after the history and a careful neurological examination. Many physicians in other fields don't have that luxury, and must rely heavily on ancillary radiological and laboratory information.

In our man's case, we then went directly to a myelogram. By knowing precisely where to look for the pathology, we would not only confirm our diagnosis, but any additional radiological information obtained would later aid us in performing the operation. Accordingly, the compressed right C8 nerve root sheath failed to fill with the injected contrast material, confirming the presence of a ruptured disc between the C7 and T 1 vertebrae.

The operation was performed through the front of the neck. Under magnification and fiber-optic illumination, a large disk fragment was, indeed, found compressing that critical C8 nerve root— the major component of the "musician's nerve." All disk material was removed, and a bone graft taken from his ilium inserted for fusion. All of this sounds very straightforward, but because he was a highly visible city official, it of course had to be more difficult than usual. The disk herniation was low in his neck, and because he was both husky and "barrel-chested," I was working within a very deep cavity just above his breastbone (sternum). Furthermore, I felt the eyes of the medical staff (the entire community for that matter) looking over my shoulder.

Parenthetically, there is an important message to be delivered here: As a professional, much like an NFL field-goal kicker trying to win a game in the midst of a large roaring crowd, the surgeon learns to dismiss any adversities or distractions while concentrating solely on the work at hand. The operation ultimately went well and, within days, our man began to move his fingers once again. A more grateful patient I have never had, as he made a full and lasting recovery in the facile use of his dominant hand. Long after both of our retirements, we continue to meet at the annual hospital Christmas party, always cordially greeting one another with a firm handshake, and reaffirming a lasting mutual respect and friendship resulting from that challenging experience we faced together so many years ago.

~~~
~~~

A small segment of our neurosurgical practice consisted of rather unusual interesting cases. Because of our extensive referral area, there was always an "at-random" chance that something out of the ordinary would cross the threshold of our clinic.

Early one Sunday evening at the farm, I was attempting to finish up harrowing out some nuisance field vegetation. Frank had covered the practice over the weekend and was scheduled to leave town Monday morning. Because we didn't have cell phones in those days, his nurse had to call a neighboring farmer to fetch me. Upon returning her call, she told me that Dr. Davis had scheduled me to perform a brain tumor operation at 7:30 in the morning. Apparently, a late middle-age man had presented himself on Sunday afternoon with signs of increasing intracranial pressure. Dr. Davis proceeded with the angiogram, which demonstrated what he thought was a very vascular meningioma (a benign brain tumor) beneath the frontal lobe of the patient's brain. It became essential that I get to the hospital very early the next morning. Not only must I make rounds on all of our common patients, but also needed to both examine the new surgical candidate and review his x-ray findings in preparation for what was expected to be a very challenging operation. Needless to say, I hurriedly increased my pace that night to finish the fieldwork before driving 20 miles home for supper and bed.

Upon examining the new patient early the next morning, I found him awake and alert, but complaining bitterly of headache. When specifically tested for the sense of smell, I found him totally lacking in that modality, but he had no other abnormalities on his examination. When I put his angiogram upon the x-ray view-box, I was impressed by the extreme vascularity of the tumor. The contrast material within the arteries and capillaries supplying and staining the tumor took on the resemblance of a dimly-lit light bulb. It appeared typical of a meningioma in that region, insofar as the blood vessels feeding the tumor coursed up to it through the floor of the skull. And to make matters even more challenging, the tumor had appeared to have broken through the skull base and into the frontal sinuses of the man's forehead as well.

In the operating room, we began by turning a large bifrontal bone flap to approach this lesion which, after arising from the bony floor of the anterior cranial fossa, was growing upward beneath and between the cerebral hemispheres. As my assistant, I had one of our skilled ENT surgeons, Dr. Robert W. Snyder, standing by. Upon entering into this rather soft tumor with a small biopsy instrument, I found it extremely vascular. When the pathologist called me over the intercom with his microscopic report, I was quite surprised when he told me that it was not a meningioma after all. It was a most unusual tumor known as an esthesioneuroblastoma. This is a very long word with a simple meaning: It is a primitive nerve cell tumor derived from the nerve cells (neuroepithelium) of the olfactory mucosa of the nose. Later I was to find out just how rare these neoplasms really were. In reviewing the subject at the time, only a scant few had been reported from a select group of the larger medical centers throughout the country, the Mayo Clinic being one of them.

Although constantly hemorrhaging, the tumor, being quite malignant, necrotic and friable, was conducive to a total gross removal from the frontal fossa. Realizing that there was a rent in the frontal bone with tumor invading the nasal cavity and sinuses, I rotated a vascular pedicle graft of fibrous tissue to construct a watertight closure of the intracranial cavity. This was carefully done in an attempt to prevent future spinal fluid leakage, a subject previously discussed.

In a later operation, this time through an osteoplastic frontal sinus flap, Dr. Snyder was able to radically remove the remaining tumor from the paranasal sinuses. After six weeks of expected wound healing, any remaining small deposits of this malignant neoplasm, generally considered very radio sensitive, were subjected to a full course of external beam irradiation therapy to the entire tumor bed.

The man survived his ordeal, and years later I lost him to follow up. In a recent telephone conversation with Dr. Snyder, he informed me that the patient had lived for several years after his treatment. He went on to say that he had later run into the patient's son who remarked, "I don't know what Dr.Geissinger did to my father, but he had always been a real son-of-a-*! But since the surgery he turned out to be a halfway decent guy."

~~~

Despite major advances in the surgery of intracranial aneurysms, each case remains unique and may harbor hidden potential dangers. Such a patient presented at a time when we were feeling very confident about the outcome in most instances.

A young lady in her early to mid 20s was struck down with a very severe headache, which promptly led to the diagnosis of a subarachnoid
~~~

hemorrhage. Despite the intensity of her headache, she was fully alert and neurologically appropriate in every way. Her arteriogram clearly demonstrated the offending aneurysm, which had a well-defined neck. This aneurysm occupied one of the more common sites on the circle of Willis, and there were no unusual anatomical circumstances; any contemplated surgery appeared straightforward. Of paramount importance, the arteries of the brain otherwise looked perfectly normal.

Because she was so alert and intact, we felt that she was a candidate for early surgery to obliterate her aneurysm, thus obviating the ongoing risk of a second bleeding episode. On the day following her contrast studies, she was taken to the operating room where the customary small right frontotemporal craniotomy was performed. As we dissected our way down to the site of the aneurysm, the subarachnoid blood from her hemorrhage two days previously was gently removed with copious gentle suction-irrigation. Under continued magnification with the microscope, both the approach to and the dissection of the aneurysm neck were carried out uneventfully. Once the geometrical relationship between the aneurysm neck and the parent artery was ascertained, a clip of appropriate size and angle was prepared on the applier. That critical moment all neurosurgeons face when applying the clip was short-lived; the device was methodically placed in the intended position, and released without any physical movement of the vascular structures involved. Clip placement having been deemed "optimal" there was no need whatsoever for re-positioning or manipulating it. The wound was irrigated and closed in the usual fashion. After such a smooth procedure, there is always a welcomed "sigh of relief" by the entire operating room staff.

It is a very gratifying moment, indeed, when the neurosurgeon greets the family in the waiting room to give them the good news: Their loved one's life has been spared by a potentially hazardous, yet successful operation.

The young lady did very well after the operation, promptly awakening from the anesthetic and was alert and neurologically intact. In keeping with our standard protocol, a postoperative angiogram was done the following day both to evaluate the position of the aneurysm clip and to assure ourselves that the sac itself was completely obliterated. The study confirmed that all was well concerning the aneurysm, and the surrounding vasculature appeared normal.

We ordinarily kept our patients in the hospital for at least six days postoperatively at which time the sutures were removed prior to discharge. Her Friday operation allowed a projected discharge the ensuing Thursday. She did well over the weekend. On Monday her condition was such that she was moved out of the neurological special care unit (NSCU), and transferred to the neurological wing of the hospital where she was later ambulated. This gregarious, young lady enjoyed her visitors, TV and the company of other hospital personnel and patients with each passing day. Early on Thursday morning rounds, I removed her scalp sutures in anticipation of discharging her home. However, in conversing with her, she just didn't somehow seem as alert and affable as she had been. I therefore decided to keep her just one more day to be on the safe side. Early Friday, I found her clearly worse; she was slow in her verbal responses, and hinted of a blunting of her emotions. I felt that we needed to repeat her angiogram, concerned over the possibility of late arterial vascular spasm. A carotid angiogram was done that morning; the chilling results demonstrated our worst fear—diffuse severe arterial spasm. In view of her abrupt neurological decline, and recalling what had happened to my partner a few short years previously, I became fearful of a disastrous outcome.

While we briefly touched on this subject of arterial spasm as a cause of my former partner Bryan's demise, it is apropos to elaborate on the condition at this time. Arterial spasm, for many years, had been a well recognized complication of subarachnoid hemorrhage secondary to ruptured aneurysms. Because it is seldom significant within the first few days of the hemorrhage, but more commonly so during the second post-hemorrhage week; it was the consensus of most neurosurgeons and researchers to be the result of one of the chemical products of the late breakdown of blood in the subarachnoid space, serotonin being one such substance. However, despite a wealth of research on this subject, a satisfactory drug had not been found to consistently break the spasm once it was present. According to one report, over 80 agents had been tested, but with only nine inconsistently showing any promise of lasting benefit in this condition. Some of the patients will recover on their own with minimal to no deficit providing the spasm is minimal, and the hemorrhage has not been severe as visualized on the CT scan. To the contrary, those patients with large amounts of subarachnoid blood and severe spasm often fare very poorly. If because of the diminished caliber of the arterial vessels, the cerebral blood flow should fall below half of the normal value, and the perfusion pressure becomes inadequate to supply oxygen to the tissues, it may result in neuronal death (infarction) with the end result being either severe neurological deficit or death.

Immediately upon returning our patient to the NSCU, we began her on intravenous medications to both counteract the effects of serotonin and to block calcium influx into the cells in an effort to relax the smooth muscle of the arterial walls. Despite our treatment, by Saturday there had been distinct worsening; she was becoming deeply lethargic and was manifesting an early paresis of her extremities. Additional pharmacologic agents with different actions were administered by intravenous drip while, in addition, she was made both hypervolemic and hypertensive in an effort to break the spasm and perfuse her brain. Despite our aggressive treatment, her condition relentlessly deteriorated, and we helplessly stood by witnessing her decline. I desperately queried neurological colleagues at a few university research centers, among them being the Mayo Clinic in Rochester, to enlist their thoughts and assistance. One such researcher and friend, a professor and chairman of neurosurgery at a large university in the South, was actively engaged in research at the time on this very subject of arterial spasm.

But nothing we did worked. To see her slip away from us day by day, despite the uneventful operation to clip her aneurysm, was almost more than anyone could bear. Ultimately, she became brain-dead and life support was terminated. After her passing, we requested that family and friends contribute to my neurosurgical colleague's research fund involving spasm. Many generously did.

This case, as much as any, attests as to how trying neurosurgery can be at times. When I first began my training in Chicago, I thought that the end result in any given aneurysm case was heavily predicated upon the judgment and skill of the surgeon and his staff. While indeed those are very important factors, there are others that can determine the final outcome in any given case.

~~~

We shall now move to entirely different subject matter in describing a high school teenager who one day began having headaches, followed several days later by an elevated fever. In retrospect, several weeks prior to the onset of the headache he had complained to his parents about pain and "stuffiness" in his right ear. Because of worsening symptoms his parents took him to the family doctor who began treatment of a chronic
~~~

ear infection and also ordered a CAT scan. After receiving the radiologist's report the boy was soon referred to my office. Upon examining the lad, he appeared very dull and blunted both in his emotions and responsiveness to questions. There were no other localizing neurological signs. However, upon examining his eye-grounds with an ophthalmoscope, I noted swelling of the optic nerve heads (papilledema) from increased intracranial pressure. The parents then handed me the scan which they had brought to me from the radiologists' office. The CAT showed a large mass in the right temporal lobe of the brain. As a result of the x-ray technician having administered contrast material prior to the scan, there was "ring enhancement" of a capsule surrounding the mass. This almost certainly represented a brain abscess, the bacterial source most likely extending from the right middle ear infection. After explaining the serious nature of this condition and the rising pressure within the brain, we recommended immediate surgery. He was promptly admitted to TMH where he was closely monitored for any change in his status, while being prepared for urgent surgery.

The reader will recall the earlier discussion of a frontal lobe brain abscess, which we initially drained and, months later, excised its capsule. In the case at hand, we planned to deliver the entire mass much like one would a superficial tumor. In so doing the challenge was to remove it intact without violating its capsule. Spilling purulent material into the cranial vault could likely touch off fulminant bacterial meningitis. Dr. Raimondi, years previously at Children's Hospital in Chicago, had demonstrated to us the surgical technique in accomplishing this. Once the skull had been opened and the dura mater reflected, a judicious incision through a "silent area" of the boy's non-dominant temporal lobe was made. Using careful dissection and the frequent insertion of protective cotton paddies, the incision was carried down into the white matter adjacent to the abscess capsule. Then after working circumferentially around the mass, always careful not to penetrate it, we enlisted the aid of the anesthesiologist. Of relevance at this point, the reader will recall our previous discussion of cerebral blood flow as a function of blood carbon dioxide content. By having the anesthesiologist carefully decrease the ventilatory rate, the patient's CO_2 began to rise, and with the commensurate increase in blood flow the brain began to expand. The abscess tumefaction then gradually began to extrude itself from the brain as we proceeded with our dissection. To safely accomplish its removal, the surgery was done in a very slow, methodical and controlled manner. The end result was the total removal of an encapsulated, un-violated abscess the size of a large egg which was sent to the pathologist for bacterial culture and microscopic examination.

This proved to be a very gratifying case, for the young man's temperature promptly returned to normal, implying no intracranial bacterial contamination. He subsequently left the hospital neurologically intact after a 14-day course of appropriate intravenous antibiotic coverage based upon bacterial culture material.

Brain abscess in years past has carried a high mortality rate, but with the advent of computed tomography and improved antibiotic therapy, it has been reduced considerably.

~~~

Discussion of yet a different type of abscess is now in order. Scarcely had I met Ray, who at the time was the most recent orthopedic surgeon to join our medical staff, when he urgently consulted me late one afternoon regarding a case causing him great concern.

It appeared that his young female patient had initially become ill with the insidious onset of upper back pain, malaise, and low-grade fever. Sometime later she began to notice weakness in both legs, initially more evident when arising out of a chair, but later when walking. By the time Ray was asked to see her, the young lady was unable to walk at all, being densely paraparetic. In addition she had an associated loss of bladder function. Alarmingly, her symptoms had progressed very rapidly during the 24 hours prior to the orthopedist's evaluation.

In view of the rapid progression of the patient's neurological deficit, I was asked to manage the case from that point forward, Ray standing by if needed. My examination corroborated a dense paraparesis, and an associated sensory loss (pain and temperature) in both lower extremities extending proximally to mid-thoracic levels. Also noted was significant percussion tenderness over the spinous processes of the thoracic vertebrae roughly corresponding to the sensory level.

In view of the constellation of symptoms including: a rapidly progressing paraparesis, spinal tenderness, an associated sensory level, plus the constitutional symptoms of malaise, fever and an elevated peripheral white blood count — this was a spinal abscess until proven otherwise. The plain x-rays of the spine were normal and therefore
~~~

unhelpful. The definitive radiographic localizing test at that time was a myelogram.

The patient was taken to the x-ray department where a lumbar puncture was done, fluid removed for analysis, and contrast material instilled. The x-ray table was then tilted with the patient's body inclined head down. Upon doing so, the flow of contrast material in the subarachnoid space abruptly ceased at the suspected mid-thoracic level; this is referred to as a complete myelographic block. This inferred that some type of obstructing mass was compressing the spinal cord at that level, and secondarily prevented the upward flow of spinal fluid. We then had to establish the upper limit of the blockage by instilling contrast material through a high cervical needle puncture, after which we tilted the table with the feet down. With these two maneuvers, we had defined the limits of our surgical incision and the extent of our laminectomy. By this time, the laboratory results of the spinal fluid analysis revealed the presence of many white blood cells, thus confirming the diagnosis of an infection rather than a tumor as the source of the blockage. These cases of spinal epidural abscess must be treated as emergencies of the first-order, not only because the delicate cord is under direct pressure, but also because the blood perfusion to the structure is compromised. Of equal importance is the fact, that there is stasis of blood in the draining veins of the cord with impending thrombophlebitis and additional circulatory compromise. All things considered, there was a critical time frame of irreversibility which we were either within or rapidly approaching.

Our patient was prepared for surgery immediately after the myelogram, and was taken to the operating room that night. A multilevel mid-thoracic laminectomy was performed. Upon entering the epidural space after incising the yellow ligament, there was an egression of purulent exudate (pus). The dura mater was beefy-red from the inflammatory process, but in view of the purely extra dural nature of the abscess, the dural covering over the cord was not opened. In point of fact, great care was taken not to inadvertently violate the potentially friable dura mater in the slightest way, fearing spread of the infection into the subarachnoid space.

By this time all bacterial culture material had been taken, and a shield of continuous intravenous antibiotics begun. Once the upper and lower limits of the blockage were decompressed, a small red rubber catheter was used to irrigate the epidural space, grossly removing additional infected material. The wound was closed loosely using heavy gauge stainless steel wire sutures after temporary drainage catheters had been placed.

It was pleasing to us all when she began to show neurological improvement within hours of her operation. During the ensuing days, as her convalescence continued, she was begun on physical therapy. After several weeks of treatment, the patient made a full and lasting recovery resulting in normal leg strength and bladder function. In retrospect, it was fortunate for this patient that both her original referring physician and Ray had recognized the problem early, and acted with such commendable urgency. I have often thought that had the treatment been delayed even six hours longer, the outcome could easily have resulted in permanent paraplegia.

Over twenty years later and long after my retirement, I went to see Ray regarding a rotator cuff problem in my shoulder. During the course of that examination he said, "Jim, do you remember that first case that I sent you concerning the woman with the spinal abscess?" No matter how long one practices medicine, certain cases stand out above the rest, and this happened to be one of them.

~~~

In the same manner that I diversified my own adult life, let me now divert the reader's attention from the hospital to the outdoors. After several years of searching for relaxation by driving out to my farm, I became tired of finding it in an ever-deteriorating state. The dairy farmer leasing the property was a sordid man always wearing a three day growth of beard and dirty overalls. My kids even likened him to one of the characters seen in the weekly TV series, "The Dukes of Hazard." He had originally told me that he wanted to lease my fields to raise corn and sorghum for his cows, yet he would plant the fields and never harvest them. They were always shoddy with dead stalks and weeds. It was clearly evident to everyone that he was playing the subsidy game by scattering a few seeds and then ignoring the fields. To that extent, he was receiving a government check for the use of my land. To make matters worse, the fields were rarely cultivated and virtually never fertilized, thus becoming severely depleted in minerals as later shown by soil testing. Adding to the problem, those areas not under lease by Charles were in equally bad shape. There were fallen trees, eroded gullies and an overgrowth of what I called "man eating weeds." These prickly,
~~~

vine-like plants with woody stems would entangle a man trying to negotiate a trail through them, and would have him screaming and cursing while trying to extricate himself. Some of the more densely wooded areas resembled a jungle, with extremely thick plant undergrowth laden with insects and poisonous snakes, and hanging from the canopy of tree branches were thick vines that would trip anyone trekking through. Because these vines could support the weight of a heavy man, I used to call them "Weissmüllers," named after the heroic star of the epic Tarzan movies, who would gracefully swing from one to another as he traversed the jungle. If one should venture into one of these heavily wooded, thorny, low-lying wet areas, he was lucky just to get out of there in one piece!

To tame this place, so primitive with such dense foliage and crawling animals, seemed a daunting task. But obsessed with the idea of someday having a well fenced cattle ranch, complete with healthy, attractive animals grazing in open green fields; it was all the motivation that I needed.

Realizing from the onset that if I were ever to tackle this gargantuan task, I was going to need both expert outside advice and knowledge gained from intense study. In essence, I envisioned becoming a self-taught, competent rancher. I did question how this could possibly be accomplished while jointly holding down a large practice of neurosurgery. My wife, having grown up on a northern Illinois dairy farm, knew very well that it would take both inordinate amounts of time at backbreaking work as well as a barrel full of money. With the passage of time, as she watched me get deeper and deeper into all of this, she started becoming disenchanted. But like other people with ambitious undertakings, my passion was unwavering, and I enjoyed every aspect of the toil involved. And to my wife's credit, she was right there at my side, participating in the arduous work.

Things had to begin with my establishing some type of water source. We had no electricity out there in those early years, but there was a natural spot for a pond to be nestled within the woods. The state water-management people came out and studied the landscape. They subsequently told me where to cut a swath through the woods in preparation for surveying a site for a dam. The state engineers would then draw up the formal plans for my dam and pond, and because it was a water conservation project their work was to be done free of charge. The plans also contained the design for a deep-water-release, which would both oxygenate the water for fish and also provide a means of draining the water from the impoundment.

Never to be forgotten was that unbearably hot, humid, summer weekend during which Robbie and I spent hours upon end with machetes and a chain saw, slicing through the trees and underbrush while clearing that swath. Drenched with sweat, never seeming to have enough water on board, and constantly swatting insects, we continued forward, totally exhausted, and with no end in sight. If there was ever brutal "chain gang" prisoner work, this was certainly it! But with steadfast perseverance, we eventually succeeded, and pulled through a dragline, marking the way for the state surveyors.

Once the plans for the dam were completed, I hired the best bulldozer man in the county to do the job, and a good one he did! The core of the large dam was clay, the base being very wide and the length being about 120 yards. Once the various pipes had been laid, and the entire project finally completed, the three natural springs began filling it up. It was because of these springs that my pond would never run dry, even during times of severe drought. Because Mr. Slater, the bulldozer man, had churned up the boggy land in both digging the pond and constructing the dam, snakes were frequently seen. I remember one evening as I was walking the perimeter of the freshly excavated site, mesmerized by observing the rising water level; something caused me to suddenly look down at my feet. Words can't describe the sudden fear and disbelief as I came within 8 inches of squarely planting my foot down on an enormous Eastern diamondback rattlesnake. It looked like a large fence post, perhaps 6 inches in diameter. I summoned Mr. Slater, far off in the distance on his bulldozer, and while he pinned down the giant reptile's head with a forked stick, I beheaded it with my machete. This formidable serpent was 6'2" in length by direct tape measurement, and possessed 13 rattles. While this was my first experience with a venomous snake, it was only the beginning. Throughout the years, we encountered not only many rattlesnakes, but also a substantial number of water moccasins as well. And on one occasion in the woods, I was surprised to see the rarely visualized, poisonous coral snake.

Once filled, the pond was nearly four acres in surface area, and was 12 feet deep at the deep-water release. Prior to the construction of the dam, my daughter and I had laid down galvanized pipe which was later to serve as a natural source of water to the gravity-fed livestock tanks situated further downgrade from the reservoir. Years later we experienced a major hurricane in which the power to the entire area was out for over a week. While my friends had to hand-carry water to their livestock, our animals were well provided for in that regard. After nine months the aquatic ecosystem in my pond was such that I could then stock it with catfish, bluegills and large-mouth bass. For years the entire family enjoyed fishing, both from the bank and from a canoe. One such memorable occurrence was on a weekend evening when I took my little boy, Roger, with me camping. By then there was an abundant growth of grass on top of the dam— a splendid place for a tent. We spent the evening fishing and then proceeded to build a fire and cook our dinner. Many years later as an adult, Roger recalled the enjoyment we experienced that warm, summer evening. He also reminded me that I had killed a cottonmouth moccasin at the edge of our campsite.

Much to my dismay, after several years the neighbors began getting word of our well-stocked pond. After that it didn't take them long to figure out the doctor's routine work schedule in Tallahassee, whereupon they soon took it upon themselves to cleverly sneak onto my place during the week. In a short time they had fished us out. Raised to be an honest person myself, I could never understand how people could justify their right to trespass, uninvited, onto your property, and harvest your fish and game. I re-stocked the pond on three subsequent occasions with all of its incurred expense and work, only to have them clean me out each time. Despite posting signs, and even at times trying to frighten them off by various means, they kept coming back to help themselves when I wasn't around. Admittedly, this later became a great source of bitterness. It was a very negative aspect of this beautiful place in which I had invested so much time and effort. I had always envisioned it as a miniature state park not only to be enjoyed by my family, but to be passed on to my heirs.

The next item of farm business was the prospect of fieldwork. My primary advisor was my farmer friend with the brain tumor, Terry, who drove out with me and looked the primitive place over. I can remember his telling me, "Doc, if you are going to do this all by yourself you will need a lot of big equipment." Naïvely, I didn't really know exactly what he meant until he called me one day at the office, and told me to meet him at the John Deere dealer's in Cairo, Georgia. Terry had worked out a potential deal with the proprietor in which I would get a three-piece package of used, heavy equipment. Included were a three gearbox mower and a harrow, each being 14-feet wide, plus a dual-wheel 4430 John Deere tractor complete with a cab and an air conditioner. In view of my limited time, Terry's reasoning was that in order for me to be able to mow down and harrow any given 20 acre field on a weekend myself, I needed wide, heavy, durable equipment. I proceeded to buy those three pieces of impressive equipment, learned how to use and maintain them, and eventually became the master of my land. A year later when it came time to erect extensive rows of fencing, I needed an auger to dig the post holes, a device which can be fitted to the rear PTO (power take-off) of the giant tractor. I called the John Deere dealer again in Cairo, and told him what I wanted. He said, "Doc, what you need is a post-hole driver, not a post-hole digger." I in turn said, "But Sonny, you don't understand… I have large areas of rock-hard clay on my farm." He then replied, "Doctor, this machine will drive a large post through the asphalt of a parking lot!" Heeding his advice, I purchased the heavy driver, and used it for the ensuing twenty years in constructing literally miles of fence, driving countless inverted wooden posts firmly into the earth, much like gigantic nails.

Over the next two years we were able to design, fence-in, cultivate and plant seven independent fields, five of them providing access to water without the need for electricity. Robbie's father was also very helpful to me in getting the ranch started. Among many other things, he showed me how to build something as simple as a "fence stretcher", which we used in erecting thousands of feet of taut barbed wire and/or woven field fence. We also had a large metal barn constructed on the hill of what was to later become our 20-acre hayfield planted in Bermuda grass. Behind the barn I both configured and constructed a versatile multi-pen corral, complete with a heavy-duty steel squeeze-chute and scales in which to later work the cattle. All of this was done with the assistance of my wife and our older son, Jeff.

Our initial animals consisted of a handful of Nubian goats which we found to be gentle companions, much like dogs. They were easy to manage and perfect for testing the integrity of the fences and the gravity-fed watering system.

The overall project is best described as a monstrous task, which took several years to complete, and while it was by no means easy, it ultimately gave us an enormous sense of accomplishment and satisfaction. I often used to think of the early pioneers in our country who homesteaded and built their own farms out west, and how proud they must have been.

The farm was also a good reprieve from the weekly routine of medicine, and I think it provided a much needed balance in my life. I have often said that after a long weekend of work while toiling in that dusty, hot, humid, oppressive Florida atmosphere, it was refreshing to find myself in a cool, clean operating room on Monday morning. With added endurance, I felt that I was rejuvenated to tackle the most challenging surgical task that might confront me.

~~~

In returning to medicine, one of my favorite subjects of study is the pituitary gland. This structure is a 12-millimeter endocrine gland located between and beneath the anterior portion of the cerebral hemispheres. Suspended by a functioning stalk, it sits in a cusp of bone called the sella turcica within the base of the skull. In front of the stalk are crossing neuronal fibers (optic chiasm), which contribute to each optic nerve, occasionally limiting but not precluding surgical access to the area. This tiny glandular organ receives both chemical and neural signals from the brain, whereby, through its own release of several different hormones, it targets various tissues and other endocrine glands throughout the body such as the thyroid, sex and adrenal glands. When it is affected by disease, especially primary neoplasms, it may secrete either an excess of a given hormone or be rendered deficient in all of them. When considering surgery on this master endocrine gland, we may approach it in one of two ways. If the tumor is very large or extends far laterally to the sella, it is best decompressed from the top of the skull through a conventional frontal craniotomy. On the other hand, if the tumor remains primarily in the mid-line, it may be dealt with from below; a procedure alluded to during my early training at the Evanston Hospital. This is called the transsphenoidal approach. And finally, when the gland contains a microscopic hormone-secreting tumor, it can only be dealt with through the skull-base approach. I shall describe two interesting such cases.

The first patient was a 16-year-old boy, who had not only lagged far behind his peers in body stature, but had also failed to develop normal secondary sex characteristics, causing him great embarrassment in high school. In addition to those stated signs and symptoms, I found a boy with a moon-shaped face and a buffalo type of obesity ordinarily associated with a condition known as Cushing's disease. The cause of that disorder is usually a tumor of the pituitary gland which secretes an unregulated excess amount of ACTH. This hormone in turn stimulates the adrenal glands to discharge dangerous quantities of cortisol. This
~~~

illness must be treated in order to avert a shortened life span from its complications, particularly diabetes and hypertension. Excess cortisol in this child, which we were able to demonstrate, also suppressed the release of other hormones resulting in his stunted growth and sexual development. Although we suspected a tumor of the boy's pituitary, it could not be visualized radiographically, even with the most refined techniques using the latest generation of CAT scanners. We thus had to rely solely on laboratory studies reflecting cortisol overproduction. We found that he had extraordinarily high early morning and evening serum levels of cortisol, which did not follow the normal diurnal variation. Most conclusively, his 24-hour urine production of free cortisol, also alarmingly high, was diagnostically suppressed with the oral administration of a potent synthetic cortisone product. Because of these abnormal values and with a high index of suspicion, we felt that this teenage child most certainly had a microscopic ACTH secreting tumor within his pituitary gland. These important laboratory tests are presented not only as evidence supporting the clinical diagnosis but serve to emphasize our justification of a major intracranial operation in a child with normal radiographic imaging.

We necessarily operated upon him through the skull base using the transsphenoidal approach. This surgical pathway through the nasal cavity originates below the upper lip, and entails the separation of the leaves of the mucosal lining from the cartilage of the nasal septum. A small portion of the septum of the nose is then removed, providing direct access to a mid-line sinus (sphenoid) at the skull base. Once within the sinus, the floor of the sella turcica housing the pituitary body is visibly at our disposal to enter and explore. Using the surgical microscope, we then opened a tiny window within the bone of the sellar floor. After then opening the dura mater, we were faced with what initially appeared to be a normal pituitary gland. Upon closer scrutiny, however, under very high magnification a small area of grayish discoloration was observed on the surface of the gland. Using a 2 mm. micro-dissector, we found a nice cleavage plane around a tumor estimated at 1.5 mm. in diameter and removed it. The specimen was so minute that the pathologist was unable to successfully mount it on a glass slide for examination. It defies the imagination that a tumor that small could possibly cause so much physiologic disruption to the body. We closed up the wound, and the boy appeared to emerge from all of this uncompromised. We repeated his serum cortisol level during the first postoperative week, and, much to my dismay, it remained very high. I was extremely distraught, thinking that we had mistakenly left secretory tumor tissue behind and had totally failed in our operation. I was seriously contemplating re-operating upon the child, but backed off after conferring with my fellow endocrinologists on the case. They felt that we should give it a few more days for the extraordinary high preoperative serum cortisol levels to fall to normal. After repeating all of the laboratory tests 14 days later, we were ecstatic at the values obtained. The cortisol levels had not only dropped precipitously, but his growth hormone levels were no longer suppressed. Within months after hospital discharge, the boy began to both grow in stature and develop sexually. We were later to publish this informative case in the neurosurgical literature (13). From a professional standpoint, this was a most interesting and challenging case for us.

The second illustrative case involved a middle-aged, married female accountant, who was infertile, but strongly desirous of having children. On her work-up she was found to have a microscopic prolactin secreting tumor of her pituitary gland. Because these particular tumors suppress ovulation in the female, they are a major cause of infertility. We were able to remove her secretory tumor in a manner similar to the boy's, and she also fared well. Upon follow up she had successfully become pregnant upon two separate occasions, and each time delivered a healthy baby.

These are but two examples of the many hormone-secreting pituitary tumors that my partner and I had operated upon throughout the years. When addressing the non-secretory pituitary tumors, the majority are not cancerous in the true sense of the word, but they may enlarge to the point of causing serious disability or death if left untreated —recall our discussion of the young male patient who went blind from pituitary apoplexy. To the contrary, if diagnosed and treated in a timely fashion, the results are among the most gratifying of all neurosurgical cases.

~~~

A totally unrelated, yet thought-provoking, philosophical subject relative to most surgeons at one time or another during medical practice is a discussion concerning "surgical pride" or the loss thereof. Cases such as the child in whom we first diagnosed and then removed the 1.5 mm. hormone producing pituitary tumor— something unthinkable 15 years previously—is a very rewarding, if not an exhilarating experience. After all, the opportunity to treat such patients was the very reason
~~~

prompting most of us to enter this challenging specialty; it enables us to bear witness to the wonders of science and the fruits of our labors in treating unusual maladies of the brain. This brings me now to revisit those important tenets offered by Sir William Osler — equanimity in success as well as in failure.

It is befitting at this time to recount the Greek myth of Daedalus and Icarus. Incidentally, I have seen this myth referred to on several occasions both within our specialty of neurological surgery and outside of it (27).

Daedalus was an Athenian craftsman of the highest order, but during an instance of blind envy he threw his apprentice off of the Acropolis. The court sentenced Daedalus to exile on the island of Crete under the service of King Minos. The king constructed a complicated palace whose corridors formed such an immense labyrinth, that it was impossible for one to find his way out. Into this labyrinth, which had no roof, was placed the horrible Minotaur which fed on human bodies. For years Daedalus tried to figure out how he could possibly escape. In the meantime, he had a son, Icarus, from a slave girl. The father and son, now both captive within the labyrinth, desperately needed to escape. Daedalus finally came upon a solution — they would fly out. So one day he stuck feathers to both Icarus and himself using wax, and with that they ascended. Daedalus then wisely warned his young naïve son that during moments of exhilaration he should fly neither too high toward the sun, lest the wax would melt causing him to plummet into the sea, nor too low near the water, where his wings would become wet and heavy, resulting in a similar fate. But the over-confident son flew higher and higher ultimately resulting in his demise (36).

As surgeons we must also control our hubris if we are not to exceed our limitations. Sometimes after having enjoyed a long streak of successful cases, we may feel that we are safely beyond ever again having an undesirable result. We may then, for instance, over-schedule our elective surgical load in the operating room, making the day a "race against the clock." Unfortunately, it is often under these circumstances that adverse events occur. If, for instance, one happens to be dissecting out a complicated aneurysm or tumor, and runs into an unexpected anatomical complexity, he shouldn't be worrying about the rest of the day's cases lining up in the hallway and angry relatives in the waiting room. Years ago a scholar wrote in direct reference to an older, nationally prominent surgeon, "If while driving, one continues to take corners at very high speed — sometime a wheel will come off." We have herein emphasized Osler's "equanimity in success," lest we fly too high and fall into the sea. Below we shall address the antithesis — "If we should fly too low."

It was late one spring Sunday afternoon, as I was winding down a relatively slow weekend on-call, when the telephone rang. This time it was the emergency room physician, not the nurse, who was to be the bearer of news defying the wildest imagination. Dr. Dan Jones, not only a medical colleague but a friend, was to tell me that he was currently looking at a patient brought in by ambulance from a nearby town, who had the handle of an ice pick sticking out from the back of his neck immediately below the skull. Allegedly the young man's wife, while in a state of rage from his infidelity, sought to take revenge. While he was in a deep slumber lying on his stomach, she silently approached him, and very slowly and methodically slid an ice pick all the way home into his head.

Fully expecting the patient to be moribund, I asked Dan what kind of shape he was in. Much to my surprise he replied, "His eyes are open and he is awake." On my way to the hospital I couldn't imagine what I would find awaiting me, but within a few minutes I was astonished at the reality of it all.

On the emergency room gurney, sprawled out prone, face straight down, and arms positioned at his sides against his body, was a young man in his early twenties. He was lying in deep repose — quiet and afraid to move a muscle. Large droplets of sweat were building up on his forehead, and he was verbally silent. At the junction of the foramen magnum of the skull and the cervical spine, while precisely within the midline, was the brown handle of an ice pick — shoved in clear to the hilt. As I stood looking in disbelief at this terrified young man, my mind was trying to comprehend this horrific medical dilemma with which I was faced. How would I begin to approach this complex problem? Additional history regarding his symptoms would have been helpful, but the man was afraid to talk. Ordinarily, we would perform a neurological examination, but I didn't want him so much as to flinch. Based upon the alignment of the handle, the ice pick visually appeared to be impaling his upper brain stem, and possibly more. I could not examine his cranial nerve function, because he was face down. I did not want to disturb him in any manner whatsoever. Facing the chilling stark reality that the shaft of the instrument was directed far intracranially, it was imperative that I obtain a radiograph to ascertain its position. We quickly summoned the x-ray technician to bring over his portable machine for a lateral projection. During that five minute interim, while awaiting his arrival, my mind was attempting to sort out this anatomical dilemma. Ordinarily, when operating upon the posterior fossa, I would sit the patient up for adequate exposure, but in this case I could not maneuver him to position him in that fashion. As an alternative I could operate in the semi-prone position, but again — for adequate entry— I would need to flex his neck, which I could not begin to do (nor could the anesthesiologist extend it during the process of intubation). My conclusion was to leave him in his present prone position, and do the best I could at nibbling off the bone of the posterior rim of the foramen magnum. But the hazardous part would yet remain to follow. Upon exposure of the tool's shaft entering the brain substance (providing I could even visualize it), I would still be left with the formidable task of extracting it. The dire consequences would include not only hemorrhage but the phenomenon of pulped brain exuding from the track and the reactive edema (much like the little girl we described with the lawnmower-projectile injury), but in this case almost certainly resulting in a fatal issue.

As I bent over once again attempting to talk to the man, I found him by this time extremely pale and perspiring profusely, whereupon he anxiously cried out, "I'm going to throw up!" My thoughts of surgery were promptly erased, for in the flash of the moment, I felt certain that the violent retching from his vomiting would alter the position of the anchored pick within his head most certainly resulting in his demise. Without time for further thought I attempted to extract the instrument without altering its trajectory. Moments after removing it, and to my horror, he stiffened, jerked once, and died before me from abrupt brainstem failure.

In all of my years of surgical practice I have never experienced anything even close to this. Admittedly, we neurosurgeons have all lost patients from diseases, injuries or attempts at treatment, but this incident was one of a kind. Here was a man who was alert and responsive, but in reality he was probably a dead man from the moment his wife directed the ice pick into his head. Dr. Jones said as we both left the room devastated — "Jim, we didn't put it there." A post-mortem examination revealed not only the expected brain injury, but evidence of extensive hemorrhage into all major intracranial compartments, both above and below the tentorium. His wife was later tried in a court of law during which I gave testimony of the facts as presented here. She was convicted of murder.

Throughout the years I have re-revisited this case in my mind time and time again and have discussed it with close medical friends and neurosurgical colleagues throughout the nation. Everyone with whom I spoke was in agreement that this young man, with a high degree of probability, presented with an untreatable condition and was destined to have expired as a result of it, irrespective of any intervention, immediate or delayed. But that is of little consolation to me, since it was my patient who died. An experience such as this bears down heavily on any surgeon's soul. It causes him to second-guess himself, to re-think his judgment, and ultimately try to shed off the melancholy associated with such a horrific, fateful event. Like the case of the Greek myth— our wings come close to touching the water.

Soon after that happened to me, I was contacted by a colleague practicing elsewhere who had recently had a similar experience and was deep within the depths of despair. He had undertaken an extensive cervical spine operation to decompress the spinal cord from cervical spondylosis. Upon awakening from the anesthesia the patient, for reasons unknown, ended up permanently quadriplegic. When confiding in me with his head hung so very low he said, "I went into this surgical specialty to help people, and not to have things like this happen. I'll never perform that operation ever again." And he hasn't!

From time to time throughout the book, I have alluded to others who have been devastated by adverse surgical outcomes. For the prospective student entertaining surgery, one must be he prepared to deal with such adversity, always trying to embrace Osler's— "equanimity in failure."

~~~

Thus far we have said nothing about childhood spinal trauma. Because of high risk-taking, the majority of spinal injuries occur in males aged 18 to 30. Automobiles, contact sports, skiing and diving accidents are ranked high as being environmentally conducive to such injuries. Pediatric injuries stemming from similar sources would be considered rare. In addition, there has been much written about the flexibility of the young spine. Because of the relative laxity of the numerous spinal ligaments, the range of motion in flexion-extension of the pediatric spine may exceed that of the adult's, resulting in unusual injury patterns.
~~~

One week day I was called to the emergency room to see a 10-year-old boy brought in by ambulance from a nearby county. The history given was that of a fall during recess from the old sturdy metal slide, familiar to so many of us, on his school playground. Fortunately for the child, the school personnel would not allow him to either move or be moved because of his complaints of neck pain. The emergency medical technicians, arriving soon on the scene, carefully fitted him with a firmly supportive cervical collar and moved him onto a spine board. When seen by the ER physician in Tallahassee, the boy had a normal examination, but because of his neck pain cervical spine x-ray films were ordered. While no abnormalities were really anticipated on the radiographs, the staff was surprised when the radiologist told them that the child had a severe fracture-dislocation of his upper cervical spine. My findings on his neurological examination were unequivocally normal. However, in view of the unstable spine coupled with any degree of neck movement, he was at serious risk for a spinal cord injury. We inserted the Gardner-Wells tongs into his skull using a local anesthetic and implemented cervical traction after transferring him to the recently acquired automatic rotating bed. Follow-up x-ray films the next day showed his dislocation to have been totally reduced, and perfect spinal alignment restored. We then fitted him with what we call a "halo vest." This is nothing more than a stabilizing device rigidly fixed at four points to the skull, and firmly mounted on a series of metallic adjustable struts, which in turn are conjoined into a stout vest fitted to the upper torso. Keeping the patient in such an apparatus disallows any movement of the cervical spine during the period of healing. But equally important is the patient's ability to remain otherwise perfectly mobile; namely, he may negotiate getting into and out of cars, beds, etc. In this case it enabled him to attend school soon after discharge from the hospital.

Upon leaving the hospital in less than a week he was neurologically intact, had perfect alignment of his spine on his x-ray films, and was ready to return to school. After four months, bone healing was complete, and spinal mobility was normal on follow-up dynamic radiographs. The irony of all of this was the fact that I distinctly recall having mentioned to a nearby staff member when the parents had originally left the hospital ward, "I hope these people do not even think of suing the school system for this." One year later, I received the expected word that these people did, indeed, file a law suit against the school. Once I heard that this had transpired, I made another prediction that recreational slides would be removed from all of the school playgrounds in the entire area. This also came to pass; disquieting, indeed.

The ultimate legal ramifications regarding the school in this case have to this day been a source of great consternation to me. In retrospect, there was no negligence on the part of the school. To the contrary, the boy had received optimal treatment beginning with the school's staff watching over him, this probably having been the major factor in preventing paralysis. Furthermore, he made a full recovery without any neurological deficit. Simply stated: "There were no permanent damages!" In mulling this case over, I have frequently asked myself, why should not only our children but our grandchildren be deprived of a source of fun previously enjoyed for generations because of the self-serving greed demonstrated here? Our great society is slowly being stripped of its freedoms as legal pressure insidiously eats away like a cancer, encouraged by allowing a relative few to line their pockets. The only way for businesses, institutions or individuals to economically survive is to avoid any circumstance, whatsoever, that might result in a financially devastating lawsuit. I have known truly good, reputable people who have lost nearly everything they have worked for in life because of this reprehensible activity. This topic will be revisited later in the book.

~~~

On an upbeat note, one of the things that originally attracted me to Tallahassee were the beautiful woods, rivers and lakes, a paradise for the outdoorsman. My friend, Terry, was to introduce me to the sport of deer hunting. As mentioned before, my love for guns began at about age 9, when I received my first two 22-caliber rifles as successive Christmas and birthday gifts. Years later, when in the Boy Scouts, I earned several of the NRA shooting medals of which I was always quite proud. Marksmanship was not only an acquired childhood skill, which I would enjoy the rest of my life, but as a youngster, it also served to enhance my ever growing self-confidence. Thirty-five years later I constructed a shooting range on my farm, while subsequently teaching my entire family not only the safety rules of handling firearms but good marksmanship as well. My first deer rifle was a 30-30 caliber Marlin lever-action model with which I became reasonably proficient on the target range. I felt now was the time to take my skill to the next level.
~~~

Reading everything I could about deer hunting soon became a passion and instilled in me the challenge of outwitting the animal, the ultimate goal being to land him in my freezer.

One day during an office visit, Terry and I began talking about the up and coming deer season. Because he managed a large southern plantation teaming with deer, he invited me to prepare myself to get one. Soon after the season opened, I gave him a call with my license in hand and my Marlin sighted-in. We decided on an evening hunt, and after meeting him at his home he drove us into the thick woods of the plantation. Terry had me climb up perhaps 20 feet into a permanent tree stand, which he had erected in a huge oak. The stand overlooked a small clearing, planted with beautiful green ryegrass, the perimeter of which was surrounded by a forest of trees and thick underbrush. He left me on my high vantage point as he then drove off to another distant site. It was a cool evening as I watched the sun setting before me on the west side of the clearing. A gentle breeze blew against my face, keeping my scent away from the area of interest. This was a magnificent, peaceful embrace with nature, its silence interrupted only by an occasional rustling squirrel in the woods, or the distant call of an owl. As the sun fell below the horizon, the increasing sounds of the wilderness replaced its fading visual splendor. After a couple of hours I began to accept the fact that the rookie was about to be shut out and began anticipating Terry's return. Visibility became obscured, and the faint dark images of the trees began to blend together. Suddenly appearing like a ghost, the dark figure of a deer silently moved into the clearing at a distance of perhaps 50 yards. I dared not move a hair as the animal froze for a moment, ears and nose up to dismiss any danger, before bending down to graze the ryegrass. At that point I carefully and very slowly lifted the Marlin into position, while cocking the hammer. This is the moment of excitement that every hunter experiences for the first time. The stark reality of my confronting my prey was upon me! Now— what was it that the book said? Ah, yes— the book warned about what is known as "buck fever." That serious condition reflects the anxiety overwhelming the rookie hunter, brought on by a surge of adrenaline which often causes him to forget what he has read and learned. The hunter beset by that fever, while in his haste to bring down his first deer, will recklessly jerk the trigger, causing him to wildly miss his game. The latter then promptly scampers off into the woods with its white tail upright, never to be seen again. Not to be seized by this anxiety-charged condition after so many months of preparation, I tried my best to remain calm. Despite my heart's beating like a triphammer, I now had the deer firmly aligned in my unwavering sights and began slowly squeezing the trigger. At the moment of the rifle's booming discharge, the deer appeared "stunned", momentarily buckling, but promptly recovered to limp off into the woods as the last vestige of daylight vanished.

Within minutes Terry drove up with the lights on in his truck, as I sheepishly climbed out of the tree. Embarrassed by my miscue, I told him the story. Flashlights in hand we walked to what I thought was the impact site, but nothing was found. It was at that moment that I came to realize what an astute, experienced hunter my friend really was. Very much like an Indian, he began slowly following the flashlight beam, while looking for anything suggestive of a deer... a bent piece of brush, disturbed earth, or better yet — a track. For 10 or 15 minutes we searched around in vain; then, Terry abruptly stopped, and bent over touching a wide blade of grass holding a tiny drop of fresh blood. He said... "Doc, you hit him — now let's find him...." For the next 30 minutes we pursued our wounded game through the dense forest while following disturbed underbrush, tracks and spatterings of blood. With steadfast perseverance, we ultimately found ourselves standing over my first deer. Even though it was not an instant kill shot, a significant wound was found in the abdomen, certainly enough to bring down my prey. Together we dragged the animal back to the truck through that thick underbrush and, after loading it, drove to Terry's place. He then demonstrated firsthand to me the skills of skinning and field- dressing a deer. Upon arriving at home late that night, I wrapped my game in a wet sheet and hung it from the rafters of my garage in the cool autumn night air. The next day it was taken to the butcher, who then nicely packaged the meat for our freezer.

Throughout life I, like so many others, have enjoyed very much the challenge of learning new skills. Whether it is catching that first fish, skiing or completing a somersault off of a diving board — these are treasured memories never to be forgotten. I have tried to share many of these experiences with my children. While my sons both later became avid hunters and fishermen, my older son, Jeff, was to later become a much more accomplished hunter than I. His passion for hunting has led him into much bigger game in the Pacific Northwest — elk, bear and moose

~~~
~~~

1983 was a year introducing many significant changes at the hospital, both in the physical environment and the manner in which we practiced neurosurgery.

Tallahassee Memorial hospital (TMH) had for several years been involved in a series of new construction projects which would immensely improve the way things would be done in the future. An entire new wing had been added to the facility which provided dedicated floors for the specialties of radiology, neurology, coronary care and pediatrics. Also incorporated into the latter three specialty floors were provisions for their respective intensive-care units. Before construction ever began, I recall a conversation I had with the medical director at the time, Dr. I. B. Harrison. As a spokesman for our group, I asked him the feasibility of our having our own neurological intensive-care unit. He requested that I submit to the hospital a formal letter stating the need for such a facility. There was no problem in my formulating that letter, simply because the facts spoke for themselves. I can recall listing the following data: Arguably, 70% of all medical illnesses have been known at some time to have had some manifestation of nervous system involvement, stroke remained the third leading cause of death in the country; and finally, 70% of multiple-systems injury from roadway accidents have head / spinal injuries. Furthermore, there was a substantial routine elective neurosurgical load. The hospital's response honored our request for the intensive-care facility to supplement the planned neurological / neurosurgical hospital wing on the second floor of the new addition. The neurological special care unit or NSCU was a 10-bed facility, each cubicle with glass frontal enclosure. Collectively arranged in a circumferential manner, each individual unit was clearly visible from the central nursing / monitoring station, the entire ensemble containing state-of-the-art patient-monitoring equipment.

By the late 1970s, neurosurgery had more than proven itself to be a major specialty in the overall scheme of healthcare delivery in our multi-county region. Thus, when the surgical operating room suite was renovated, we gave our own important input for its design as well. We were accordingly provided with two spacious, adjacent surgical operating rooms, the larger one having been conjoined to a small observation room complete with writing surfaces and dictation equipment. As an added convenience, we no longer had to negotiate annoying electrical cords or anesthesia hoses on the floor while moving about in the operating room, for all of these conduits now descended from ceiling-mounted outlets.

By this time the Robinson Neurological Foundation was fiscally sound and able to fund for us a large ceiling-mounted, superbly-balanced, Zeiss surgical microscope. The optical equipment was thereafter always conveniently available whenever needed, eliminating the hassle of rolling the old microscope out of a distant store room and down the hallway to our operating room. The optics and maneuverability of the new microscope were unsurpassed by any other in the land at that time.

For years TMH had also envisioned a professional office building (POB) contiguous with the primary facility. Since our neurological group had committed to the hospital as a reliable rental occupant, our needs were respected. The architects, expanding upon our own sketches, factored in our needs concerning the future neurological clinic suite. It was also important that in order to meet the demands of the increased patient population by the late 1970s, we recognized the need to add several new neurologists to our clinic. Since these men were also trained in electro-diagnostic testing, we needed added laboratory space for both electroencephalography (EEG) and electromyography (EMG). Because of the additional square-footage requirements of the neurologists, coupled with the fact that their practice was office-based (in contrast to the hospital-based practice of neurosurgery), we elected to compartmentalize. As neurosurgeons we envisioned a much smaller, yet efficient, office with our own staff, but would share common waiting and file room space with the neurologists. Thus, our own Department of Neurosurgery, while still under the umbrella of the Tallahassee Neurological Clinic (TNC), could manage its own personnel and lesser overhead expense. By having been able to work the design out to everyone's satisfaction, we not only kept the group together, but continued to enjoy close proximity for either brief informal consultations or extended referrals. The availability of such expertise merely a few steps down the hallway enhances the capabilities of the entire group, and provides for more expedient, better, patient care. Ours might even be considered a good model for any large group neurological/surgical practice.

As an added practical feature to all of this new construction, the Neurological Foundation funded an “in-house” television / audio monitoring system between our new operating room suite at the hospital and the POB office facilities. When one neurosurgeon was operating on a complicated case, his partner, while in the office, could switch on the monitor to see how the surgical procedure was progressing. This conveniently enabled him to better estimate when he would be needed to assist in the operation. It not only improved our efficiency, but kept us in close communication throughout any procedure. Also, the referring neurologist on the case could merely step over from his nearby office (as opposed to donning scrubs in the operating room) to observe the pathology firsthand. This entire scheme provided an academic, university-like atmosphere in which to practice, and was conducive to a free exchange of information.

In addition to the physical changes in the hospital and office, we also reorganized our office staff. Since the office was designed with three neurosurgeons in mind, we wanted to utilize the entire space efficiently. By taking full advantage of all of the examining rooms, one neurosurgeon would work on alternating days with his own nurse (also trained in surgery) in seeing patients; meanwhile, the other surgeon and his nurse would work in the operating room at the hospital. Because of her invaluable knowledge of both the medical and business components of the practice, Jenny was moved from the nursing role to our office manager. From that point forward, not only was the office practice more efficient, but also the preoperative preparation and surgical procedures themselves progressed much more smoothly.

We learned to rely so heavily upon our nurses that we often felt that an optimum result in any given complicated surgical procedure largely depended upon them. This reliance upon our nursing staff is best illustrated by the following case.

One Friday evening a middle-aged lady, the wife of a prominent physician on the hospital staff, was brought into the emergency room after having been seized with a severe headache. She was perfectly alert, the only abnormal physical finding on her examination being a stiff neck. The bloody spinal fluid found upon lumbar puncture substantiated the presumptive diagnosis of a subarachnoid hemorrhage. She was directly admitted to the NSCU as a probable aneurysm rupture, that diagnosis soon confirmed by cerebral angiography. We heavily sedated her and maintained her blood pressure on the low side, hoping to reduce the chances of a second hemorrhage. Mindful that it was "after-hours" on Friday night, Frank's nurse was on vacation, and my nurse, Nena, was unavailable; I had an important decision to make. I was left with the uncomfortable choice of either proceeding at that time with surgery, while using hospital personnel unfamiliar with both the preparation of the microscope and the complex instrumentation used in aneurysm surgery, or deferring surgery until a later time. Merely opening the large case containing a confusing array of assorted aneurysm clips and appliers might boggle the mind of the unfamiliar instrument nurse at a critical moment in the operation— potentially contributing to a suboptimal surgical result.

Earlier in the book, I touched briefly on the importance of surgical judgment. Considering the circumstances just described, I felt that in my best judgment the doctor's wife stood the best chance of an optimal result by my foregoing surgery until Monday morning when Nena would be available to set things up and hand me the instruments. As I have already graphically described, the overall outcome of any given aneurysm case is predicated upon many factors, some of which being beyond our control. We must therefore be compulsive in every detail, and ready to respond to any unexpected event. I sat down alone with the husband-physician and explained everything, clearly emphasizing the risk of hemorrhage while waiting, as opposed to taking a chance with immediate surgery under less than favorable conditions. I recommended deferring the operation, and he respected my judgment.

The patient did remain stable over the weekend. Early Monday morning with my nurse now present, and everyone rested and fresh, we successfully clipped Nancy's aneurysm. She went on to make a full and uneventful recovery without any neurological sequelae. Having endured that harrowing weekend so many years ago, while anticipating his wife's surgery, Don has remained both grateful and proud to show me how well she has done whenever we cross paths at a social event.

~~~

By this period in time, there had been significant further major technical advances in neurological surgery. One of them was the advent of ultrasonography. Improved radiological imaging techniques, especially refined CAT scanning, had afforded us the ability to accurately localize sub-cortical mass lesions (tumors, hematomas and abscesses) on film. However, once the neurosurgeon removes the bone flap over the appropriate area, he might well be looking at a cerebral cortex of normal color and consistency. Heretofore, often in order to make a rational cortical incision under such circumstances, the surgeon had to either gently palpate the brain surface with a sensitive finger in trying to discern the location of the underlying pathology or had to pass an exploratory trocar into it. And if neither was helpful, there was no
~~~

other recourse than to make a judicious exploratory incision into a brain sulcus. The foregoing attests to the value of initially being able to locate the lesion with a surface ultrasound probe before going directly to it through a safe, well-placed incision into a "silent" area of cerebral cortex.

There was yet another major scientific advance in our specialty by 1983, the development of the surgical laser. To the laymen this device may imply the sensational, storied exploits of the legendary postwar comic book hero, "Flash Gordon", who would "vaporize" his enemies. As we have done with other major innovations, a brief description of the laser is in order.

Many have been taught that an atom may spontaneously release a packet of energy in passing from a high-energy state to a lower one until such time that it is "grounded" and can go no further. The packet of energy spontaneously emitted is a photon, the electromagnetic waveform of which produces light. Conversely, if a medium containing atomic particles already residing in a low-energy state is given an energy boost (such as an electrical charge), those particles convert from a low to a high-energy state.

Given a group of these now recharged and energized particles in the high energy state, one of the atoms may then, as previously stated, <u>spontaneously</u> decay to a lower energy level while emitting a photon; i.e., $E_2 – E_{1+\text{Photon}}$ (described by Albert Einstein in 1917). This emitted photon in turn can strike yet another high-energy atom, this time <u>stimulating</u> the emission of a second photon. At this point we now have two photons passing through the medium chamber. These two photons may then strike two more high-energy atoms, again stimulating the emission of two more photons, the resulting total now being four. One can well imagine that in a chambered laser medium (e.g., carbon dioxide) with reflective mirrors, a very large population of photon waves may be rapidly generated. Furthermore, these electromagnetic waves are both coherent (same wavelength) and collimated (parallel). If allowed to escape through one end of the lazing chamber, an energy beam is produced which, because of its organized nature, can be controlled by the surgeon. After what has just been described, the acronym "Laser" becomes meaningful: Light Augmentation by Stimulated Emission of Radiation.

Once this intense beam is generated, let us now discuss how it is used in surgery. What is called the "power density" of the laser beam is expressed in watts/cm^2. The numerator (wattage) of this equation is a function of the laser machine itself, while the denominator (expressed in cm^2) relates to the spot size of the laser beam. The latter is a function of the focal length of the microscope's lens. Finally, the element of time enters into the manipulation of this energy source. Reason tells us that the longer the time interval of energy exposure, the more extensive the tissue damage. If we may now summarize: High wattage associated with a small spot-diameter yields a high power-density, and when using a long time-interval can lead to extensive tissue destruction. Such settings might be employed in surgically debulking a large tough fibrous tumor. To the contrary, a low power density as produced by low wattage and a large spot size, while generated in short time bursts, allows highly regulated, extremely delicate tissue removal. This ability to precisely control tissue removal (vaporization) to such a fine degree through the magnification of the microscope is what makes this machine such a splendid surgical tool. It allows a "hands off" dissection without the need to physically touch neural tissue.

Frank and I independently learned the use of the laser by taking a comprehensive, instructional, hands-on, course at the University of Tennessee Medical Center in Memphis. This well contrived, well taught course covered everything from the physics of the laser to its use in live experimental animals. Without the latter we could not have possibly developed a "feel" for the various power densities and the integral time factor of the laser on living brain tissue. Nothing less than this would have been acceptable before using this powerful device on humans. Our training was in the use of the carbon dioxide laser, that particular laser medium being best suitable for neurosurgical work. After returning to Tallahassee, the hospital purchased a quality, high wattage machine for our use. For the safety of others, we also formed a Credentials Committee, which established criteria for the use of this modality, assuring future patients that any surgeon utilizing the laser had been properly trained. The preceding discussion on the laser should be comforting in serving notice to the public of the care that goes into bringing highly technological advancements into the operating room, always with consideration of both quality and safety issues in the patients' best interest.

The value of the laser during intracranial surgery is best illustrated by the following two examples of tumor removal.

We have previously discussed the pituitary gland as a structure sitting within the sella turcica of the skull. On the most superior aspect of the anterior wall of the sella is a tiny excrescence of bone called the tuberculum sellae. Above and behind it are the aforementioned crossing fibers of the optic chiasm, and straddling it from above are the two optic nerves. This tuberculum is the location of 10% of intracranial meningiomas. Meningiomas are considered benign brain tumors, and with few exceptions— if they are totally grossly removed— the patient is cured. However, there are certain inherent characteristics in these lesions which can prove a challenge to the surgeon. First, they are known for their vascularity, and hemorrhage at times may be profuse. Second, they can be firm, rubbery lesions attached with a broad base to bone. And finally, they may be surrounded by delicate structures. In the case of the tuberculum sellae meningioma, it may have both a firm wide bony attachment and a tendency to splay-out the optic nerve elements embracing it from above. It is to be strongly emphasized that the optic nerves when under tension by the underlying tumor cannot be retracted, for in so doing, there is the risk of irreversible damage to them. I have often remarked that the carbon dioxide laser seemed tailored to remove this particular tumor. Under magnification a totally "hands-off" approach may be used both to totally obliterate this neoplasm and control any associated bleeding — a very satisfying operation, indeed.

In a previous chapter we referred to the acoustic neurinomas of the posterior fossa as being considered by many to be the "queen" of neurosurgical operations both in technical difficulty and hazard during their removal. We emphasized that the facial and acoustic nerves were often splayed out into a thin veil by large tumors, their presence being difficult to discern even under high magnification. Under these circumstances the facial nerve often could not be salvaged in the past, necessarily leaving the patient with a paralysis of one side of the face. The acoustic nerve (hearing) could almost never be preserved. Currently, in the large neurinomas the laser becomes a valuable addition to the surgical armamentarium. I can recall instances in which, after gross intracapsular tumor debulking, we brought in the laser for the fine work. By using a very low power density, tumor tissue could be removed from the facial nerve literally one cell-layer thickness at a time, conducive to preserving the nerve.

Several additional technical points deserve comment. As opposed to the early days of attacking these tumors when the illumination was poor and magnification not available; the microscope has not only addressed both of these issues, but has afforded us the coaxial laser beam as well. Also, the development of a highly refined, multi-jointed, self-retaining cerebellar retractor has allowed gentle, sustained retraction of the overlying cerebellum away from obscuring the surgeon's line of vision. Something as simple as a retractor can make an immense difference in the outcome of an operation. Finally, advanced imaging techniques with the third-generation CAT scan now allowed us to diagnose very small acoustic nerve tumors confined within the bony internal auditory canal. This afforded us the opportunity to remove some of these neoplasms before they attained a large dangerous size. Under these circumstances total removal of the tumor with preservation of the facial nerve became the rule, and I can recall two cases in which we were able to preserve a minor degree of hearing as well. Nowhere is the importance of radiological and surgical advancement over the previous two decades better illustrated than what we have just discussed concerning acoustic-nerve tumors. While still a very challenging procedure, science and engineering have made it much safer for the patient and easier on the surgeon.

~~~

While there was an ever-changing environment in which we practiced surgery, I was also moving forward in the future development of my cattle ranch. The acquired goats helped to keep the place cleaned up, but if I was ever going to replace them with cattle I needed to provide sustainable plant growth to carry me through any given year. In this regard the University of Florida provided indispensable help to me in many ways. Through its Institute of Food and Agricultural Sciences (IFAS), I acquired the equivalent of a textbook of knowledge concerning forages in Florida, raising cattle and the inter-relationship between the two. In addition, an annual two-day seminar appropriately called the "Beef Cattle Short Course" was held in Gainesville. It was a very informative, well organized conference with contributing professors and experts from throughout the southern U.S. participating. Each year there was a central theme, an example of which being "Forages in Florida and factors concerning weight gain in cattle." My home library was replete with agricultural textbooks from the University, and ranged from soil chemistry to animal genetics and husbandry. Over the ensuing 20 years of both study and experience, I felt that I had probably attained the equivalent of a college degree in agriculture, albeit self-taught.

When the casual highway observer drives by a well fenced farm, and marvels at those beautifully nourished cattle with sturdy calves at side
~~~

grazing on the rich green pastures, he can't begin to comprehend the extensive planning, study and work that had contributed to such a tranquil scene. No longer do most knowledgeable, small-scale ranchers merely cast their animals out on the land and hope for the best. If one should neglect testing the soil regularly or adding important nutrients, yet allowing the animals to graze the grass too low, the soil not only becomes rapidly depleted of critical elements, but it precludes acceptable animal growth and productivity. In converting plant to animal protein, science can now tell us rather precisely how many pounds of beef per acre can be produced, given a certain species of grass with appropriate fertilization. In my case all pastures were planted in either Pensacola or Argentine bahiagrass, which both grow well on the porous sandy soils in Florida. And the hayfield was sprigged with Tift-44 bermudagrass.

Once the hayfield was established, I needed to acquire some equipment to harvest it. A flat multidisc hay-cutter was purchased for attachment to my giant tractor's three-point hitch. As opposed to a standard mower which grinds and fragments the grass, this machine crisply slices the base of the stems, laying the grass down in flat shocks. The second-order machine needed was a hay-tedder, a device with twin rotors, each harboring revolving tines. It is pulled by the tractor and mechanically-driven by its power-take-off (PTO), the revolving shaft extending from the rear. The tedder not only breaks apart the shocks of hay and scatters them, but fractures the stems, allowing for more expedient drying of the grass. This becomes very important in curing the hay as quickly as possible before any rain ruins it. Wet hay, even after it ultimately dries, has had much of its nutritional value leached out. During the next step the hay is raked into windrows in preparation for baling it.

The days of the small square bales have greatly diminished on cattle ranches, where large quantities are needed, and storage space is at a premium. Furthermore, whereas it takes at least two workers to bale, stack and expeditiously store the small bales, one man can easily wrap and gather up the large round ones. What's more, tightly wrapped, large round bales may be stored outdoors until used, even if not ideally covered. After diligently doing my research and shopping around, I purchased a New Holland chain-driven baler directly off of the show room floor at one of the large farm dealers in Georgia. New Holland has always been recognized as a leader in farm equipment. Like everything else, there was a learning curve in becoming proficient in its use; specifically, it was important to avoid inadvertently "over-sizing" the bail, and jamming the machine. I can recall more than once trying to extricate a 1,500-pound, jammed bale, when working alone in the hot sun racing to beat the forecasted showers. Once I was no longer intimidated by the uncertainties of all of these potentially dangerous new hay-making machines, it became fun.

For anyone contemplating future farming, I cannot begin to over-emphasize the safety precautions in using farm equipment. Years ago we lost a prominent, well-liked local physician in a nightmarish tractor accident. And just recently while writing this portion of the manuscript, I learned of a retired prominent major league baseball player who lost his life after having been caught up in the PTO of his tractor. In neurosurgery we are all familiar with de-scalping injuries caused by people with long hair getting caught in a revolving PTO. These are ghastly, terrifying accidents caused by powerful machines designed for tearing up hard earth and torquing monstrous loads — nothing stops them if it gets in the way!

I'll never forget the end of that very first summer's hay experience when, despite the newly planted grass being very sparse, I was able to bale up 10 rolls of hay. I was so proud of that accomplishment that everybody in the office heard about it on Monday morning. While using proper management in the years to follow, that quantity escalated to well over 100 bales per cutting per 20 acres, and it was nice quality hay. Like one of my hay-farmer friends once said, "At the end of a long, hot summer day as you stand looking at the edge of a large field full of round bales, you feel like you have really done something!"

~~~

I have described many of the technical advancements in neurological surgery through the years and the greatly improved outcomes in many of the more difficult cases, especially with regard to aneurysms. But I have mentioned nothing concerning the natural history of this condition, and our rationale with regard to surgical intervention. Many people are very much aware of the fact that, at any moment, either they or someone close to them could be snuffed out in the blink of an eye with a subarachnoid hemorrhage (SAH) from a ruptured intracranial aneurysm. Most have either read about someone of national prominence dying from one of these vascular crises, or have known of such an event within their own community. As a result, some of the questions asked to me by those
~~~

folks concerned about aneurysms are: the incidence of these lesions in the general population, the probability of their rupturing, and if so — the likelihood of death. In answering these questions let me cite two unique case histories, preceded by a few important statistics.

Based upon postmortem material and clinical studies, it has been estimated that 2% of the population-at-large may harbor an intracranial aneurysm. The risk of hemorrhage in those having an aneurysm is on the order of 2% to 3% per year; consequently, during any given person's lifetime, his cumulative risk may become quite significant.

With regard to the mortality rate in those untreated patients who have ruptured an aneurysm, we may refer back to the landmark Cooperative Study at the University of Iowa. The mortality rate during the first 24 hours after a subarachnoid hemorrhage from a ruptured aneurysm is 10%, but after seven days it escalates to 27%. Furthermore, nearly half of the untreated patients in the Iowa study had expired by one month after their initial hemorrhage. These are dismal statistics, and leave little doubt that urgent therapeutic intervention must be instituted to alter the natural course of this deadly condition.

As we have already seen, even if the patient makes it to the operating room, there are other factors dictating the final outcome in any given case. Among these we might include: the size and location of the aneurysm, the age and condition of the patient, the degree of hemorrhage and subsequent vascular spasm; and finally, the skill and experience of the surgeon.

Headaches, invariably present to some degree in a SAH, are one of the most common general complaints encountered by both the general practitioner and the emergency room physician. The critical issue is to recognize when they may signal a serious problem. The following case well illustrates this diagnostic dilemma.

One of the neurologists in my group was eventually asked to see a woman in her early fifties in the emergency room subsequent to two previous ER visits over a span of several hours. On each of the two previous physician encounters, the headaches were thought trivial, and she was sent home on pain-relieving medications. The neurologist, based upon his detailed history and a careful physical examination which revealed nuchal rigidity (stiff neck), strongly suspected a subarachnoid hemorrhage and recommended an immediate lumbar puncture in the emergency department. Bloody spinal fluid proved his diagnosis correct, and the patient was admitted to the NSCU. To our surprise, an ensuing diagnostic arteriogram revealed not one but two intracranial aneurysms. By using several criteria as we studied the angiogram, we were able to determine which one of the aneurysms had bled. It was the larger of the two, and possessed a ragged, irregular dome. In addition, the vessels within its close proximity had begun to show early minimal signs of vascular spasm. Fortunately for the patient, this offending aneurysm was located in the anterior region of the Circle of Willis, an area where I felt confident operating. Its fellow, on the other hand, was located at the tip of the basilar artery — a more formidable location — which neither I nor my partner were comfortable in handling. We have already addressed the fact that the surgeon must always be cognizant of his limitations, and place the patient's safety first. As is so often the case, we were again confronted with a critical judgment issue, the logistics of which were discussed with the patient and her husband. Simply stated— with some added risk to the patient —we could have flown her out of Tallahassee to a referral center in order to have both aneurysms secured. This would have entailed several patient-transfers and some unavoidable jostling around during the process, highly undesirable factors when trying to maintain a sedated patient and a stable blood pressure to preclude another hemorrhage. Alternatively, we could urgently proceed with operative treatment of the more dangerous aneurysm which had already bled, keeping in mind that only a small residual clot within the dome of that aneurysm was preventing another hemorrhage. This procedure could easily be implemented in our own facility, and the incidental aneurysm dealt with at a time and place later to be determined. The patient and her husband preferred that we proceed with the surgery at TMH in an effort to immediately obliterate this lesion, which statistically ran a 27% chance of taking her life within the ensuing six days. Accordingly, we proceeded with her craniotomy the next morning, and were successful in excluding the offending aneurysm from her circulation. She recovered nicely without any incident.

We were then left with the problematic, incidental aneurysm. There was no doubt in my mind that she needed the second aneurysm treated. In support of my opinion, the majority of neurosurgeons at the time were recommending operative treatment of most incidental aneurysms, providing such treatment didn't pose any undue risk to the patient.

Parenthetically, I would like to interject a very salient feature regarding our specialty. Neurosurgeons represent a small percentage of the total physician population. Because we are such a small group, each of us at one time or another has become acquainted with many of the neurosurgeons (both within and outside of the academic community) throughout the United States. Conferences and small luncheon discussion groups at national meetings have afforded us the opportunity to know many of our colleagues on a first-name basis. Because we have remained such a closely affiliated group, we all freely communicate and may consult with one another from time to time for the benefit of our patients. An expert on any particular facet of neurosurgery is but a phone call away.

One of the more nationally prominent neurosurgeons, whom I had happened to meet several years before, had just published in the *Journal of Neurosurgery* his excellent surgical results on a small personal series of aneurysms of the basilar artery. In view of my firm opinion that we should not put our patient at risk of hemorrhaging from her incidental aneurysm during the ensuing thirty years by ignoring it, I again met with the patient and her husband. My recommendation was to send her across the country to Dr. Charles Wilson, the author of the aneurysm journal article, at the University of California at San Francisco. After my having successfully clipped her ruptured aneurysm, they confidently accepted my recommendation without hesitation. I then merely picked up the phone, and within minutes was discussing her case with Dr. Wilson. I can recall our conversation which ended with his saying, "Jim, I'll be more than happy to make arrangements out here to operate upon her if the family so decides." Without elaborating any further, Dr. Wilson did a magnificent job in handling a very difficult, potentially dangerous, vascular lesion; and when all was said and done, she was free to live out the rest of her life without the constant, justifiable, anticipation of another dreadful aneurysmal hemorrhage.

Another entirely different, yet interesting, point should be made concerning intracranial aneurysms. People often ask if they are hereditary. While extremely rare, familial aneurysms do make their presence known from time to time. They are so unusual that unless another sibling or a parent-sibling have a documented history of an aneurysm, we don't usually recommend routine screening of family members. To adequately rule out an aneurysm in years past meant to perform extensive (four-vessel) pan-cerebral angiography with its inherent expense, discomfort and small risk — none to be taken lightly.

Another one of my associate neurologists, who was a consultant in a nearby town, asked me if I would perform an angiogram on a lady with recurrent headaches who was obsessed with the thought of harboring an aneurysm. It seems that she had a distant relative who had met his fate with an aneurysm rupture. I told him that the woman should not worry, for her chances of having such a lesion were extremely unlikely. My opinion only pacified her temporarily, for each time that Bill would see her in his clinic, she remained unrelenting in her quest to persuade him to exclude the possibility of an aneurysm located somewhere in her head. This went on for months, possibly as long as a year. Finally, after this obsession was beginning to take an emotional toll on her daily life, she insisted that if our neurology group didn't perform an angiogram, she would go elsewhere to have it done! Somewhere along the line in my medical training, a professor once told us that there are times, contrary to one's own medical opinion, that you should "listen to the patient." Rather than having our lady deteriorate further into an emotional wreck, I finally consented to perform the arteriogram. This vascular study was done without any undue complications, and, much to our surprise, she proved correct in her intuition —a sizable incidental aneurysm was indeed present! Because she was a young individual, the cumulative risk of her rupturing that aneurysm was well over 50% during her remaining lifetime. Needless to say, we operated upon her, not only excluding the aneurysm as a threat to her life, but also eliminating her obsession as well. My professor had certainly been correct in this case — "Always listen to the patient."

~~~

One day in late 1983 I received a formal letter from the American Board of Neurological Surgery inviting me to appear on the oral examination board as a guest examiner in May 1984. In a previous section of the book, I had discussed in detail the requirements necessary to become board-certified as a neurosurgeon, while relating my experiences at the time in achieving that status. Now I was extended an invitation to sit on the other side of the table as an examiner. This was, indeed, an honor.

Several weeks after I had accepted the position, I was sent the details of the protocol concerning the examination process. The board examination that spring was scheduled to be given where I had studied the laser several months earlier, the University of Tennessee Medical Center in Memphis. I was expected to arrive on a Saturday, and was scheduled to meet with the board officers and the other examiners on Sunday for formal instruction. The examination itself was scheduled to run the better part of the week. My role as an examiner was to prepare a
~~~

series of individual neurosurgical cases, divided evenly between spinal and cranial neurosurgery. Keeping in mind both the number of candidates to be examined, and also the fact that the cases themselves could not be repeated, it translated into a modest amount of material. Understandably, because this was a unique opportunity for me, I had an obligation to uphold the highest standards in the process. Therefore, my effort in preparation entailed reaching deep into my bag of experience to provide a good mix of material. This included both routine common cases seen in everyday practice and requiring a basic fund of knowledge of neurosurgery, plus an assortment of the more unusual, difficult, yet interesting cases as well. My office manager, Jenny, pulled the patients' charts, and the radiology department made copies of the appropriate radiographs and CAT films for me. One of the pathologists graciously supplied me with several selective photomicrographs of various tissue preparations which I had submitted to the department over the years.

Once the case material was organized, I then broke each one down into a series of questions of increasing difficulty, in anticipation of leading the candidate into academic discussions of diagnosis and treatment. Although not anywhere near the volume of material covered when I took the oral examinations nearly twelve years previously, I found myself being every bit as meticulous in preparing to give it to others.

Upon arriving in Memphis, I was pleased to see that several of the examiners were neurosurgeons whom I already knew. Dr. David Kline, the chairman of the board, had been a friend of mine for years, having been over to Tallahassee for a visit with Frank and me in the early 1970s. As for the other examiners, Dr. Kline included, it looked like a "Who's Who" in neurosurgery. The majority of them were in academic institutions throughout the land, some being heavily involved in research, others having been authors of important neurological and neurosurgical textbooks, but virtually all of them nationally visible in our specialty. Later in the week while riding en route to one of the elegant evening dinners provided by the Board, I was privileged to sit beside and visit with Dr. Richard C. Schneider, professor of neurological surgery at the University of Michigan. I not only related to Dr. Schneider that I had read most of his important landmark books, such as his authoritative book on *Head and Neck Injuries in Football*, but also expressed my respect and gratitude to him for his life-long contributions to our specialty. I considered it an honor, indeed, just to be sitting next to this well-respected neurosurgeon and teacher.

The long days of the examinations were challenging, occupied as they were by intense, well-directed thought throughout that entire week. We attempted to discern who was of such proficiency in their knowledge of neurosurgery that they could be entrusted to the public as "board-certified." By far the majority of the candidates did very well, and I personally felt that it was a pleasure to have examined them. A select few eventually proceeded over the ensuing years to attain national prominence as heads of high profile, neurosurgical departments at universities.

This section was entered into this book not merely to reflect my personal experience as an examiner, but also to provide insight to the reader regarding a mere fragment of the extensive, arduous, process of physician training (in this case a highly technical specialty) in offering our patients the best and safest care possible. The media are very quick to provide us with information concerning isolated misadventures in medicine, but little is written relevant to the intensity of education and the collective efforts of a multiplicity of institutions, teachers and formal examination bodies which ensure quality physicians and surgeons.

In closing, I would have to say that I was deeply humbled by this entire experience. It was indeed an honor to have been chosen, as a community neurosurgeon, to sit on the board as a guest examiner amongst such a prestigious group of academic neurosurgeons and neurologists. As I have said to those close to me, "I feel that the week in Memphis was probably the academic high point in my professional career as a neurological surgeon."

~~~

With the ever-increasing workload at the hospital, it became even more important that I maintain the farm as an outlet, a place in which to give the mind a respite from treating the endless flow of broken bodies and disturbed souls. It afforded me great peace of mind when savoring the beauty, fresh air, and tranquil solitude one finds only in nature. Moreover, by indulging in the persistent, heavy, outdoor work, it helped me to remain not only physically fit but mentally sound. I am confident that I was a better surgeon as a result.

Because the fields were both thriving well and luxurious by the fall of 1984, I was anxious to begin my cattle herd. For those unfamiliar with the beef cattle business, there are two major subdivisions: the
~~~

commercial beef cattleman and the purebred breeder. While the commercial cattleman, many with enormous herds grazing the open-ranges out west, supply our dinner tables with beef, the purebred group basically raises and sells seed stock for genetic infusion into those commercial herds. There are any number of different breeds of beef cattle (a few of them being very large animals, some even considered "exotic"), each being selected for specific traits, often to include color and appearance. In our particular case, I felt we were better suited as breeders of seed stock. To have a small quality registered heard, which I could constantly try to improve upon, seemed to make sense, simply because I lacked the acreage for a cattle operation mandating large numbers of animals for volume marketing at the feedlots and stockyards.

After rather extensive research on the subject, and after having spoken with others knowledgeable in the field, I learned of a breed of cattle called the "Beefmaster." The roots of this interesting breed date back to 1908, when Mr. Ed C. Lasater first began breeding Brahman with Hereford cattle in South Texas. However it was his son, Tom Lasater, who in 1931 began the three-way cross of superior Brahman, Hereford and Shorthorn cattle which led to the recognition of the Beefmaster as a breed by the Department of Agriculture as recently as 1954. By combining the genetics of the Brahman (½), Hereford (¼) and Shorthorn (¼), he was able to produce a very hardy animal which with the Brahman influence could better tolerate the hot, parasite-laden, drought-prone southern U.S., yet maintain the characteristics of the heavy carcass, milk-producing English breeds. During the course of my reading, I have seen reference to him as having been considered a genius in conceptualizing and implementing this genetic cross. But he never ceased to stop improving the breed, continually emphasizing that Beefmaster cattle should not be bred purely for looks in the show ring but rather for what he called, "reproductive efficiency." Color or the absence of horns means nothing when it comes to the bottom line of survival and beef production. He conceived of breeding these animals based solely upon his "Six Essentials," these criteria continuing to be the basis for Beefmaster breeding to this day. The Lasater Six Essentials include: Disposition, Conformation, Weight Gain, Milk Production, Fertility and Hardiness. If these criteria are continually strived for in the breeding process, it becomes automatic that, as his son once said, "A bull will look like a bull and a cow like a cow." If I were writing this for prospective breeders, I would go into greater detail regarding these Six Essentials which, for current purposes, I think speak for themselves.

When it came to culling the undesirable individuals not meeting these stringent criteria, Lasater's self-discipline in removing them from his herd appeared to other people as almost merciless. For example, a first-year heifer must wean a calf by 25 months of age or be culled for the stockyards. In essence, her subpar genetic constitution was not to be perpetuated in the breed. Similarly, a mama cow should wean a healthy, robust, well-conformed calf every year or likewise be sent to slaughter. He also felt that Beefmaster cattle should be genetically fit to survive the elements whatever they may be. Instead of being taken-down during a coyote attack, they should kill the coyote if they are to remain in the herd. Each Beefmaster breeder is expected to follow these strict guidelines of the selective process to ensure breed improvement. In being willing to stand behind his effort, each of his cattle must therefore be branded to identify him as the breeder (24).

The entire concept of the Beefmaster breeding program was very intriguing to me, and I began looking into how I might get started. As good fortune would have it, Fred Thompson, of the Thompson Cattle Marketing Company, had his office just up the road from me in Pavo, Georgia. Fred was among those at the top as a market-manager for the premiere Beefmaster cattle sales throughout the Southeast. I gave him a call one day from my clinic office, and he certainly sparked my further interest in the breed. Subsequently, he invited me and my wife to attend a large southeastern Beefmaster cattle sale in Jackson, Mississippi, in September. Robbie and I meanwhile agreed that this sounded like the right breed of cattle for us. We envisioned raising exemplary seed stock to produce quality Beefmaster bulls, which we would then sell to the commercial cattleman in our area to breed with their herds. By following those Six Essentials laid out years ago by Tom Lasater, I proposed striving for those genetics in my bulls that would not only produce calves of high weaning weight, but also calves that would continue optimal weight gain and continued fertility under adverse range conditions, including extreme drought. The bottom line of this "reproductive efficiency" concept is to then enable the commercial cattleman in turn to produce more beef and realize higher profits. My proposed marketing strategy, like that of the Lasaters, was not only to have prospective buyers "look" at my bulls, but also to invite them to examine my statistics on raising them. Therein lies important information such as their weight gain and the reproductive history of their respective parents.

We departed from Tallahassee two days prior to the big sale in Jackson, anticipating arrival there well in advance in order to evaluate the cattle prior to the auction. We envisioned buying a group of female "base-cows" with high-end genetic backgrounds which would be the foundation for our own sound herd. By the time the Saturday morning auction rolled around, we had decided on the six lots we hoped to purchase. We would attempt bidding on six "3 N 1's", which in layman's language means: a quality mother cow confirmed as settled (pregnant) by a good bull, and nursing a calf at side.

On the day of the big event, Robbie and I were among the first to occupy choice seats at ringside. We grew increasingly more excited as the crowd began filling up the arena. The well-lighted arena, complete with its rich-looking red dirt floor, the scent of freshly-cut hay permeating the air, and the bellowing sounds of those magnificent animals in the hidden background pens, provided a compelling backdrop for what was to follow. Fred Thompson, who sat facing the audience above and behind the ring, was the sale-master who would introduce the various lots as they were individually led into the arena and circulated about the ring by a cowboy. At Fred's side was the auctioneer who would begin barking out the bids over the erratically crackling, yet booming, loud-speaker, while the cows and their calves nervously pranced about the arena under the close scrutiny of the cattle buyers. Occasionally during the auction, one of the animals would abruptly turn on the defenseless cowboy, and while furiously snorting and pawing the earth, would cause him to dart behind a protective shield-like barrier as the crowd moaned. From beginning to end, this event smacked of a rodeo-like atmosphere. The ring men (auctioneer's assistants) were constantly on the move through the arena's aisles amongst the buyers, while loudly shouting and relaying the bids to the auctioneer himself. I'll never forget one such ring man who reminded me of "Hoss" in the old TV series, "Bonanza." Although similar to Hoss in stature, this man did not reflect his gentle disposition. This large burly fellow with his ten-gallon hat had a deeply resonant, loud, booming voice and was right up in your face shaking his large, meaty finger at you while trying to elicit an ever-increasing bid. Once these ring men gain insight into the buyer's intent, they act as catalysts in generating higher and higher bids. That is their profession, and this aggressive guy was good at it. As an admonition to anyone contemplating delving into this business, one must decide well in advance of this emotionally-charged, noisy event— when initially examining the cattle in their lot pens — just what they are worth and the limit as to what one is willing to pay for them. Don't let this "Hoss" of a man empty your wallet. Despite any negative inferences regarding what I have just written, there are few situations in life which are more exciting than an auction for high-quality, showcase, purebred cattle.

It was indeed a very exhilarating and momentous hour, my wife and I both realizing at the time that we were buying into a well respected, highly sought-after breed of cattle. It was quite evident that those animals we had picked were also on the list of many others as well. The bids for them had escalated higher and higher, and everyone's emotions reached a fever pitch. By the end of the auction I sensed many mixed feelings pervading the group, but think very few folks left disappointed. Robbie and I ended up with six highly regarded, pregnant females with good-looking calves "at side." After writing the auction check for our initial base herd, arrangements were then made to have the cattle shipped back to our ranch in Monticello— the ranch we had worked so hard to develop for this moment. The rest of the day and evening was quite festive both in meeting the sellers of our cattle, representing ranches from Texas to Mississippi and Georgia, and enjoying good food and drink. On Sunday, while still energized, we pointed the Oldsmobile back toward Florida, and, during the drive home, made further plans on both naming our ranch and deciding upon our own brand.

EIGHT

The Era of Magnetism in Medicine

~~~

The year 1985 saw the introduction of magnetic resonance imaging to the medical community of Tallahassee. Interestingly, the basic concept for MRI, while not destined for clinical use until much later, was developed long before the CAT scan. In 1946 Felix Bloch and Edward Purcell each independently discovered the magnetic resonance phenomenon which led to their both being awarded the Nobel Prize in 1952. A select group of scientists during the ensuing thirty years, by gaining additional experimental insight into the physics of this phenomenon, were eventually able to consummate their efforts by displaying an image of tissue.

Relevant is our earlier discussion of the CAT scan in which the reader will recall that different tissues possess different coefficients of x-ray absorption. This physical characteristic may be represented numerically in a defined volume (pixel) of tissue, which is then run through a computer, thereafter producing a digital representation. Those tissues with high x-ray attenuation, such as bone, are represented by high numbers, and those with low coefficients of absorption, like water, have low values. These numbers are then represented in a matrix, and are assigned various shades of gray (the extremes being white and black) depending upon their values. The visual image that we then observe is derived from that matrix.

In the case of MRI, the digital-imaging process is much the same as it is in the CAT, but those unique physical properties of the tissues imaged are entirely different. Instead of measuring the propensity of an x-ray beam to be absorbed in passing through a given tissue, as in the case of CAT, the MRI measures the response of that tissue when placed in a magnetic field.
~~~

The body is composed of 70% water, which most people know is represented by the molecular formula H_2O. It follows then that each molecule of water contains two hydrogen nuclei, each of which possesses a single positive charge (+); in essence, each is a proton. These protons independently spin randomly about a vertical axis like tiny tops. In so doing, each one generates a magnetic field that has a vector (denotes both magnitude and direction). If subjected to a powerful external magnetic field (which also has direction), the vectors of the majority of these protons align themselves both parallel with and in the same direction as the external field. In that arrangement, they are described as residing in a low-energy state. To the contrary, the remaining protons align themselves in the opposite direction, existing in a high-energy state. Given time, those in the high-energy mode will reorient themselves in the opposite direction to join those within the low-energy group, all now aligned in the same direction as the external magnetic field. This process is called magnetization.

Interestingly, this system can also be manipulated by the machine operator, who may deliver a pulse of radio-frequency (RF) energy into it. This serves to orient all of the protons in the direction of the high-energy state. As they then begin to reorient in the direction of the external magnet (low energy), they release energy in the form of electromagnetic radiation, the signal of which may be captured by an external antenna. Both the initial signal and those signals released during the reorientation process (decay envelope) are unique to disparate tissues. Furthermore, the operator may "fine tune" the signals released by controlling the RF excitation input process at various points in time. This allows precise differentiation of tissue types as finally represented by shades of gray on the digital image (3). For example, a minute focus of myelin breakdown in the brain of a patient with multiple sclerosis, while perhaps unresolved on a CT scan, may become clearly visible on the MRI when the operator maximizes tissue differences.

There are other positive attributes to the MRI as well. In the case of spinal imaging, CAT scanning is basically limited to cross-sectional (axial) images of the spinal axis, whereas the sharply defined MRI images in the sagittal plane are now considered indispensible. The MRI, most will agree, is more sensitive in demonstrating small brain contusions and plaques of demyelination, and in determining the age of intracranial hematomas. Now MRI angiography has in large measure supplanted the arteriogram in the diagnosis of aneurysms. Finally, this procedure does not subject the patient to potentially harmful x-rays, the effects of which may become cumulative over a period of time.

On the other hand CAT scanning is considered the diagnostic procedure of choice in several other conditions, including spinal fractures and other maladies involving bone. Furthermore, CAT is more readily available, especially in smaller towns, and is less expensive to maintain. Most physicians see these diagnostic modalities as being complementary and, not infrequently, a patient may have both procedures done before a definitive diagnosis can be made.

In conclusion, we have come a long way since the early days of my residency training, during which we frequently had to drill exploratory burr holes on an emergency basis to rule out surface hematomas from head injuries, or instill air into the brain ventricles to diagnose either hydrocephalus or intracranial mass lesions. Not only has there been a revolution in the manner and accuracy with which we are able to diagnose diseases within the CNS, but we can now spare the patient the misery and potential complications from injecting foreign substances into the head or spinal canal.

~~~

The reader will recall that in 1976 we had performed our first superficial temporal artery-middle cerebral artery (STA-MCA)) bypass procedure in an attempt to prevent a major stroke. Although postoperative angiography confirmed patency of the bypass graft with its supplemental blood flow to the brain, that particular patient failed to show any clinical improvement after the procedure. During the succeeding ten years, my partner and I performed a number of these operations, and while our postoperative angiograms documented a very acceptable patency rate, the clinical results in our combined patient population were variable. I can't recall any of our patients having been made worse by the operation, nor were there any deaths related to the procedure. Surgeons by nature seem to recall most vividly either their best (or worst) cases after any given operative series. My last microsurgical bypass procedure aptly fits into the “best” category and serves to illustrate several important points.

The neurologists referred to me a man in his early sixties, who they felt might be a candidate for a bypass graft. His primary neurological deficit consisted of ongoing weakness in all four extremities. His paresis
~~~

was much greater in the legs than in the arms, so much so, that although he could move his legs, he could not bear weight and walk. Furthermore, his lower extremity weakness appeared accentuated when he was in the upright position. Clearly the nature of his paraparesis was neurological in nature (in contradistinction to primary disease of the musculoskeletal system) as evidenced by his very brisk deep tendon reflexes and the presence of bilateral Babinski signs, both indicative of long-tract disease affecting the pyramidal cells originating in the cerebral cortex.

During his work-up with the appropriate neuroimaging studies, we excluded cervical spinal stenosis and/or spondylosis (arthritic spinal canal narrowing) as possible causes of cervical spinal cord compression and myelopathy. The existence of cerebral infarction (stroke) was also eliminated with CAT and MRI scanning of the cerebrum. The neurologists also assured me that they found no evidence of complicating systemic disease to account for this patient's fluctuating weakness.

We thus proceeded with the definitive procedure of cerebral arteriography to evaluate blood perfusion to both cerebral hemispheres. Our findings indicated that, while he lacked a total occlusion of any major arterial vessel, there existed a very high-grade stenosis of the internal carotid artery where it penetrated the skull base through what we call the carotid siphon. Beyond the siphon there was but a scant trickle of blood into the middle cerebral artery, and even less perfusion was visualized into the distal anterior cerebral artery supplying the motor "leg" area of the cerebral cortex. Compounding the problem was an equally severe stenotic lesion of the contralateral carotid siphon, and there was virtually no cross-filling through the anterior circle of Willis.

Because this patient had exhibited an erratic, fluctuating lower extremity weakness for several weeks, we thought it quite likely that his condition was indicative of what is known in neurological parlance as the "idling neuron." We surmised that the meager blood flow to the leg area of his brain was merely enough to keep those neurons alive but insufficient to allow normal physiologic nerve conduction activity on a volume scale. This was further corroborated with increased weakness when he would try to assume the vertical posture with its concomitant drop in blood pressure and brain perfusion.

After further discussion with our neuroradiological colleagues, we elected to operate on him in an effort to augment his cerebral blood flow. I accordingly planned staged, bilateral, STA-MCA anastomoses, the operations being separated by an interval of six weeks. In each instance the operation was subsequently carried out without any complications. Equally important was postoperative angiographic documentation of the patency of each graft between the external carotid and the internal circulations of the brain.

Postoperatively, over the course of several weeks, in contrast to his long-term preoperative debilitative status, this man showed a remarkable and sustained improvement in his leg strength. Under the guidance of the physical therapist, he first began to bear weight and later ambulated with the aid of a walker. Months later, he moved about independently of any stabilizing devices. The happy conclusion to the story entailed his walking down the aisle during the ceremony of his second marriage.

There was absolutely no doubt in either his mind or any of his physicians that the bypass operations had been a therapeutic success and had richly improved this gentleman's life.

Throughout the 1970s and early 80s there were reported, throughout the world literature, numerous neurosurgical series of cases comprised of patients such as the one I have just described. Workshops in microsurgery such as Dr. Al Rhoton's at the University of Florida were available to most neurosurgeons. Instrument-makers provided us with magnificent, miniature, well-constructed devices to engage in this fascinating world of microscopic vascular surgery. Needles with swaged-on suture material, nearly invisible to the naked eye, were so exquisitely crafted that they could be passed cleanly through delicate, translucent tissues without tearing them. In laboratories throughout the world, sophisticated scientific research methods and angiographic studies seemed to eliminate any doubt that the blood flow to the brain could be enhanced with the EC-IC bypass procedure. Pure logic alone seemed to tell us that this well-conceived, incredibly delicate surgical procedure, requiring both a degree of refined surgical skill and certainly a steady hand, should go a long way in helping to salvage the potential stroke victim. However, there were growing concerns as to just what type of patient would consistently be a candidate for this procedure, and whether the operation really did, indeed, prevent stroke. These fundamental questions still needed to be addressed.

In 1977, the International Cooperative Study on Extracranial-Intracranial (EC-IC) Arterial Anastomosis was organized to statistically evaluate this surgical method in augmenting the circulation to the brain in patients with surgically inaccessible atherosclerotic lesions of the internal carotid and middle cerebral arteries. If one carefully reviews this large clinical project, one will find that it was an extremely well designed study, involving nearly 1,500 patients from participating centers in North America, Europe and Asia. The 1,500 patients, each one of them meeting the established criteria for surgical intervention, were then randomized by chance into two separate groups: Those who had the STA-MCA bypass operation and a second equivalent group in every way except that they were treated only medically with aspirin (a substance well known to inhibit blood coagulation). It is to be emphasized that a purely random study of this nature eliminates any bias whatsoever (as opposed to alternate or matched controls), and has often been referred to as the gold standard in clinical scientific analysis. The duration of the study (1977-1982) entailed meticulous follow-up on each and every patient with frequent examinations by unbiased neurologists (31).

The conclusion of the Cooperative Study in answering the question — "Does the EC-IC bypass reduce the rate of stroke and stroke-related death in symptomatic patients with appropriate atherosclerotic cerebrovascular occlusive disease"— was no! It goes without saying that the neurosurgical community was stunned in disbelief at the conclusive results of this study. What we had been endeavoring to accomplish had made so much common sense, appeared to be backed by sophisticated laboratory data, and was supported by the world neurological literature replete with positive clinical results. There were those who were quick to criticize various aspects of this International Study, but the latter appeared flawless and inviolate in every respect to most. Even when examining various subsets of the patients, the surgical group often fared worse than its medical cohorts. Until more is known about the natural course of this illness, medical therapy appears as good as anything for treating atherosclerotic occlusive disease of the intracranial carotid circulation and its derivatives.

In conclusion: There remains a body of positive information to carry away from nearly two decades of this microvascular cerebral bypass surgery. First, the procedure can still be utilized in other surgical situations such as, for example, when a critical vessel might need to be sacrificed in removing a giant aneurysm or tumor. Secondly, the precision of the technical discipline learned in performing this operation can only serve to enhance the skills of the neurological surgeon. And finally, it is laudable that our specialty engaged in the task of self-evaluating some of our work, namely, an operation that seemed so biologically sound and logical. It is difficult to comprehend the fact that our last patient would have fared just as well on an aspirin each day, ultimately enabling him to walk down the aisle to take his bride. Nonetheless, we must show confidence and respect in the scientific method by abandoning the operation altogether. We owe it to our future patients not to impose upon them either the risks or the unnecessary costs of the procedure. As we shall see later, in view of the rapidly inflating and uncontrolled costs of medical care, it would be prudent for future generations of physicians and surgeons to apply the lessons learned from this international study to other procedures of unproven value.

~~~

Earlier in the book I mentioned that soon after my arrival in Tallahassee my partner and I were asked to assume the responsibility as neurological consultants for the mentally ill at the Florida State Hospital in Chattahoochee. We subsequently provided this service for well over twenty years. On a monthly basis, with few exceptions, one of us would attend a clinic and would examine patients referred by the hospital medical staff. While most of the cases seen entailed medical neurological entities, occasionally we would encounter a client requiring surgery, in which case we would transfer him to our hospital in Tallahassee.

The small panhandle town of Chattahoochee is thirty-five miles northwest of Tallahassee, near the Georgia state line and the headwaters of the great Apalachicola River. I always enjoyed a break from our medical routine in Tallahassee when driving through the colorful countryside along the narrow, two-lane highway en route to this little town off of the beaten path.

After parking my car upon arrival, I would ascend the steps of the old familiar clinic building, always anxiously wondering what was in store for me. Immediately upon entering the large door of the state hospital's medical facility, one's senses alert him to the fact that he is in a totally different environment, one typical of a state hospital. The air circulating in the wide, light-colored hallways with the tall ceilings is permeated by the odor of disinfectant reminiscent of the old hospitals of the 40s. The walls themselves were spotless, as if recently painted, void of any pictures or decorations, and the floors always appeared recently waxed. With instruments in hand as I strode down the hallway toward
~~~

the clinic, I heard echoing in the distance the clamor of the clients as they awaited my arrival. Upon rounding the final corner I encountered them sitting on old wooden benches and chairs, not infrequently in wheelchairs — some totally silent, always a few who were mumbling to themselves and still others shouting nonsensically. Most were well behaved, but upon occasion an unruly inmate would require firm restraint and/or removal by the hospital attendants.

As I entered the examination room with its centrally placed 1930s-vintage, heavy, flexible, steel, examining table, I was greeted by Ginger, an extremely pleasant, well-organized registered nurse whose help and efficiency in setting up and running the clinic was indispensible. Not a minute was ever wasted, nor patients ever lost to follow-up. Charts, radiographs and the results of all laboratory work were always right at hand.

On one such day in the early 1970s, the attendants escorted into the examining room a tall African-American man in his early sixties, unsteady of gait while sliding his slippered feet, and who was totally void of both speech and any emotional expression. He uttered not a sound during the entire examination, but in no way resisted it. His charted history, as recorded by the hospital physicians, indicated that he had been institutionalized at FSH in 1937, the year of my birth, for some undisclosed mental abnormality, and he had been incarcerated there ever since. Somewhere along the line he had developed the semblance of a clinical state which we term "akinetic mutism." That is to say, although ambulatory, he needed help with activities of daily living, and had not only become totally flat in his emotional affect but had also quit speaking altogether. Several days prior to my seeing him in the clinic, a member of the house staff had peered into his eyegrounds with an ophthalmoscope, and thinking that there was swelling of the optic nerve heads referred him to me. My examination, in addition to several other neurological abnormalities, did indeed corroborate the presence of florid papilledema. This finding of increased intracranial pressure demands urgent attention, as we have previously emphasized.

In a case of chronic increased intracranial pressure without a history of trauma, one must first think of an intracranial tumor. I recommended that they transport the patient to Tallahassee as soon as arrangements could be made for a neuroradiological workup in full anticipation of probable surgery. Ginger got right on it, and the patient arrived at TMH within twenty-four hours.

Of little surprise upon CAT scanning was the presence of a frontal brain tumor, but of great surprise was the immense size of the mass. It occupied the greater portion of the entire frontal fossa, and its slow centripetal upward growth had compressed the overlying frontal lobes of the brain into a mere shell. Cerebral arteriography verified the diagnosis of an olfactory groove meningioma with its characteristic blood supply emanating from the skull base and its strong capillary blush. Such an enormous, slow-growing benign tumor, displacing the brain as it did, had to have been there for many years, indeed. If this man had instead resided outside of the walls of the state hospital during the years of protracted growth of this tumor, others undoubtedly would have noted long ago progressive changes in his mental status, thereby leading to an earlier diagnosis and treatment. But confined within this isolated world of abnormal behavior, he blended imperceptibly with all of the others.

Several days after having totally and uneventfully removed this man's "grapefruit-size" intracranial mass, he was returned to the Florida State Hospital. His recovery was nothing short of amazing over the months to follow; he metamorphosed from what had been a "zombie-like" habitus into a normally acting human being. He resumed all normal activities of daily living, regained full cognition and speech, and became emotionally appropriate. In short, he was to later achieve a state of mental wellness that nobody in the state hospital had ever previously observed in him.

Eventually, we had a social worker see this affable man in hopes of releasing him in the future into the outside world. But this proved fruitless. After several months of attempted rehabilitation, it was concluded that his extended period of incarceration had ingrained in him a total dependence upon the hospital environment. He was ill-equipped to survive in the demanding society outside of those walls— in a world he had long since forgotten. In short, he was woefully deficient in the social and educational skills necessary to earn a living and live independently. The analogy, of course, is likened to raising an orphaned wild animal to adulthood, and later returning it to the hostile jungle in hopes it would survive.

I have often reflected back on this case, wondering whether the neurosurgeon who freed this man from the bonds of his tumor had, ironically, been born the very year that its early anlage first began encroaching upon the base of his brain.

~~~
~~~

Stepping briefly again outside of the halls of medicine, let me return to the outdoors, where I found solace through a much-needed change in scenery and redirected thought. In a previous chapter, I spoke of a hunting adventure with my friend, Terry, when we dragged a deer out of the woods in the middle of the night. Before bringing to conclusion my hunting endeavors, I should like to relate my challenging experiences using a primitive weapon.

As most students of American history are aware, many of the brave men who pioneered our country forged their way using muzzle-loading black powder guns. The tradition of firing such rifles has since endured as a sport enjoyed by many outdoorsmen today. In my particular case, I purchased a .54 caliber muzzle-loading rifle built by Thompson/Center Arms Corporation. To say that it is a beautiful, well made, superbly balanced firearm, simply is an understatement. As most know, the measured black powder charge is emptied down the barrel before the patch and lead ball are rammed home. The charge is ignited by an explosive cap mounted firmly onto a nipple protruding from the breech when it is struck by the hammer during the pull of the trigger. Even though the gun had no scope, I found the open sites surprisingly accurate when first sighting in the weapon at the shooting range on my farm. Always when using the gun, I would also carry, slung across my shoulder, a small pigskin leather bag called the "possible bag", a pouch which contained various tools, powder charges and lead balls for the reloading process.

One of the emergency room doctors at the hospital and I became seriously interested in black-powder hunting, and were intrigued with the possibility of successfully bringing down a deer with one of these primitive weapons of old. We even went so far as to make our own ammunition. I can recall once having procured a discarded lead box used in the nuclear medicine department at the hospital for the storage of radioisotopes. While listening to a Seminole football game one Saturday afternoon, we melted the lead in preparation of casting the .54 caliber balls with a ladle and the appropriate mold. Years later, we learned that it was probably a dangerous thing to do because of the inherent exposure to the fumes of that toxic heavy metal.

Dick and I both preferred to hunt from a tree-stand because of its superior visual advantage, while at the same time reducing the likelihood that the deer could pick up our scents. Always on the day prior to the hunt we would scout out a likely site in the woods (usually on a state-designated hunting preserve) based upon deer sign. Once such a site was found, we would designate a strategic tree at the fringe of the area from which we could hunt the following morning. After thoroughly familiarizing ourselves with the landscape, we would return in the total darkness of the early morning hours the following day.

I would pick Dick up in my truck as early as 3A.M. on the day of the hunt, and after leaving the vehicle parked at the edge of the preserve, we would trudge through the woods to find the respective spots we had staked out the previous afternoon. Things always seem to appear different in the shadows of the flashlight, but usually we were able to find our choice vantage points —safely well out of each other's range. After identifying my predetermined tree at the edge of the clearing, I would scale perhaps twenty feet up with my portable tree-stand. Once I was sitting comfortably in the stand, the rifle and little bag were then hoisted up by a rope. To keep from drifting off to sleep and tumbling out of the tree, I would firmly harness myself to the trunk with a seatbelt. Then began the long wait in the coolness of the early morning. While listening to the animal sounds and awaiting the first glimmer of sunlight, I would eagerly anticipate the appearance of a dear venturing into the clearing below.

Although considered grown, allegedly sophisticated men, we were youngsters at heart by the challenging prospect of outsmarting a deer and bringing him down with a single shot from a muzzle-loading rifle. My physician friend, Dick Camberg, and I would sit in those tree stands at intervals for entire weekends at a time during hunting season. We would try anything to lure in an unwary buck during rut. I can recall rubbing fresh apples all over my body to extinguish my scent just before leaving home. One time Dick purchased a product derived from doe urine that allegedly contained female hormones which he sprinkled around his legs for the benefit of the male deer in a sexual frenzy. To his dismay, one night while up in his tree stand in pitch darkness, Dick accidentally spilled the entire bottle of potion all over himself. Later that morning with his dry sense of humor, he said to me in his usual drawl, "Jim, I was afraid to climb down the tree in fear of being raped by a buck."

Then one day, I was invited by yet another hunting friend, Ron Moody, to join him for an afternoon hunt on a large piece of property which he leased annually. Ron, incidentally, is considered both a seasoned hunter and an expert, having felled animals both in the western United States and on the continent of Africa. In one of the rooms in his house, all of the wall space from ceiling to floor is covered with mounted trophies.

It was a bright sunny late-afternoon in the fall when Ron pulled up beside a permanent tree stand and let me off. While carrying my muzzleloader and toting the "possible bag," I climbed into the stand which was perhaps fifteen feet from the ground, and located right on the edge of a clearing with a good stand of ryegrass.

After I had waited for roughly an hour, a buck ventured into the clearing perhaps sixty feet from me and began consuming the lush foliage. One is always mindful that in the muzzle-loading game, you have only a single shot to bring down your prey. If you should miss,… the deer will scamper halfway across the county before you finish fiddling around dropping powder charges and patched lead balls down the barrel. Keeping that firmly in mind, I took a few deep breaths and calmly sighted the animal in. I felt I had this one already bagged as I gently squeezed the Thompson's trigger. A few moments later, the hammer struck the cap, but it resulted in a mere "click" rather than the loud explosion and strong recoil usually anticipated. The animal promptly raised his head, ears rotating like antennae, and nostrils flared to sense out a predator. I froze in the shooting position, held my breath and didn't move even an eyelid for several seconds. Satisfied he was not in harm's way, the deer again began to graze, whereupon I lowered the gun in total disappointment and utter disgust. I couldn't believe that my trusty weapon had misfired after all of these months of preparation. What could have possibly happened! After regaining my composure with heart still pounding, I could only assume that the nipple port and breech were fouled with gun oil. To rectify it meant to disassemble the rifle. With a deer only sixty feet away, I deemed it impossible to clean my gun. Nonetheless, I decided to attempt it in micro-steps while not taking my eyes off the deer for even an instant. First, by using the sense of touch only, I removed the forend wedge, which allowed me to separate the barrel and breech from the stock. The deer looked up; I again froze. He then resumed grazing, freeing me up to resume my critical work with the gun. From the possible bag I grasped my nipple wrench, and was able to unscrew the nipple and clean-out plug from the breech. A small copper wire was then passed through the nipple, and a dry patch used to clean out the port of but a scant amount of oil. I then set forth to reassemble the firearm in long intervals, interrupted when the deer would momentarily look up from his meal, always reassuring himself that he was safe. This entire process proved both methodical and time-consuming. The initial powder charge and lead ball in the barrel itself, of course, needed not to be disturbed. Once everything was reassembled, I again carefully raised the gun and took aim. In doing so I thought it extremely unlikely, despite what I had already accomplished, that I could position the gun without the insatiable buck sensing my movement. But this time after the hammer fell, the gun bellowed, and with the clearing of the large plume of smoke— the deer lay motionless upon the earth.

Ron drove up a few minutes later, listening intently as I told him the unbelievable story. Deer, by their very nature, possess extremely acute senses alerting them to danger, and are normally very skittish animals. They are ordinarily very quick to pick up motion, sound and dangerous scent in self-defense. My friend proceeded to examine the deer which had sustained a kill shot through the heart, then saying, "Jim, this is a textbook shot." Coming from this expert hunter, I took that as a real compliment.

Twenty years after the fact when we were together one evening, Ron recalled that unique fascinating experience. In retrospect, it is one that I probably should have published in a sporting magazine such as *Field & Stream.* This incident certainly supports the adage that one should never give up, even when the odds are heavily stacked against you. In this particular case, perhaps the deer was just plain "dumb" or, possibly, I was simply lucky. It was probably a little of both.

~~~

The year 1986 ended on a bad note for me personally. My wife of 26 years took my children and left me to move far away. Although it left a terrible void in my heart, served to forever disperse our family, and had far-reaching consequences; many years later in life, my children and I were destined to again become closer than ever before.

~~~

Because the emergency department in the hospital is such an important part of a surgeon's practice, a few additional points bear mentioning. Whenever a physician is called upon to provide coverage for an emergency room, irrespective as to whether he is a general practitioner, a well-trained emergency-room physician or a specialist, he may be called upon to treat any conceivable condition at any given moment. Although not often talked about, this can cause a great deal of stress. We had a very popular, conscientious, ER doctor in our hospital, who took great pride in his physical state of health. He was a good athlete, didn't smoke, and was of lean body stature. The medical staff was shocked the day they heard of Michael's untimely death from a massive heart-attack shortly after he had turned fifty. Having known him very well, I will always be convinced that the stress of his job was a major factor in our losing him at such a young age.

The subtle, yet ever-present stress agent under these circumstances concerning emergency medical practice is the "fear of the unknown." Questions a young physician might frequently ask himself are: What is the next crisis that looms around the corner? Will I be up to the task? After several successive days (and nights) of hard work, will I even have the endurance to measure up? After so many years covering a busy emergency room, my answer to those questions has always been to remain both physically and mentally well-rested, and above all— to be academically prepared for any eventuality. This means remaining current on the medical literature, attending national meetings, looking up unfamiliar material in the textbooks, and even asking colleagues in advance how they would handle a given situation. The incident below illustrates many of these points.

At about midnight after a long day's work, I was called urgently to the emergency room to see an automobile accident victim who reportedly was in very bad shape. Upon entering room number thirteen (where they always placed the bad ones), I found a late middle-aged man who was deeply obtunded and harbored a right hemiparesis. The history at hand was that he had been involved in a single-car accident. He allegedly had been the sole occupant of the car, and seriously lacking were any other details or witnesses. Other than the stated neurological findings, he also had an unmistakable contusion of his scalp.

We rushed him on over to the x-ray department, and transferred him into the CT scanner. Of no surprise to anyone was the presence of a large acute, left frontotemporal subdural hemorrhage. Little time was lost shaving his head before wheeling him to the operating suite.

What initially appeared to be a routine trauma case was about to become a surgical nightmare. To begin with, it was by now nearly 2 A.M., and conditions were suboptimal. My only surgical assistant was one of the hospital's night-shift surgical technicians who, as I have noted earlier, was lacking in her fund of knowledge of both the neurosurgical instruments and the procedure. Expeditiously I reflected the bone flap, and, upon incising the underlying tense dura mater expecting to find strictly a surface lesion, I was confronted not only with a large hematoma but also a torrential flow of bright-red blood. The anesthesiologist immediately hung up cross-matched blood and began literally pumping it in to keep up with the harrowing loss. Try as I might, I could not initially find the source of the bleeding within the dark shadowy depths of the intracranial cavity. Both the overhead surgical light was insufficient, and the suction apparatus ineffective in evacuating the swirling pool of arterial blood. I rapidly donned the fiber-optic headlamp, and asked the circulating RN— a well-seasoned, "cracker-jack" nurse, who functioned superbly under stress— to quickly get me another large-bore suction apparatus. All of that having been done, I was then able to carefully work down the Sylvian fissure of the brain toward the source of the hemorrhage. The totally unexpected cause of the bleeding proved to be a ruptured aneurysm of the middle cerebral artery! While the element of time precluded my setting up the microscope, I did the best I could with my light source and without the aid of an angiogram in securing the aneurysm neck with an appropriate clip. Upon closing the wound, I felt very lucky to have gotten this critically ill patient off of the operating room table alive. In retrospection I believe that this man probably lost consciousness from the aneurysm rupture and then sustained a secondary head injury when wrecking his car.

Postoperatively, the patient had a crippling neurological deficit from the combination of the bleeding aneurysm, compressing subdural clot and vascular spasm. He was both aphasic and had a dense right hemiparesis. Follow-up postoperative angiography indicated less than ideal placement of the aneurysm clip. To make matters even worse, the patient was found to have two additional incidental aneurysms. A second craniotomy was performed a week later using the microscope, thereby enabling us to optimally clip all three lesions. Although this man did ultimately show some recovery of his speech and his hemiparesis, he was still left with a lasting severe neurological deficit, rendering him unable to work.

Worthy of emphasis: This patient with multiple intracranial aneurysms (20% of the aneurysm population at large) presented as an emergency head-injury case with what appeared to be a straightforward subdural hematoma. Keeping in mind the annual bleed rate of 2-3% with incidental aneurysms, all of the lesions in this patient were ultimately and effectively treated, despite the near fatal initial presentation. Again, as stated at the onset of this section, one must be prepared in advance for the unexpected, and must utilize his training in a composed manner while attacking the problem as it unfolds. Interestingly, soon after I had treated this patient, a small series of ruptured aneurysms presenting as acute subdural hematomas was published in the neurosurgical literature.

~~~

Throughout the years, pediatric head injuries comprised a very significant segment of our practice. The following case is presented to drive home a very important point to anyone involved with pediatric trauma.

One afternoon I was called to the emergency room to see a four-year old boy who presented in a stuporous neurological state, allegedly after a fall. His understandably concerned parents were standing nearby during the course of my examination. Overlying contusions of the child's scalp were noted, but his general physical examination was otherwise normal. Because this was obviously more than a trivial head injury in view of the child's altered level of consciousness, a CAT scan was immediately requested. An acute subdural hemorrhage was disclosed. We proceeded with a craniotomy, and evacuated the clot from the underlying swollen and contused brain. We have previously cited the high mortality rate associated with this condition, but happily, in this instance, the small boy stabilized. Under the close, watchful eyes of our dedicated, pediatric intensive-care nurses, he survived what appeared to be a very serious injury. After several days in the hospital he was dismissed home.

Upon subsequent office visits, he followed a progressive road to a complete recovery with absolutely no neurological residue. With each succeeding clinic visit as the brain proceeded to heal, little "Sammy" began to display an absolutely delightful childhood personality. He would race across the room and literally "spring" into my arms, giggling with joy to see his doctor. I don't recall much about his mother, because his stepfather usually brought him in for his follow-up visits. He too was always glad to see me, and appeared to genuinely love this little kid with such an unparalleled magnetic personality. When entering the door he would energize Sammy by telling him, "There is your doctor." With each succeeding return visit all of the office personnel, upon seeing the day's schedule, would anticipate with glee seeing little Sammy and his
~~~

smiling "dad." Finally, after perhaps three months, we dismissed him from our care and were somewhat sad that the two of them would no longer be coming back to "lighten up" the rather mundane, daily office routine.

Then one day about a year later, we were to find out that one of the general surgeons had encountered an emergency in which he had to operate upon a little boy, who went into shock from a ruptured spleen. The child tragically didn't survive the incident. His name was "Sammy." Yes— this regrettably proved to be the same, cute little boy we had come to cherish in our office. As things began to later unfold, the "concerned" stepfather was arrested for child abuse, and was later convicted of manslaughter. We had not picked up on that abusive home environment at the time of the child's initial head injury one year previously. There were no other bits of physical or familial evidence to suggest it. A young newspaper columnist was quick to research this tragedy, and proceeded to write some scathing things about me in the local newspaper for not having originally picked up on the abusive nature of this family. Perhaps she was justified in doing so.

Because child abuse has in recent years become recognized as being rather prevalent, injured children are frequently scrutinized for other physical evidence of previous bodily injury and are screened with radiographs of the chest and long bones to exclude old fractures of the ribs and extremities, respectively. Also, social workers are frequently called upon to investigate the family environment. Had we done these things, perhaps we could have spared further suffering and the early childhood death of this cute little boy with the "elfin" personality.

~~~

I consider it very important at this juncture to devote a few words to my family of origin. Sadly, my mother passed away in 1985 and my father followed shortly thereafter in 1987. I think that the tragic aspect of their lives is that neither had ever achieved any lasting true happiness, and for that I will forever be sorry. My parents ultimately had three sons, my being the oldest. The second son, Richard, was a bright individual who, like my youngest brother, Gary, always had a bent toward electronics. Both of them later became amateur ham radio operators. After his time in the Air Force, Rich was snatched up by IBM, trained in
~~~

their school in New York, and subsequently became a successful technical engineer with that company.

My brother Gary, who is fifteen years younger than I, initially received a BA degree in music with honors from the University of Colorado. Not satisfied that music would fulfill his permanent vocational interests, he shortly returned to the university, and again graduated with honors, this time with a degree in mathematics. Blessed with a very bright, innovative mind, he was well-suited to work with a prominent aerospace company. His initial job, among many other things, entailed working on the navigational guidance system for the space shuttle. Several years later, Gary went to work for Digital Globe Corporation, a leader in satellite imaging of our planet, eventually becoming its chief electrical engineer. As most people are aware, this company provides quality, high-resolution imagery of the earth for the Federal Government and for Google Earth, among other customers. Gary, while already an established scientific leader in the space industry, continues in his academic pursuits. He has been asked to teach several courses at the University of Colorado, has received a master's degree in electrical engineering from that University, and is currently working on a doctorate, all while fully employed with the preeminent satellite imaging company. I've always been extremely proud of both of my brothers for their accomplishments.

~~~

We have previously discussed cases demonstrating the value of the correlative neuroanatomy of the spinal cord, but have made little mention of the brain in that regard. When evaluating a patient for the first time, most neurologists find it academically challenging to establish a likely presumptive diagnosis following a careful history and a detailed neurological examination. The various scanning modalities and other laboratory tests are then used to confirm (or negate) the clinical impression, often adding important anatomical details as well. Allow me to review two very rare syndromes, each emphasizing the value of the initial neurological examination. The reader will also appreciate how precise functions can be localized to specific regions of the brain at the time of the bedside examination.

The first patient was a late middle-age man who was sent to me by a concerned local family physician. He had been having headaches for
~~~

several weeks, and, according to close family members, seemed to have been experiencing other rather protean mental deficiencies as well. Upon examining some of his higher cortical functions in the office-setting using simple "bedside" testing methods, I first discovered that he appeared to have trouble writing, an abnormality known as dysgraphia. In addition, despite being an educated man, he could not perform very rudimentary calculations (dyscalculia). By this time it was clearly evident that I was onto something quite unusual. In continuing, I was to soon find out that he was perplexed in differentiating right from left. For instance when I would ask him to identify the correct side of one of my bilateral symmetrical body parts, he would invariably point to the incorrect side (left-right disorientation). Finally, I asked him to identify his index finger, which he didn't recognize as being his own (finger agnosia). Specifically, when I asked the patient who the finger belonged to, he appeared puzzled and couldn't answer me, much like the boy described earlier in the book who denied the existence of his left arm. These four components make up a well-known neurological syndrome familiar to most neurologists— the Gerstmann's syndrome. It is the result of a lesion of the angular gyrus, a cortical area bordering the parietal and occipital lobes of the dominant hemisphere. In this man's case, because of the insidious onset and slow progression of symptoms, a brain tumor was a likely tentative diagnosis, its epicenter being in that dominant left angular gyrus.

A CT scan with enhancing contrast material confirmed the presence of a malignant glioma in the suspected region of the brain. A craniotomy was subsequently performed, and because of the eloquent area of the cerebrum involved we were limited to only a brain biopsy. The pathologist corroborated the preoperative diagnosis of an anaplastic (malignant) glioma. Despite a full course of whole brain irradiation therapy and follow up chemotherapy, the prognosis remained very poor.

The second case involved a man in our town in his late fifties, who had been a healthy, very successful small business owner until the recent onset of symptoms. Because he was having increasing difficulty with his eyesight, uncorrectable by glasses, he was sent for a neurological evaluation. This patient also had an extremely interesting constellation of symptoms which, even to this day, is considered both unusual and reportable.

On examination he was perfectly alert, very intelligent, fluent in his speech and had no paralysis of his extremities. He did, however, have what we call a right homonymous hemianopsia; namely, his right visual field in each eye was severely impaired. This implied a destructive lesion of the visual cortex within the left occipital lobe of his brain. When testing his higher levels of cortical functioning, I also determined that the patient could no longer read (alexia), this occurring despite his being able to clearly identify objects presented to him through his intact left field of vision. The following interesting fact remained: He was still both able to write and clearly speak the language. Moreover, when asked to write down a specific word, he could promptly do it — but couldn't read what he had just written.

In analyzing his case of alexia without agraphia (not able to read but retaining the ability to write), we suspected that his lesion was in the left occipital lobe; moreover it had probably extended forward into and destroyed the posterior portion (splenium) of the corpus callosum (the great commissure connecting the two cerebral hemispheres). In essence, that information which he gleaned from visualizing the written word with the right side of the brain (through the intact left visual field) could not be transmitted to the language area on the dominant left side; more explicitly, the left side of his brain could not vocally express what the right visual cortex was seeing. This represents what is known as a disconnection syndrome. A CAT scan was done, confirming our clinical impression.

A left occipital craniotomy was performed, and, after a confirmatory biopsy, a total left occipital lobectomy was carried out. As expected, we had to stop short of entering the corpus callosum where residual tumor had to be left behind, thus precluding any hope of a surgical cure. The histopathology of this neoplasm was that of a malignant lymphoma. Because the tumor was both radio-sensitive and slow growing, this well-liked man was able to anticipate enjoying his retirement and family for several years thereafter.

As I have reiterated many times throughout the years to others and to the readers of this book, the neurological clinician, while utilizing his knowledge of neuroanatomy and neurology, has a distinct advantage over many of his medical colleagues; he is often able to make a surprisingly accurate tentative bedside diagnosis— certainly in terms of location, if not also in etiology.

A few years ago I was asked by Dr. Charles Ouimet, professor of neuroanatomy at Florida State University College of Medicine, to give a lecture to a special-interest group in neurology of sophomore medical students. In closing, I told the students that Dr. Ouimet had given them a "gift" by having taught them the subject of neuroanatomy. For someone going into one of the neurological fields, this is the most important item in his bag of tools.

~~~

At the time that I was beginning to write this chapter, the television and newspaper media again reminded us that celebrities are by no means immune to the tragedies that may confront the average citizen. A prominent, attractive young movie actress was injured in a collision during a skiing accident in Canada. Although the details of the injury were never released, allegedly she was initially shaken up, yet remained alert and talking immediately afterward. While advised at the onset to see a doctor, she preferred not and was able to walk back to her hotel room. An hour later, after developing an intense headache, she agreed to go to the hospital, which unfortunately was many miles away. Her condition thereafter rapidly deteriorated, and, tragically, she expired before emergency surgical intervention could be obtained. Her final diagnosis of an extra-dural hematoma is by now familiar to the readership. Time and again, I have emphasized the extreme urgency in treating this condition. Any delays in treatment, whether they are either due to patient noncompliance or problems accessing medical care, reduce the patient's chances of survival. Keeping in mind both of these factors, I am reminded of a case of my own.

Late one spring afternoon, I received a call from a concerned referring physician in a town forty-five miles from Tallahassee. Sitting in his office at the time was a twelve-year-old, Little League baseball player, who had been struck in the side of his head by a sharply driven baseball. While the boy had not lost consciousness, he did complain of an unremitting headache. The physician had obtained a plain skull radiograph in his office, which disclosed a linear fracture of the thin temporal bone, an anatomical point we have previously addressed as particularly significant. Because we were the nearest neurosurgical facility available to treat the child, I urged them to promptly transport him to Tallahassee.

Even though this alert, normal-appearing boy had no neurological findings when seen by the doctor, we were to presume that he was developing an epidural hematoma until proven otherwise. I therefore had my nurse begin preparing the operating room for emergency surgery and alerted the radiology department to have available a vacant CAT
~~~

scanner at the time of his arrival. Everyone was sitting on "go" when the little kid arrived in the emergency room an hour later. I don't recall much about the neurologically intact child other than his complaints by now of a very severe headache, but I could sense a problem with his understandably concerned, yet extremely aggressive mother. I immediately encountered a totally unexpected resistance from her, despite my explaining the strong probability of a blood clot causing pressure on her son's brain. Because of his intensifying headache and the skull fracture, I emphasized the urgency of getting him over to the x-ray department for a CAT scan. Instead of being cooperative, she was contentious and determined to engage in an adversarial dialogue concerning lengthy, irrelevant details for which we had no time. Despite this encounter, the nursing staff promptly transported the boy over to the CAT unit, while I was trying to reason with the mother.

As the scan films were ejected out of the processor, what had been my deep concern suddenly became a fearful reality, for they did, indeed, demonstrate a potentially life-threatening extradural clot. It goes without saying that we didn't wait for the rest of the unprocessed films, as I helped to lift him onto the gurney in preparation for directly transporting him to the now-ready operating room. In the meantime, the emergency room nurse had prepared an operative consent form for a craniotomy for the mother to sign. As I pushed the cart down the hallway with the mother briskly walking at my side, I explained to her what we must urgently do— but the mother obstinately refused to sign the operative permit! Ordinarily in this litigious society in which we live, physicians may have no recourse but to obtain a court order for necessary life-saving treatment under similar circumstances. But in this case there simply wasn't enough time to even discuss bringing a judge into this. I sternly told the parent that her child needed immediate surgery or he could soon very well die. I was then further adamant in telling her that I would not allow that to happen, whether she signed the permit or not. From past experiences, I knew very well that my decision and actions would be upheld by a court of law. Apparently she then became perceptive enough of both my concern and intent that she finally did reluctantly sign the form.

This story had a happy ending for everyone concerned, as we were able to evacuate the clot in time to avert a catastrophe. This is in stark contrast to the tragic case of delayed treatment concerning the movie actress. Six weeks later the little ball player was again on the field.

The message in this case history is an obvious one: Because we are dealing with a condition carrying a mortality rate of 35 to 40%, there can be absolutely no delays in treatment. The surgeon's judgment and experience must prevail under such dire circumstances.

~~~

The majority of craniocerebral injuries treated by the neurological surgeon are either secondary to blunt trauma or to penetrating wounds of the head. But I shall never forget an unusual case involving a deep thermal injury.

One cold winter night, a local middle-aged lady consumed an exceedingly large (nearly lethal) quantity of alcohol during a drinking binge. Because it was such a cold evening, she was sitting alone beside her open fireplace. Overtaken by sedation from the alcohol, she lost consciousness, toppling forward— face-down— on the fiery, hot surface of burning coals. Historically, in the early days of surgery the spirits of alcohol were actually used as an anesthetic agent, although the "dose" required for a reasonable anesthetic was nearly killing. This woman, having remained in that undisturbed position for a lengthy period of time, her face burning in the coals, attests to the effectiveness of alcohol as such an agent. Suffice it to say that her entire face was consumed by deep, even greater than third-degree burns, since the underlying bone structures were themselves directly involved as well. She was destroyed beyond recognition, but incredibly survived. After having been discovered by a family member, and subsequently brought to TMH by ambulance, she came under the care of one of our excellent plastic surgeons, Dr. Charles Moore. The irony of this case is the fact that, despite the horror of it all, the actual burned area was disproportionately small compared to the total body surface, and therefore was a potentially survivable wound— although without a face!

As a testimonial to Dr. Moore's skill and assiduous care, she did indeed recover from this horrific injury. Over the course of many weeks, the patient underwent numerous surgical procedures, first for débridement and later reconstruction of her entire face. Initially in this long process, Dr. Moore asked me to assist him with the débridement of the bones of the orbits and skull, since he suspected that these, like the other bones of her face, were no longer viable.
~~~

On the day of our combined surgical effort, we were overwhelmed by the sickening, "sweet," stench of gas ordinarily associated with anaerobic bacterial infection. Over the better part of an hour we worked in piecemeal fashion, cutting away successive layers of bone from the upper half of the face, these being charred, soft, and impregnated with the odor-producing bacteria of gas gangrene. The globes of the eyes were necessarily sacrificed, being no more than shriveled, grape-like structures in the dark depths of the eye sockets. The damage on the left side extended up to include the devitalized left frontal bone of the skull. Realizing this dead bone needed total removal, I proceeded to cut a frontal bone flap with the air craniotome. Upon elevating the bone plate, we unexpectedly encountered an extra dural collection of putrid, thick purulent abscess material, later identified by bacterial cultures as being produced by the organism causing gas gangrene— Clostridium perfringens. While initially reluctant to open the dura mater, there was substantial evidence that it too had been violated by both the burn and the infection. We were forced to proceed yet further. Inspection of the underlying brain did, indeed, reveal charred, cavitated areas of cerebral cortex with interspersed abscessed pockets, which we unroofed and flushed with antibiotic solution.

It was a morning in the operating room over which Dr. Moore and I have often reminisced throughout the years. The sight was ghastly, and the odor obnoxious, the latter translating into an ineradicable sick-sweet taste lasting for days. The process of removing someone's face led to a hideous, terribly dehumanizing image, one that would rival the most frightening of Hollywood productions.

Although I never did seem to find the time to research the literature on the subject, I don't ever recall having read about a Clostridium perfringens epidural abscess, and can only imagine that they must be very rare. Dr. Moore and I talked about both publishing this case and presenting it at a meeting of the American College of Surgeons, but unfortunately, never seemed to find the time to do so.

From the onset, the attentive plastic surgeon nurtured the patient through this devastating injury. She was maintained on a ventilator for weeks and fed through a tube for months, while all the time being treated for recurrent infections until final wound healing beneath the flaps of her reconstructive operations had matured. After what seemed like endless months of medical-surgical treatment, help with ambulation (both eyes as stated being totally absent) and strong psychological support from both the medical staff and her daughter, she reached a point when discharge from the hospital was feasible. She had a good beginning to the semblance of a face with a new nose and mouth, and in a little more time could look forward to a reconstruction of eyelids and "glass-eye" prostheses. Amazingly, she appeared quite content to sit quietly on her front porch, her dog in her lap. And then the irony of ironies occurred: About four weeks after her discharge, she was found dead on her porch— from a pulmonary embolism.

~~~

I began this chapter by discussing the MRI machine, truly a magnificent device in improving our diagnostic capabilities of neurological disease. I should like to end with brief mention of the improvements in lumbar disc surgery.

In a previous discussion, I spoke of the ruptured disc as being a herniated fragment of cartilage impinging upon a nerve within the bony spinal canal and causing pain. When first learning to operate upon these lesions during my residency training, I was taught that after exposing the disk rupture deep within the surgical wound, the first order of business was to "pack off" the epidural veins spanning the disk capsule. This was an essential maneuver in an effort to prevent intra-operative hemorrhage, which can seriously obscure vision while removing the offending disc fragment. Alternatively, any attempt at electro-coagulating these epidural veins was fraught with the possibility of injury to the adjacent nerve root itself, because of the uncontrolled spread of current and heat from the monopolar coagulating forceps. Usually the bleeding was controlled with direct pressure from judiciously placed cottonoid and hemostatic gelatin sponge material. Meanwhile, the surgeon was not infrequently working in a very deep wound with limited depth visibility, and an overhead surgical light that invariably never seemed focused in the right place. While our results were generally satisfactory for that era, I am firmly convinced that many of those cases of "failed back pain" could have been prevented by addressing these issues. More specifically, any postoperative bleeding from torn epidural veins serves as a source for later scar tissue formation and nerve root entrapment leading to subsequent pain. At a national meeting in the early 70s, I can recall having been on a committee, during which a group of experienced neurosurgeons gravitated to the subject of failed back cases. I learned that in many instances these patients represent a universal dilemma for
~~~

everyone treating them. Patients would pass from one major institution to another, seeking relief of their back and leg pain, and in so doing underwent sometimes multiple surgical procedures. Over the years I operated upon many "re-do" cases which were initially treated elsewhere, and I had no delusions in thinking that some of my back patients with poor results never ended up in another facility.

There were three major innovations which have immensely helped to improve disk surgery in general. First, there was the advent of magnification and with it the second factor— improved lighting. The microscope was one such method used. While my partner used the microscope regularly and had excellent results, I preferred to use the combination of modern, customized, magnification loupes (glasses) in conjunction with a high intensity fiber optic headlight producing a strong focal beam illuminating the wound. While I employed the microscope myself for all intracranial work and spinal tumors, I felt more comfortable in navigating the operative field of a deep disc wound with the devices mentioned. This was true of cervical disc work as well. The third factor improving surgery on intervertebral discs was the development of the bipolar coagulating forceps. In contradistinction to the spreading current/heat of the monopolar unit described above, coagulation with the bipolar is induced by the precise control of current flowing only between the tips of the forceps. These forceps in turn are both bayoneted and available in different lengths, such that the visual line of sight is not obscured during their use.

In marked contrast to the disk surgery of years past, the surgeon can now make a smaller incision; retract the muscles with improved, stronger and smaller self-retaining retractors; and can readily visualize those often imposing, engorged epidural veins from the onset. With magnified, well-illuminated visibility, the veins could individually be dissected and coagulated with the bipolar forceps, and thereafter cleanly divided with microsurgical instruments. The disc itself is then easily removed in a bloodless field, and the epidural space secured from later hemorrhage, particularly worrisome with the patient straining upon awakening from the anesthesia. Simply stated— this was all that was necessary in treating the simple lumbar disk rupture, uncomplicated by arthritis, instability or fracture. There was no need for extensive bone fusions, plates, screws or artificial discs, which could only serve to increase the expense and morbidity (especially infection) of the procedure. Such was the general feeling of most neurological surgeons in the late 1980's and into the nineties.

As a concluding statement: Lumbar disc surgery, like most of our procedures, had become safer, more expedient and more effective than it had been 20 years previously.

~~~
~~~

NINE

Arrival at the Summit

~~~

1988 was the year in which we brought stereotactic neurosurgery to Tallahassee Memorial Hospital. This facet of neurosurgery, which certainly captivated my interest throughout my years of training, should prove both educational and of interest to most readers. A brief history and overview of this unique subject is thus included.

In the latter part of the nineteenth century, British surgeons undertook the bold venture of opening up the human cranium to treat abscesses and tumors. Because radiographic imaging was yet to be developed, their operations were predicated upon localization of the pathology by means of the history and the neurological examination.

Mindful of the complexity of the brain's anatomy, they were well aware of their limitations as to where and how far they could probe into this mysterious organ. Man could only imagine the possibility of pinpointing and treating a small, if not minuscule, target deep within the midst of surrounding delicate normal, brain matter.

One such surgeon, Sir Victor Horsley, and his associate, R. H. Clarke, developed an apparatus in 1908 which enabled them to accomplish this feat in experimental animals. In aiming for deep brain structures in cats and monkeys, they navigated their way using the Cartesian tri-coordinate system (17).

Today's high school solid geometry students soon learn to locate a point anywhere within a cube by defining its position common to the X, Y and Z axes. So it was with Clarke's frame which was rigidly affixed to the animal's skull, and a probe passed to the pre-determined point. Although quite successful in animals, only cranial bone landmarks were used for reference, thus precluding its safe use in humans. However, this experimental animal work provided the foundation for stereotactic surgery as we know it today.
~~~

In 1947 Spiegel and Wycis employed this method in bringing stereotactic surgery to human beings. Their device, based on Clarke's principles, referenced the proposed deep brain target to normal structures within the fluid filled ventricular system as outlined by injected contrast materials (37). When first learning the principles of stereotaxis at Northwestern University as a neurosurgical resident, I assisted in the use of Spiegel's apparatus in the treatment of the tremor of Parkinson's disease and in a restricted group of patients with psychiatric disorders poorly amenable to psychotropic drugs.

In the early 1970s the use of stereotactic methods for treating psychiatric disturbances, such as obscessive-compulsive neuroses, fell into disrepute. However, there has always remained an interest in treating involuntary movement disorders, such as the often incapacitating tremor of Parkinson's disease and other flailing or dystonic maladies, by either stimulating or destroying deep brain structures using radiofrequency methods. Other applications for stereotactic brain surgery include: obtaining biopsy material, depth-electrode recording, draining abscesses, implanting radioisotopes, or even transplanting neural tissues into brain regions unapproachable by other means.

As early as 1984 I began exploring the possibility of bringing this technology to our hospital. One of my friends and colleagues, Dr. André Olivier, a neurological surgeon at the Montréal Neurological Institute, invited me to Canada to spend a few days visiting and learning the stereotactic system utilized at his institution. At that time Dr. Olivier was a leading world investigator in using stereotactic implantation of recording depth electrodes into the brains of patients with intractable epilepsy in order to identify foci which could then be surgically excised. The stereotactic apparatus he used was a modification of the arc-radius frame devised by Leksell (25). In this instance the frame, having first been rigidly affixed to the skull, and after defining the target point with the three (X,Y,Z) coordinates, is then fitted with a revolving arc. The established target point may then be re-defined as the center of a circle (or sphere) constructed from that arc. Again in referring to our geometry, a line drawn perpendicular to a tangent to the arc of a circle at its point of tangency — if continued to the center— will follow the path of the radius. The point of tangency of course may be anywhere along the 180° course of the arc. In addition the mechanical arc may be rotated on gimbals, thereby establishing a new plane of entry. With this degree of latitude in establishing our trajectory, we not only maintain our defined fixation point, but can also avoid transgressing eloquent brain tissue when approaching any given target, the latter always residing at a known position and depth upon following the line of the radius. Then by inserting a probe in following the path of that radius, we may guide its tip to the target.

In more recent years these stereotactic frames were made both CAT and MRI- compatible. Moreover, computer software had become available such that our intracranial targets could be defined and referenced without the unpleasant, time-consuming task of instilling either air or iodinized contrast material into the ventricular system as in years past. This is much better for the patient and shortens the time of the operation.

After approval by both the hospital and the Federal Drug Administration, our precision arc-radius frame was constructed and sent to us by Tipal Instruments LTD in Montréal, Québec. However, this was only the beginning of a long process before we could safely employ this operative technique on our patients.

We first mounted our frame on an actual dry-skull with implanted targets and accessible burr holes. The skull was first scanned with its attached frame and fiducial markers. This having been done, the disc of the CAT images was downloaded into a computer, and the coordinates visually identified. Jeff Long, our radiation physicist, was indispensable during this phase of development, and was always present for future work. Once the coordinates were defined, the arc was applied, the coordinates mechanically set on the device, and the depth probe guided through the burr hole toward the target. After a successful series of "dry runs" with the skull, we then turned our attention to yet another experimental model. We injected a tiny bolus of radio-opaque material, as a proposed target (which could be visualized on a CT scan), into a life-size Styrofoam manikin head mounted in the stereotactic frame. In this instance, after defining the target coordinates on the CAT scan, we injected a minuscule amount of colored dye through the stereotactic needle probe.

Accuracy was then checked by sectioning the manikin. The probe was consistently placed within 1-2 mm. of its target, confirming our entire system as being both accurate and safe. Finally, after thoroughly and repeatedly educating the respective staffs both in the operating room and also in the radiology department, we were prepared to schedule our first patient.

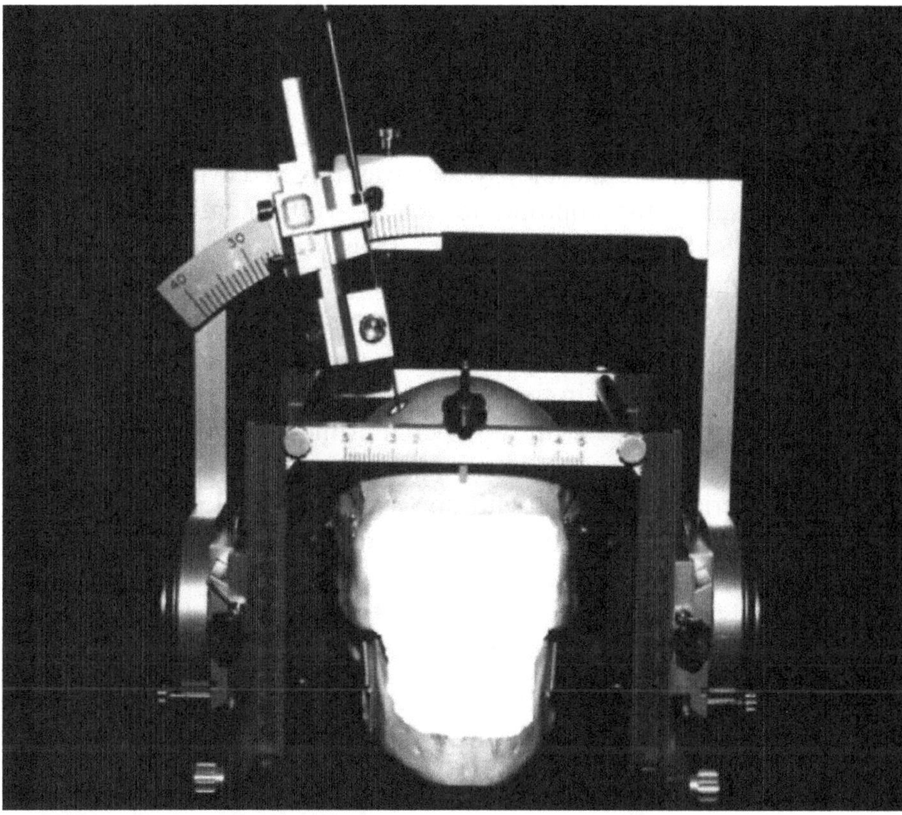

The first stereotactic frame used at Tallahassee Memorial Hospital

Note the probe passing through the burr hole in the skull directed to its pre-determined target.

The patient who was in need of a brain biopsy was referred to us by Dr. Charles Maitland, one of the neurologists in our clinic group. She was initially taken to the operating room where, under sterile conditions and under local anesthesia, the frame was rigidly mounted to the skull. The lady was then transported to the radiology department, where the frame was secured within the gantry and the CAT scan done. She was then returned to the operating room after all calculations were computed and the coordinates determined. The scalp was prepared, the patient surgically draped and the burr hole made under local anesthesia. After setting the coordinates on the frame, and re-checking all geometric points and calculations, the biopsy site was targeted with a large bore needle probe set to the appropriate depth. Instruments, milled to fit concentrically within the probe, were then passed to obtain biopsy material. After diagnostic confirmation of the retrieved tissue by the pathologist, the small burr hole incision was closed, the frame removed and the patient returned to the NSCU overnight for observation. She was then discharged home in forty eight hours.

Our initial experience with the operation included drainage of deep brain cysts, biopsy of inaccessible brain tumors and acquisition of diagnostic material in patients with non-surgical neurological disorders, such as multiple sclerosis and AIDS. Future applications of stereotactic techniques for which we were preparing included surgery for Parkinson's disease and other involuntary movement disorders, and depth electrode recordings as a prelude to corrective surgery in certain cases of epilepsy refractory to conventional medications.

~~~

While visiting at the Montréal Neurological Institute regarding the stereotactic program, I also had the opportunity of touring the PET (positron emission tomography) scanner facility, and visiting with the physicist in charge. Because the PET scan was also an important scientific innovation during my generation of medical practice, I consider it timely to discuss this interesting diagnostic modality.

Before any further discussion, it is important to emphasize that the PET scan is a physiological diagnostic tool rather than an anatomical one. In contradistinction to the CAT scan, where we have shown that the tomographic pictures ultimately reflect the coefficients of absorption of externally directed radiation through disparate tissues, the radiation
~~~

quantitatively measured in PET scanning emanates from tissues containing parenterally administered radiopharmaceuticals. The isotopes in these radionuclides have a short half-life, and must be produced on site before being synthesized into the appropriate pharmaceuticals, such as glucose. The physicist with whom I spoke first showed me the cyclotron where the isotopes were made, and later discussed the scanning process itself.

When viewing the brain from purely a metabolic standpoint, only oxygen and glucose are the substrates utilized for energy production; accordingly, radiopharmaceuticals containing these substances are conveniently utilized. Once parenterally administered to the patient, the products of radioactive decay released during metabolism are captured by the scanner's paired opposed detectors, and are fed into a computer, which, like the CAT, then formats the tomographic images.

Simply stated, the basal metabolic rate (measuring utilization of oxygen and the radioactively tagged glucose) of a particular neuronal cell population is first ascertained, and subsequently compared to that same group of cells when they are aroused. The scan will "light up" in physiologically activated areas. For example, while the inactive visual cortex of the brain in a blindfolded individual residing within a dark room is relatively silent, it will then become pictorially highlighted on the scan during arousal if light were to stimulate the patient's open eyes, thus reflecting increased metabolic activity (47).

In the pathological state, a CAT scan is often concurrently performed and is used as an anatomic onlay to supplement the physiologic image of the PET scan, thus affording more precise localization. Individually, the CAT, MRI, and PET scans each provide constructs of different information even though each is represented by a tomographic picture in the final analysis. In the strictest physical sense, they are usually not substituted for one another but rather are complementary in the diagnostic information that each provides. Accordingly, there may arise complex clinical conditions in which all three studies might contribute in arriving at a diagnosis.

~~~

By the early 1980's Frank and I decided that we needed to begin looking for a third surgical partner to join us. Because our surgical practice was expanding in both complexity and volume, we were
~~~

burning ourselves out, leaving little evening time for anything else. Years later as an adult, my daughter told me she deeply resented my being gone to the hospital most of the time. Personally I was beginning to feel much like an automaton. To make matters worse, it wasn't easy finding a younger talented neurosurgeon whose personality would not only be harmonious with ours, but also someone who could contribute new advanced skills and technologies to our practice. After having had a number of potential candidates visit us through the years for interviews, we at last found a suitable surgeon with whom we began to correspond. He had come highly recommended as a neurosurgical resident from the program at the University of West Virginia Medical Center. I subsequently met him and his wife in New Orleans at a CNS meeting, and we all hit it off very well. After a visit or two in Tallahassee, he accepted our invitation to join us. Our lives were soon to change for the better with Dr. Mark Vogter on board.

~~~

One morning in reviewing my day's office schedule, I noticed that I was to see an old patient, Mr. Chad Sewell, for recurring headaches. The reader will recall that Mr. Sewell was a patient of mine back in the early 1970s. I had operated upon him for a benign brain tumor which, at the time, I felt I had totally removed.

Upon his entering the office, I found Chad to be the same astute, jovial individual I had come to know so well 17 years previously. He then related to me that he was having increasingly severe headaches and thought that I should "check him out." His neurological examination was totally unremarkable, but in view of his past history I elected to obtain a CAT scan, a test not available to us at the time of his initial hospitalization. The scan unfortunately indicated a recurrence of the tumor (parasagittal meningioma), which had grown to a size comparable to its initial presentation in late 1971. It is generally accepted that the recurrence rate of these neoplasms is roughly ten percent if they were thought to have initially been totally removed, but increases up to thirty percent if there remained tumor cells at a point of dural attachment. Despite the fact that Mr. Sewell's tumor was closely associated with the superior sagittal venous sinus at the time of the initial operation, I felt, at least to the naked eye, that I had totally excised it. The current arteriogram again demonstrated both a prominent arterial blush in
~~~

supplying this lesion and also its apparent close attachment to the great draining venous sinus, the latter being of concern to me. Those located in the parasagittal region comprise ten percent of all meningiomas, and are familiar to most neurological surgeons. My colleagues will also generally agree that under some circumstances, they may prove as much a challenge to remove the second time around. Problems encountered may include their tendency to grow into the surrounding bone, broad firm attachment to the dura mater, often pronounced vascularity, and the propensity to insinuate themselves into the dural venous sinuses— all without a clean plane of dissection.

Such was the case of Dr. Harvey Cushing's patient, General Leonard Wood, who was originally operated upon in 1910 and to whom we have previously referred. After the initial two-stage procedure, Dr. Cushing felt that he had successfully removed the General's tumor. However, 17 years later General Wood began having recurring seizures, prompting him to again seek Dr. Cushing's help. The neurosurgeon labored tirelessly in an effort to relieve the General of his symptoms by again attempting to extirpate the recurrent tumor. Despite his skill, persistence and valor, he ultimately lost the battle to save General Wood's life because of insidious, recurrent bleeding. In reading an account of this incident one can only surmise, because of the difficulty in controlling the incessant bleeding, that the source of the hemorrhage was in all likelihood somehow related to the superior sagittal sinus. It has been written that for the remaining portion of his life, Dr. Cushing never overcame the loss of this patient and blamed himself time and time again for using bad judgment in the case. He always felt that he should have backed off from the procedure at a point in time when he was both fatigued, and the bleeding was becoming excessive; namely, before he had reached the point of no return (2).

Mr. Sewell's case bears a strong resemblance to the case of General Leonard Wood in that his tumor was also a parasagittal meningioma recurring 17 years after the original operation. While the risks of reoperation were presented to Mr. Sewell, both he and I were confident that he would survive the procedure. On the other hand, I was not entirely convinced that I could safely totally remove the tumor on this second attempt. During the operation we used the very best that modern-day neurosurgery had to offer. My anesthesiologist was excellent and maintained total control over the brain edema so often associated with these operations. The overlying dural mater which was indeed infiltrated with tumor was totally excised, and later replaced with a graft, as is customarily done. The interior of the tumor was decompressed, and its capsule dissected from the overlying brain in the usual manner. Bleeding was controlled with modern-day electrocautery, the bipolar forceps and hemostatic sponge. Once the bulk of the tumor was removed we were left with the issue of greatest concern— its remaining attachment to the lateral leaves of the superior sagittal sinus. At this particular anatomical level this venous structure cannot be violated, yet we remained fully aware of the possibility of a second tumor recurrence should we leave any portion of the meningioma attached to it. This dilemma is commonplace to any neurological surgeon dealing with this particular lesion. The surgical microscope with the interfaced carbon dioxide laser was maneuvered into the operative field. Under high magnification, and using a low power density (large spot size as we have previously discussed) with brief, pulsed bursts of laser energy, those tumor cells abutting the sinus were vaporized. Again, much like the first operation, we felt that we had cured this patient of his tumor. To everyone's satisfaction he did very well after the craniotomy, and to my knowledge has yet to sustain any further recurrent symptoms.

This case is presented primarily to show how far neurosurgery had come in just 17 years since Mr. Sewell's first operation. We had yet to purchase the original EMI scanner at the time of his initial hospitalization, but by now the hospital had acquired a third-generation CAT scanner, allowing important anatomical tumor evaluation. We had better anesthesia and means of controlling raised intracranial pressure and bleeding. And, finally, we had the surgical microscope conjoined with the laser in helping us to take down the tumor so intimately attached to the great draining venous system of the brain. Dr. Cushing in desperately trying to save the life of General Leonard Wood — a patient with a similar recurrent tumor— did not have at his disposal the marvelous innovations that we are so fortunate to have today, some 61 years later.

Keeping these points in historical perspective, it was Dr. Cushing who first set the gold standard for neurosurgery. Prior to his time the skull was thought of as a mysterious closed box into which few dared to enter. Cushing boldly endeavored to save the lives of patients harboring brain tumors which, left untreated, carried mortality rates of 100%. Furthermore, his results were stupendous— even measured by today's standards. We must all remember that it was Dr. Cushing who founded those very principles which form the basis of modern day neurological surgery.

~~~

As I look at many of my cases treated throughout the years, I often think of them individually as being unique in their own right, and with something to be learned from each one.

The following case, which may at first glance appear quite mundane, best exemplifies the practice of the "art and science" of medicine, which in this particular instance had lasting heart-warming consequences.

As a background the reader will recall the prior discussion of those patients with the "failed back syndrome." Many a neurosurgeon's practice is replete with surgical patients who continue to struggle with low back pain. Collectively, these people present an economic drain as a result of one of our nation's leading causes of disability. The causes of chronic disabling back pain are multifaceted and often complex, usually beginning with a work-related injury, frequently followed by surgery, and often tainted with emotional, compensatory and litigious elements. Out of all of this there often emerges dissatisfaction and even distrust between the patient and doctor, occasionally resulting in a growing disdain, and culminating in the patient's hopping from one physician to another. For whatever reason(s), the patient may undergo multiple operations and endless trips to the physical therapist, feeling that he will never be able to work again. There are often two opposing points of view: The patient may feel that he is the victim of injustice, first, because of the initial work-related injury and later by a failed back operation— unrealistically defined nowadays as anything less than 100% successful. The other view is that of the surgeon, who, often having nothing further to offer, begins to dread the patient's return to the office time and again, often bitterly complaining of pain, and requesting ever-stronger analgesic medications. Eventually, the patient may either be referred to another doctor or shuttled off to a chronic pain clinic.

Almost as a matter of routine we would be asked to see such new patients who would often limp into the office while holding under arm a formidable stack of old medical records. Most often they were referred by either an attorney or a third-party payer, usually having had a past history of multiple back operations; and, unfortunately, they were often more interested in pecuniary compensation than an earnest medical cure.
~~~

My approach in unraveling the often multifaceted problem was simple: Did the patient have an organic basis for his pain, or was he either the victim of his emotions (i.e., depression or despair) or merely seeking compensatory damages?

One afternoon I was consulted to see such a patient. This man had been operated upon at St. Elsewhere several times by a number of different surgeons for what allegedly was a ruptured lumbar intervertebral disc. Rather than improving, he seemed to worsen with each succeeding operation. As he related all of this to me in a somewhat tremulous subdued pathetic voice, his wife corroborated his story, saying that her husband led a life of unrelenting agony with back and leg pain. Walking was nearly impossible without lancinating pain into his thigh and calf. Sitting became unbearable, and a decent night's sleep was beyond reach. He continually took medications, his appetite was poor, and he had become an emotional wreck from pain and depression. Because these cases are always so highly emotionally charged, I had learned over the years to focus on purely objective evidence of nerve damage, first demonstrated by my neurological examination and later corroborated by appropriate electromyographic and imaging studies.

The concerned physician must immediately dismiss the inherent negative bias associated with a bitterly complaining patient holding a textbook size chart containing reams of pages of often conflicting medical findings, opinions and recommendations for treatment. I have known of some very good surgeons who flatly refused to take on such patients, feeling that their time is better spent treating pristine case material. On the other hand my partner and I, as the neurosurgeons responsible for our community, looked upon evaluating them as our duty, albeit often not a pleasant one.

Days later after all of the evidence was in, I concluded that this beleaguered man probably did indeed have an entrapped nerve root in his back. The source was probably from an underlying disc herniation, later compounded by numerous operations with the inherent bleeding and secondary scar tissue formation. With this in mind, I candidly told Mr. and Mrs. Caraway that the chances of my helping him with yet another operation were exceedingly small; moreover, he could even be made worse. They literally pleaded with me to try to help him. He told me that he simply could not stand to live his unproductive life any longer with such constant, piercing pain. Just as he trusted me to operate upon him again despite so many unsuccessful previous attempts, I trusted that he was not a malingerer. To the contrary, he appeared to be a kind, sincere man living with un-exaggerated, incapacitating pain.

In retrospect after opening up this man's back, I can't recall a more challenging spinal case. To begin with, he was a very large individual, and as I worked deeper into his massive lumbar area I encountered nearly impenetrable hard, rubbery scar tissue encasing both the bony spine and its neural contents. Metaphorically speaking, it was like trying to cut into a radial tire. More than once during the case, I questioned my judgment in surgically engaging in an area where there was no semblance of normal anatomy. The operation was long and tedious, often progressing only millimeters at a time — a familiar scenario to most experienced neurosurgeons. Wide careful bone removal for exposure, sharp dissection of nerve tissue buried in scar and control of incessant oozing of blood were the initial goals of the operation. At one point during the dissection, a small rent was inadvertently created in the nerve root sheath with the immediate egression of CSF into the surgical wound. Despite the deep, confined space, we were able to protect the tiny nerve rootlets, and finalize our efforts with a watertight dural closure. Eventually the root elements were freed up from the circumferential binding scar, before a compressing fragment of disc material was, indeed, found beneath them and excised. While attempting to prevent the in-growth of future restricting scar tissue, we ensheathed the nerve root in a sleeve of fat which had been taken from the subcutaneous tissue. After several hours of work, the wound was determined free of any bleeding, irrigated with saline solution, and closed.

Mr. Caraway's recovery exceeded my wildest expectations — totally relieved of pain and without any neurological deficit. Not only was he freed from the shackles of agony that had tormented him day and night for years, but his depression lifted, and a warm smile appeared on his face. He was indeed a grateful man. There had been a mutual respect from the onset, and despite what he had been through after a number of previous back operations he had trusted me to operate upon him yet once again.

Lawton Caraway was a successful, prominent farmer in South Georgia, and for years after the surgery, he would occasionally bring his wife and sons down to my ranch to purchase my Beefmaster bulls. They were so appreciative of my surgical effort and friendship that I never failed to receive a Christmas present each year in the mail. One of those gifts was a beautiful, wide-brimmed Stetson hat, which I have frequently worn, and which I have stowed in my front closet to this day.

Sadly Mrs. Caraway subsequently passed away, but Lawton and his sons would continue to visit my ranch. Then one day a few years later, I was again deeply saddened to read in the newspaper of Mr. Caraway's death. On the day of his funeral, I drove my truck up to Hopkinsville, Georgia, and, while standing alone, paid my respects to my patient and friend of so many years. As I stood silently at the graveside listening to the pastor, I looked up to notice his grown children across the way, pointing and whispering to one another as they recognized their father's surgeon who had traveled to be at his funeral. It meant a lot to them, as it did to me. As of this writing, I still exchange Christmas cards with Mr. Caraway's son and daughter, who each year tell me how much I mean to the entire family.

This story beautifully illustrates what we mean when we speak of the total approach to a patient, looking upon him not only as someone harboring an illness to be treated, but as a human being with feelings. The very essence of being a physician during my generation was to first convey a sense of understanding and empathy to the patient, encouraging him to gain the confidence and trust necessary to better accept treatment, irrespective of the complexity or risk in doing so. The healing of both body and a broken spirit is a gift never forgotten by patient, doctor, or family.

~~~

Late one weekday afternoon a young man, as I recall in his early thirties, showed up in the emergency room. He had been escorted over to the hospital from one of the state office buildings after having sustained the sudden onset of a severe headache. Upon examination, it was immediately apparent that his sensorium was slightly clouded and his neck was quite stiff. Otherwise I found no abnormalities. Parenthetically, he was a nicely groomed, fluent, and obviously a well educated young man. The clinical history and findings most certainly suggested a subarachnoid hemorrhage. Such was confirmed by the presence of bloody spinal fluid upon lumbar puncture.

The next morning the neuroradiologist performed a cerebral angiogram which revealed a rather unusual lesion. Positioned within the left trigone (junction of the lateral ventricle with the temporal horn) was
~~~

a rather discrete arteriovenous malformation, characterized by its enlarged feeding artery and a bulbous early draining vein. There were no other abnormalities noted on the study. In view of the delicate position of this vascular mass, we were reticent to recommend surgery until his brain function was completely normal. We carefully followed him in the NSCU until he gradually improved over several days without developing hydrocephalus or any other complications. His sensorium completely cleared, heralding the emergence of both normal cognitive function and a very congenial personality. He informed us at that point that he was an accountant for the state of Florida.

Concerned that he might not survive another intraventricular hemorrhage from his vascular malformation, I recommended that we operate upon him. With full disclosure, I carefully informed the patient that, because the lesion was deep within his dominant left temporal lobe there was an attending risk of injury to his receptive speech and other important higher, associative functions during the operation. He seemed to understand the fact that the future risk of a cataclysmic hemorrhage far outweighed the risk of some operative complication. Accordingly, he requested that we proceed with the surgery so that he could return to his important work as soon as possible.

While I didn't want to alarm the patient with this fact, I would like to interject here that a massive intraventricular hemorrhage is on the relatively short list of medical conditions causing sudden death.

Although I had never previously been confronted with a lesion precisely like this one, I felt perfectly capable of dealing with it. Yet, at the same time, I saw it as a potential disaster should things go awry. I must concede that my concern over this case drove me to the point of obsession with every detail of the operation. The stakes were very high in terms of this young man's future. The night before the operation, I revisited my cadaver brain in the pathology laboratory, where I envisioned a standard low temporal surgical approach, angling toward the trigone of the ventricle. The next morning, by using the recently acquired three-point head holder we firmly locked the cranium such that I could laterally flex the neck toward the right shoulder, thereby bringing the left inferior temporal region uppermost. The logic in doing this would provide a straight-line approach to the trigone, virtually without any retraction on the dominant temporal lobe.

The next morning the operation was successfully carried out with a total removal of the AVM, and the young accountant came through it with flying colors. There were never any elements of a receptive dysphasia, and the patient subsequently returned to full work.

The reason I have gone into such detail in describing my thoughts in preparation for this case is basically three-fold: First, any well-trained neurological surgeon is certainly capable of this procedure, but, as expected, he must invest time in detailed forethought while exercising the usual surgical caution. Secondly, contrary to the general opinion of the lay public or members of the legal profession, one does not necessarily need to have performed a dozen or more of any given operation to be proficient at it. I vividly recall many years ago Dr. Sean Mullan, chairman of the department of neurological surgery at the University of Chicago and a very innovative, well-respected neurosurgeon by others in our field, having addressed this question. The analogy he used was… "To fly an airplane, one must do it correctly the first time."

My final thought entails confidence. Trial lawyers can be intimidating to surgeons, and far too many cases that could otherwise be handled locally are referred far away for therapy. This can impose considerable unnecessary cost and inconvenience to the local citizens. The young surgeon, while not foolishly bold, should step forth to provide the service for which he has been both trained and qualified by his peers. I will amplify on this subject later in the book.

~~~

On an uplifting note, I would like to share an experience I had with some very fine people, whom I had known for several years, when they visited in my office one morning. Their last name was Ward, and I had been the neurosurgeon caring for their daughter. The father was a high school football coach in Thomasville, Georgia, and at that time was coaching his son, the team quarterback. I recall his smiling and telling me, "Doctor, you need to come up to Thomasville as my guest sometime, and see Junior play." Junior subsequently proved to be the great Charlie Ward — Heisman Trophy winner and the quarterback, who was to later lead the Florida State Seminoles to their first national football championship in 1993.

~~~

The latter 1980s represented a period of major change in my personal life. After my wife had left with the children in 1986, like most caring and responsible fathers, I was devastated by the sudden void in my life. Morning upon morning after leaving my truck in the parking lot, I would tread toward the hospital with head hung low, my mind reliving the past years with my happy family, bewildered at how our lives had been so suddenly fractured. There were times when I wondered if I could even manage to get through a day's work. However, there are few, if any, people who are fortunate enough to get through life without some major family happenstance, whether it be a separation, serious accident, illness or even death.

In the months to follow, I was destined to become acquainted with an attractive, vibrant and very intelligent lady who worked over at the now-competitive, newer hospital in our town. It was an institution where my partner and I had engaged in occasional spinal work and carpal tunnel surgery. Valencia, at the time that I met her, was a surgical instrument nurse who would often assist me in some of my operative procedures. In getting to know her over the course of time, I came to realize that I had met someone in whom I could not only confide, but someone with whom I could laugh and genuinely enjoy the lighter side of life. Only she could elevate my spirits from the deep void of having had my family ultimately move so very far away. As time went on, it became increasingly evident that we shared a great deal in common, including interests in science, medicine, nature, and even ranching. We found ourselves functioning with a similar mindset with regard to intuitive thinking and senses of humor. We could communicate with a natural ease that we believed would enable us to solve any future problems that might arise. It seemed that we were destined from the beginning to be married; whereupon, we were. One of her natural talents was her versatile singing voice, a thing of beauty matched only by her face, the latter having been likened to any number of movie actresses. During our church wedding, while gazing at me with her captivating, greenish-blue eyes, she softly sang to me with such purity from her soul, that it was said ... "There wasn't a dry eye within the sanctuary." Such was the beginning of a fresh, new life for both of us.

~~~
~~~

While my personal life was destined to undergo major changes during the ensuing years, the one thing that never changed was the endless flow of critically ill patients, some cases looking hopeless from the very beginning.

One Saturday around the dangerous midnight hour, a group of three teenagers were brought into the emergency room by ambulance in the wake of a very serious automobile accident in town. I don't recall anything about two of them, or even whether they survived the crash, for my time and energy were consumed by the third member of the group. The boy was 18 years old and in critical condition from serious head trauma. He was not only deeply comatose, but had sustained an extensive disruptive scalp injury with multiple full thickness "trap-door" lacerations and widespread contusions. It looked as if someone had worked over his scalp with a meat cleaver. The scalp, being the highly vascular structure that it is, was bleeding profusely, the young man already showing systemic signs of significant blood loss. Fortunately, there was no evidence of other bodily injury. A blood sample was immediately sent to the laboratory in preparation for transfusion while I simultaneously dressed his head with a tight dressing prior to sending him for a CAT scan. By no means was I surprised at the result of the scan — he had a massive acute subdural hemorrhage. We immediately transported him to the operating room, and, while he was under controlled-ventilation by the anesthesiologist, I personally shaved his scalp with mounting concern over its continued hemorrhaging. Once the bone flap had been turned, and the tense dura mater opened, the large subdural clot jettisoned forth from considerable pressure. From that point on it literally became a marathon as we worked to staunch the bleeding from the combined hemorrhaging of the torn bridging cortical veins and the badly contused, edematous brain. The edema was quickly brought under control by the anesthesiologist using hyperventilation, but the generalized oozing of blood was unremitting. I asked the staff to quickly send another blood specimen to the laboratory for emergency coagulation studies, thinking that we might be dealing with a case of disseminated intravascular coagulation (DIC). Fortunately at that point, after having transfused him with whole blood, his vital signs had begun to stabilize.

Perhaps thirty minutes into the case, we received the results back from the laboratory which did indeed confirm the diagnosis of DIC. This malady is known as a "consumption coagulopathy" which, among other conditions, has been associated with severe head-injury cases in which there was massive soft tissue destruction. From the excessive tissue damage substances known as plasminogen activators are released into the victim's bloodstream. These ultimately activate fibrinolysis (dissolution of any formed clot), resulting in the depletion of the body stores of fibrin, the reinforcing substrate of a clot, analogous to the supporting rebars in concrete. With persistent bleeding, the body continues to synthesize fresh new blood clots but is simply unable to maintain them, leading not only to the exhaustion of its reserves of fibrin but other clotting factors as well. As one might expect, treating this condition consists of replacing the depleted clotting factors. One product used in treatment is called cryoprecipitate, a substance to replace fibrinogen (the precursor for the degraded fibrin). Once the patient's diagnosis was hematologically confirmed, we began multiple transfusions of the substances alluded to above in addition to whole blood replacement. Always keeping in mind the possibility of a recurrent subdural hematoma, I had to reluctantly leave extensive sheets of synthetic, biodegradable, hemostatic materials over large cortical areas of capillary oozing, the major torn bridging veins having previously been cauterized. Perhaps sixty minutes later, during the course of multiple transfusions and persevering to control bleeding, we were ready to close the wound.

Closure of the macerated scalp was fraught with continued oozing as well. Ordinarily the scalp sutures, when tied, will pull the layers of the scalp together staunching the flow of blood, but not in this case. All of the suture lines continued to exude non-clotted blood, having the consistency of water. Once the suture work was completed, I tightly applied a large head dressing, and proceeded to sit down to write the postoperative orders. But before I had finished writing, the patient had soaked through the generous- sized head dressing. We reapplied another, this time laying down hemostatic gauze in the suture lines. We then quickly moved him to the NSCU after a brief stop in the recovery room. By the time he arrived in the neurological unit, the dressing was again saturated, and I again changed it. Fearful that he might have developed another subdural hematoma at that juncture, we obtained one of several postoperative CT scans. Much to our relief, there was no evidence of recurrence.

And so it was through the rest of the night— we continued to transfuse him with both whole blood and blood clotting fractions to hold the DIC in abeyance, while at the same time tending to the head dressing. After changing the latter for the fourth time, I told the nurses to merely reinforce it with large sterile, abdominal pads and head dressing gauze; for each time we removed the prior dressing, we disrupted what little clot had managed to form. At that point in the predawn hours, the staff was thoroughly discouraged, as any chance of survival began to look very bleak.

Upon returning to the hospital a few hours later that Sunday morning, I was relieved to find not only a stable patient but also a large, albeit unsightly, reinforced head dressing that was densely stained with dried, dark red clotted blood. Aesthetics aside, it was a welcomed turnabout after a very tumultuous night. Follow-up coagulation studies verified adequate replenishment of blood products, and no further bleeding was to ensue.

The critically ill teenager remained deeply comatose for several days, and then to everyone's amazement, he began to show signs of neurological recovery. As the days turned to weeks, his improvement slowly, yet steadily, progressed. He proceeded to become verbally responsive, resumed motor activity upon following commands, and was eventually begun on physical and occupational therapy. Everyone on the medical staff rejoiced the day his parents finally took him home. Because of the combined effort of so many, from the ambulance driver and the laboratory technicians to the nurses and therapists, this patient was able to walk out of the hospital, talking.

As I saw him from time to time in the office, he continued to improve over the succeeding months. While inconceivable even to the most optimistic observer, the young man eventually was able to complete and ultimately graduate from high school. And now for the rest of the story—the last thing that I had heard was that he had completed his first year of college at Georgia Tech University!

In summary, there were several very good reasons why this engineering student should not have survived this violent accident with any reasonable quality of life: First, the tremendous impact to his head during the moment of the collision could itself have been fatal; second, we have previously addressed the very high mortality and morbidity rates from acute subdural hematomas and associated brain contusions; and finally, the unremitting hemorrhage which complicated his treatment.

The obvious message to be carried away from this case is that as frustrating and, at times, utterly hopeless things seemed to become, no one ever gave up on him. Moreover, to have had at our disposal the laboratory means of diagnosing and treating DIC, itself representing years of scientific research on blood coagulation, was probably the factor making the difference.

~~~

This might be an opportune time to discuss the development of injury prevention during highway vehicle crashes over the last 37 years. Most drivers are aware of the fact that when fastening their seatbelts, two things are likely: First, they won't get a citation for "not buckling up;" and foremost, they would in all likelihood survive a serious crash. However, despite the fact that we are an educated society, most of our citizens are unaware as to how seatbelts actually work to save lives. I once had a hunting companion who thought it was an utter waste of time to fasten his seatbelt— until I related to him the following information. Throughout the years I have used the following biomechanical concepts, as discussed by Paul Gikas at one of our large national neurosurgical meetings, in giving informative lectures to the medical staff at the hospital, medical students and even my family (14).

In 1970 alone, there were more than 54,000 fatalities in the U.S. from injuries sustained on our highways. Despite prior years of hopelessly attempting to educate the public, it was finally concluded: "Driver behavior could not be significantly modified to make a difference in these dismal figures." The focus necessarily had to be redirected to the environment, namely, safer highways and automobiles. Given the fact that a potentially fatal accident **will** occur, cars needed to be engineered in such a way that their occupants would be "safely packaged" within them at the time of the crash. This subsequently became the focus of intense analysis and research in the years to follow.

People by nature have always preferred large cars with engines boasting robust horsepower, translated into rapid acceleration and high velocity on the highways. Suppose for a moment that such a vehicle careens off of the roadway after its driver falls asleep, only to crash abruptly into a large oak tree. The energy dissipated during the collision will cause a collapse and deformation of the front end of the vehicle. But what happens to the driver himself? Two possibilities may result: He may be ejected from the car through any number of ports, and be propelled like a missile with the same velocity that the car was traveling at the time of the impact. Or he could remain in the car, in which case his body would decelerate against something within it, such as the
~~~

steering wheel. In either case, there is a "second collision" during which his skull (or other body part) may deform much like the front of the car by striking another object, whether a tree or culvert if ejected, or, if not— an object within the car. Assuming that the car is constructed such as to absorb the kinetic energy during the impact by deforming, and the passenger compartment remains intact (termed, "space available"); then, it becomes simply a question of preventing that second collision of the body. This may be accomplished by fastening the occupant to the vehicle with a well anchored seatbelt and shoulder restraint harness.

The formula showing the inter-related forces is depicted below:

$$g = \frac{v^2}{S.D.}\frac{(mph)}{x30}$$

Where "g" represents the gravity units of deceleration, and "S D" is the stopping distance in feet. The "30" represents a constant.

As an example: Assume for a moment that the front end of a car traveling at 30 mph is crushed-in 2-feet; g then equals 15. A 100-pound person, who was harnessed to the car, would sustain a total force of 1,500 pounds (100x15), which is well tolerated by the human body.

On the other hand, if that same person is unrestrained, and he strikes a second object with his head, whether a tree if ejected or, if not, an object within the car such as a knob or visor bracket, it will result in a deformation of the skull. Using another example, assume that his skull is crushed in for a stopping distance of 2-inches. The results of the formula are now dramatically altered. This time in substituting 1/6 for S D in the denominator; the g units become 180, and our 100-pound occupant then sustains a total force of 18,000 pounds or 9-tons—intolerable indeed.

Again assuming that there is space available left in the passenger compartment, we may prevent the second collision by implementing the proper lap belt and upper torso restraint system. This device then distributes the g forces of deceleration over a large body area, whereupon these sometimes large forces may become survivable. It has been stated that deceleration forces of up to 40-g's are well within the limits of survivability, and in one instance of a free fall, the individual survived a force of 130-g's without injury (38).

I think that the above illustrations lend irrefutable credibility to the use of these restraint systems. In addition, we have also seen other salutary developments during the course of the years: plastic knobs, collapsible steering columns and dashboards plus airbags, all designed to dissipate the energy of that "second collision." With these innovations and after having addressed other factors of concern, there has been a significant drop in the annual fatality rate on our highways. By 2009 the figure had fallen to 33,808. However, as initially stated, driving remains fraught with unchanging careless driver behavior including failure to employ the seatbelt, excessive speed, alcohol, fatigue, and a host of distractions, such as multiple teenage occupants and cell phones.

~~~

Moving away from trauma for the present time, the reader may find the following, rarely encountered, neurosurgical procedure interesting. For orientation purposes it serves our interest to briefly describe the brain's fluid-filled ventricular system. The third ventricle of the brain is a deep midline chamber which receives CSF from the paired lateral ventricles located above it within the cerebral hemispheres. It then discharges that fluid through the cerebral aqueduct (Sylvius) into the fourth ventricle within the posterior fossa below. In essence, it is an intermediary chamber within the very center of the brain.

I had just returned from a national neurosurgical meeting in which I had heard Dr. Bennett Stein, professor and chairman of the Department of Neurological Surgery at Columbia University, deliver a very informative lecture on surgical approaches to tumors of the third ventricle of the brain. Dr. Stein, considered an authority on this particular subject, has written extensively about it (40). During previous encounters within that region while using the standard trans-cortical approach to the lateral ventricle, I had undertaken the removal of an entity known as the colloid cyst, a lesion of the third ventricle which was accessible through the foramen of Monro. However, I had yet to enter the entire third ventricle via the midline approach through the corpus callosum as discussed by Dr. Stein.

Soon thereafter, I encountered a patient in whom I thought the transcallosal approach might well prove feasible. The patient was a lady in her late fifties who presented with unrelenting headaches of increasing severity but nothing more. Her MRI disclosed a solid tumor within the third ventricle of the brain. This lesion appeared relatively extensive and did not have the radiological features unique to a colloid cyst. While the
~~~

latter lend themselves to extirpation through the foramen of Munro of the lateral ventricle, this mass appeared more solid and was more posteriorly located within the ventricular chamber. We needed, at the very least, to biopsy the mass before recommending definitive treatment.

After discussing the well-recognized risks of dealing with such a lesion so deep within the middle of the brain, the family agreed to an open biopsy and surgical removal if necessary. I thought in all probability it would prove to be an astrocytoma, and we would be left with a biopsy alone followed by postoperative irradiation therapy. The corpus callosum, being a midline brain structure, was approached through a craniotomy turned across the midline at the superior aspect of the cranium. During the course of employing the surgical microscope, the corpus callosum was first identified, and the overlying trunks of both anterior cerebral arteries then gently separated. The bladed self-retaining retractors were carefully positioned over cotton paddies, and the great commissure interconnecting the cerebral hemispheres was split in a very limited fashion, and gently retracted. Upon entering the left lateral ventricle, glistening from its liquid content of clear cerebral spinal fluid, the inter-ventricular foramen of Monro was readily identified, and protruding through its orifice was the pinkish capsule of the tumor. After sending a small biopsy specimen to the pathology laboratory, I was resigned to simply prepare for closing the wound. The pathologist subsequently made his presence known over the intercom by acknowledging that this was a perfectly benign tumor. It was not a glioma after all, but rather a cystic teratoma. Although not malignant histologically this tumor, if allowed unrestrained growth over time, would likely have resulted in serious consequences. Moreover, these tumors respond very poorly (if at all) to irradiation therapy; there was no option other than to attempt removing it surgically.

Referring again to Dr. Stein's lecture, let me reflect on one of his points of emphasis. By cauterizing and dividing with impunity one of the landmark veins in the area (thalamostriate) using the bipolar forceps, and by displacing the choroid plexus (vascular structure which produces ventricular fluid), excellent exposure of the entire tumor within the third ventricle was possible. We thus proceeded with the utmost care in attempting to remove this lesion from this unusual and delicate location. Fortunately, after achieving adequate exposure, the mass was found to be loosely textured and friable making its piecemeal removal much easier. To our satisfaction, after a modest period of concerted effort, all visible neoplasm was extirpated within a relatively bloodless field of vision. In the wake of the tumor excision, only clear CSF ebbed over these vital structures bordering the ventricle. The wound was closed and the patient did very well postoperatively. She was discharged one week later, totally free of her headaches.

Aside from the interesting nature of this case, another reason for describing it is to convey the sense of accomplishment that it provided to me. I suspect that every neurosurgeon, at some point during his career, has had a pivotal surgical experience similar to what I am about to aesthetically describe: For a brief moment after having finished removing the patient's tumor, I was spellbound in viewing the magnificent anatomical structures deep within the very center of the human brain. Observing the pristine chamber of the third ventricle under magnification, glistening from the silent percolation of clear CSF and walls embraced by the mysterious and intriguing diencephalon— considered by many the seat of consciousness— is a sight to behold. In achieving this journey to a place relatively few have ventured, I could relate to the great sense of accomplishment experienced by those who have ventured into space above our planet. For each event represents the culmination of many years, beginning in early childhood, of diligent study, hard work, and perseverance under the tutelage of a plurality of dedicated mentors. Similar to the history of aviation, the history of neurosurgery has encompassed many talented and innovative minds of science and medicine. During that brief moment within that silent milieu, I humbly realized how privileged I was to have had the opportunity in life to become a neurological surgeon.

~~~
~~~

TEN

The Period of Adversity

~~~

Late one afternoon I learned that my younger daughter, Gretchen, had sustained a cerebrovascular accident and had been admitted to the intensive care unit at the private hospital. While she was still in a deeply stuporous state, we had her transferred to TMH and began an extensive neuroradiological workup. All of the specialists involved finally concurred that her stroke was most likely the result of a thrombotic occlusion of the deep tertiary arteries within the thalamus of her brain, triggered by a state of dehydration. Gretchen had been not only a scholar but an athlete as well. She had collapsed while on a 30-mile cycling trip in the hot Florida sun. Although she did eventually grossly recover from this agonizing event, her life's ambitions were seriously curtailed, and she has since intentionally secluded herself from the rest of the family as a result.

~~~

In turning our attention again to the farm, it by now was beginning to occupy even more of my time, for, by 1990, our cattle herd had grown substantially. At the time that I had entered into the cattle business, Florida, after Texas, was the second-largest beef-cattle producing state in the U.S. A primary reason was the long annual grazing season which, including two months of planted winter forage, extended for 10-months. Because I needed to reserve two of my pastures at the Monticello ranch for the winter grazing of rye grass and oats, I was then left short on space for summer grass. We thus purchased an additional 152 acres of pasture-land in Pavo, Georgia, from a friend of mine, Banner Lee, who was also a Beefmaster cattleman. Because the Georgia soil was richer and less porous than that in Florida, the fertilized grass there was very nutritious, and the cattle thrived on it. Also, because the land was low-lying, it always remained moist and productive of forage, even at times of extreme drought. This served me well when grass was sparse elsewhere. The problem facing me, of course, was transporting the herd 45 miles north every spring and back again in the late fall. Keeping in mind that the bulls had to travel alone and the cow/calf pairs together, it became problematic in segregating, loading, and, upon arriving at the destination, releasing them into the appropriate pre-designated fields.

The cyclical annual protocol called for a spring season in which the cows were bred with the bulls, followed by the nine months of gestation spent grazing in Georgia. Calving would take place in the late fall and early winter back in Florida, with subsequent cow/ calf winter grazing at the Monticello ranch.

Because I had a purebred, fully registered herd, there was no room for error in identifying which sire had been bred to any given dam, or in mistaking the parenthood of the calves themselves. Meticulous records were mandatory in this business of breeding seed-stock.

In order to maintain calf identification, a numerically designated plastic tag was clipped into the calf's ear within 24-hours of birth. To wait any longer was asking for trouble, for the calf was up and running after that time. Early in the game, I can recall many times having had to lasso a calf from my horse or to chase him down with my truck (later an ATV) and bull-dog him to the ground in order to clip on the tag. And what seemed relatively easy during the first 24-hours when the newborn calf was weak and clumsy, became, after that time, fraught not only with an active calf scampering wildly about but also with a protective and, at times, potentially dangerous mama cow storming around.

We are all familiar with the dangers of getting too close to a bear cub, always mindful that there have been a number of human lives lost by vicious attacks by the protective mothers. Although generally considered good-natured herbivores, cattle can also become quite aggressive and even dangerous under similar circumstances. Post gestational hormonal changes seem to have profound behavioral effects on them. Friends have told me of instances in which cows, upon sensing that someone was about to harm their calf, have chased them not only into open truck beds, but in one case even tried to enter the cab of the truck through an open door. Some of my cows, even with the best of temperaments under ordinary circumstances, were known to become very aggressive after having just given birth to a calf. Of greater concern is the occasional cow, merely hinting of ill-temperament under normal circumstances, which may later unexpectedly transform into a violent animal with total dyscontrol after bearing a calf. We try to cull those out, keeping in mind that one of the Beefmaster Six Essentials is "Disposition," but from time to time one slips by. To further amplify on what has just been said, I will relate the following story.

During one winter weekend morning, Valencia and I were out at the ranch routinely checking on the herd. She was in a remote back field, and I had driven my truck, while looking for any newborn calves, into a front field stocked with pregnant cows intently grazing on the highly palatable oats and rye grass. There curled up in the tall luxuriant forage was a dark-red bull calf. Standing nearby was the mother, one whom I suspected as having a nasty personality even under the best of circumstances. I remained well afar, preparing my large clip-holder with the appropriate tag. Realizing that I must remain extremely cautious not to rile up the mother, I slowly pulled my old red truck up close to the unwary calf, still moist with amniotic fluid. Leaving the truck door open, I waited for the engrossed mother to tightly wrap her tongue around a large tuft of grass before sliding out of the vehicle down beside the calf, holder in hand, and poised to quickly fasten the tag. No sooner had I raised the bull calf's ear than he abruptly jerked his head away and began loudly bleating. With that, the mother promptly stopped eating and began hastily strutting toward us, head held high and nostrils flared. Her demeanor and glazed eyes left no doubt about her protective instincts. With my heart perceptively pounding, and realizing that I must quickly seize the moment to tag the calf, I snatched it off of the ground. Wrapping my left arm around his waist, I braced its back firmly against my chest and abdomen. I had never before realized that a 70-pound calf, just a few hours old, could raise such a fuss. It bleated frantically and so loudly that it resonated like a spine-tingling alarm, signaling to the concerned mother who by now was racing toward us. I foolishly thought that I could actually clip the calf's right ear while holding it to fend off the charging parent. But this proved to be a gross misjudgment. The 1,200-pound dam butted the front of the firmly held calf with such force that it knocked us both to the ground, causing me to release the rambunctious little bull. Suffice it to say that the enraged mama cow had only begun her work, and I had suddenly become fair game. I attempted to stand, but she wasted no time attacking and striking me with head and neck extended, propelling me several feet backward and causing me to lose my balance before again tumbling to the ground. Recalling, as a child, having seen the protective clowns in the bull-riders' ring at the Colorado State Rodeo, I rolled up into a tight ball. However, she continued to effortlessly butt and roll me along the ground, all the while menacingly snorting and carrying on. Once again I attempted to get up, but with lightning speed she again confronted me. By this time she had generated such fury that she had metamorphosed into a killer. The now berserk animal was snorting very loudly, had saliva spilling heavily from the corners of her mouth, and was kicking up great clods of grass and dirt as she violently pawed at the earth in preparation for still another assault. By this time, fearing for my life, I attempted to lurch for the truck, but she headed me off — knocking me down flat on my back— and then flinging her entire body over me. In a fleeting moment, as she thrust herself over me, I thought that it was truly the end. With eyes open, I could both see and feel the hair of her abdomen smothering my face; and fearfully cognizant of her extreme weight, I felt like I was at the bottom of an elevator shaft with the elevator in a free fall. Fortunately that horrific moment was short lived. As she scooted over me, a hoof did graze my head, fair warning that I needed to do something in order to survive. After that pass I rotated my head to see her wheel around about ten feet away preparing to return. Finally realizing that she would absolutely not allow me to stand, I frantically rolled under my truck several feet away in a desperate effort to escape this beast so blinded by rage. When safely under the truck I watched her cool down and eventually amble far enough away that I was able to hoist myself into the cab. I remember that, before doing so, I experienced intense pain in my upper back and initially was afraid to move for fear that I had a thoracic fracture. On the other hand, I needed to get to the hospital and be evaluated for other possible internal injuries. Humbled by this terrifying experience I sheepishly drove my truck over to the field where Valencia was distributing hay. She took one look at me and told me to lie down in the bed of the truck; she then urgently drove me directly to TMH.

The emergency room personnel at the hospital weren't used to seeing doctors hobble in as patients, let alone one who had encountered a mad cow. Because I not only had swelling and bleeding beneath my scalp from the hoof injury but other bodily contusions, the ER doc scanned my chest and abdomen as well. How fortunate and relieved I was to have sustained only two cracked ribs and a chest wall contusion. The consulting thoracic surgeon insisted that I remain in the hospital overnight for observation, but having no complications I was discharged the next morning.

The story ends with my driving that devilish cow "down the road" to the stockyards, but not before Valencia bitterly named her — "The Angel of Death."

~~~

Valencia and I had been married just over one year when we decided to attempt having our own child. During the course of our medical evaluation, we had the customary laboratory studies performed. One week after the blood-work had been submitted, I received an alarming phone call at the office from my wife stating I had contracted hepatitis B. I was overtaken by the news, for I had no idea that I harbored that illness. My internist together with a local gastroenterologist immediately began working me up, concluding that I had enzymatic evidence of active inflammatory liver disease; meanwhile, I was carrying a significant viral load of the infectious agent. It was thus verified that I belonged to the unfortunate 10% of the infected population, who after having contracted hepatitis B, are unable to mount an effective immune response to it. Of that subset of patients, somewhere between 5 and 20% will eventually develop antibodies, ultimately eliminating the virus from their systems. The remaining individuals within this subgroup are destined to remain positive carriers for life.

When reflecting back on my surgical practice, I initially had no conclusive ideas but could only speculate as to where I might have contracted the infection. Certainly it had to have been a subclinical event, simply because I had never become clinically ill with signs or symptoms of liver disease such as jaundice. It is a well recognized fact that, irrespective of any precautionary measures taken in the operating room, surgeons frequently are inadvertently stuck with contaminated needles. This may occur when reaching blindly with the outstretched hand for an instrument passed by the surgical nurse, while remaining visually focused on the surgical field. In an effort to reduce the chances of such an incident I had even "double-gloved" for several years, but somewhere along the line, it happened anyway. Several years later after researching my past further, I did uncover the fact that I had operated upon a patient in 1981 who was documented to have hepatitis B. He was a patient with normal pressure hydrocephalus from the Florida State
~~~

Hospital in whom I had installed a ventriculo-peritoneal shunt. But there were other potential sources of exposure, including more recent cases with documented AIDS (the two diseases often coexist) on whom I had performed stereotactic brain biopsies.

My physician and friend, Terry Reisman, wanting a second opinion regarding possible treatment referred me to the University of Florida at Gainesville. It was the general medical consensus that I should be given a four-month therapeutic course of parenteral alpha interferon. Valencia, a licensed practical nurse, gave me my injections every third day before bedtime. Anything ever having been written about the side effects of this drug probably understates them. Upon awakening the day after an injection, one feels overwhelmed by the disabling feelings of weakness, anorexia and malaise so reminiscent of influenza, compounded by an overlying severe depression. There was no recourse but to take Tylenol every four hours around the clock in an attempt to allay the debilitating symptoms — just to get through a day's work at the hospital. Despite the Tylenol I remained so anorexic that I found it hard to eat anything at all. We were purchasing liquid nutritional supplements by the case. Also, I can remember many times being too exhausted to drive home after seeing patients in the office all day, and having to sleep on my examining table for a few minutes before mustering up enough energy to get to my car. I had to refer my more complicated, high-risk surgical cases to my partners, for I simply lacked the endurance for such dangerous undertakings. On day three after a dose of interferon, just as I was beginning to emerge from the oppressive symptoms and starting to feel better, it was time that night for another injection of several million more units of the drug. And so it went — by far the sickest I have ever been in my entire life— yet trying to practice neurosurgery and cover the emergency room. My partners were understanding and empathetic, but they were overburdened with work themselves. For all of us it was a tough four months and all the while I kept reminding myself that any medication that makes someone feel this bad can't help but work!

Long after the completion of the full course of interferon therapy and much to my relief, I did show seroconversion of the *Be* antigen of the virus; my liver enzymes also later returned to normal. However, to this day I have not been able to generate antibodies to the ever-present surface antigen of the hepatitis B virus and so remain infectious. Nonetheless, I continue to clinically feel very well. I consider myself extremely fortunate to have had such excellent medical care to guide me through this illness and the complications of its treatment.

~~~

Consistent with the general theme of the book, another case will now be presented to illustrate some additional points, both medical and nonmedical in nature.

As so often the case, one day I was again confronted in the emergency department by a patient with headaches. This particular time it happened to concern a 17-year-old local high school student. Apparently he had been a very conscientious, hard-working, non-complaining young man who was suddenly brought to his knees by the abrupt onset of an unbearable headache. He was quickly transported to TMH by the school officials, and his mother was soon to follow. His primary physical findings included photophobia in addition to a very stiff neck. This suspected case of subarachnoid hemorrhage was promptly documented in the emergency department by lumbar puncture. The CAT scan also confirmed the presence of blood in the subarachnoid space with strong inference that something was going on in the region of the hindbrain. Cerebral angiography the next morning unequivocally demonstrated the source of hemorrhage as due to an arteriovenous malformation (AVM) within the posterior fossa. More specifically, it was a relatively large lesion which occupied a major portion of the right cerebellar hemisphere, the primary feeding vessel being a branch of the ipsilateral superior cerebellar artery (SCA). Of immediate concern from a surgical point of view was the fact that the SCA is the most remote of the three cerebellar arteries when operating from below with the patient in the sitting position. It is also the most difficult one to expose while trying to retract a cerebellar hemisphere housing the cluster of fragile vessels comprising the malformation itself. Any mechanical distortion of this structure imposes the formidable risk of intraoperative vascular rupture. In the event that happens, what was heretofore a pristine operative field suddenly becomes visually obscured with blood. Given this catastrophe, what might otherwise have been a slow, methodical dissection necessarily becomes a more urgent one in order to secure the feeding arteries to the malformation. Until that is accomplished, any bleeding from the enlarged, thin-walled, "grape-like" veins is difficult to control, because hemostatic clips, rather than acting like ligatures, often tear these vessels. Equally important, any small arteries suspected as feeding the AVM must be carefully traced directly to it before the clip is
~~~

applied. If such care is not taken, compromise of any of the numerous recurrent branches serving to nourish the vital brain stem may occur. Over the years the literature has reported instances in which these recurrent vessels have been inadvertently interrupted, resulting in major brainstem strokes or fatalities. Any haste in trying to delineate these important arterial feeders while fighting a venous hemorrhage increases the hazard of the operation and worsens the prognosis for a good outcome.

In discussing the envisioned problematic course with the mother, I told her that we first needed to observe her son in the NSCU for any complications (including hydrocephalus), and that he should remain there until we were certain that his condition would remain stable. Without reservation I also recommended that we operate upon him in a few days to remove the AVM. Because of the imposing pathological anatomy of the lesion within the posterior fossa, I emphasized to her the delicate nature of the procedure, which was fraught with a significant risk. In point of fact, however, I could scarcely even begin to relate to this already worried mother just how very much I was concerned.

In preparing for this challenging operation, I was aware that most of the conventional textbooks in anatomy at that time didn't give enough explicit detail with regard to the arteries subserving the cerebellum and brainstem. An exception, however, was a unique book which I had purchased during the last year of my residency training. Stephens and Stilwell had published a book with photographs of human brain specimens in which major individual vessels and their remote branches were highlighted by infusing them with plastic material to produce casts (41). There is no better substitute for the neurosurgeon than to study actual human material or photographs thereof. Anything less must interject the artist's interpretation with the inherent risk of distorting the normal anatomical relationships. I spent time in preparing for this procedure by studying different projections of the cerebellar arteries as portrayed in that book, correlating them with our patient' s arteriogram. My operative plan was then solidly formulated in my own mind long before entering the operating theater. In paying tribute to my colleagues, this rather intensive preparation best illustrates how the dedicated neurological surgeon usually prepares for engaging a difficult lesion in an unfamiliar landscape.

On the day of the operation, I positioned the boy upright in the sitting position, exercising all of the usual precautions against any complications, especially air embolism. Methodically and without undue retraction on the cerebellum, we clipped the arteries directly feeding the AVM — always keeping in mind that normal anatomy so accurately depicted in the book. It took basically all day to complete the dissection, but as the late afternoon approached, the last of the pathological vessels were clipped, and the now- deflated AVM totally excised from its bed within the cerebellum. The pulsating, pink, normal-appearing brainstem suddenly became a thing of anatomic beauty. Only then was I satisfied that we had safely navigated through what had initially appeared to be a formidable procedure.

Most gratifyingly, the teenager fared well after the operation both in the short term and over the long haul. I ran into his mother 10 years after the surgery and asked how her son was doing. She softly whispered, "Just fine." I then reiterated to her what I had said to her immediately after finishing the operation and many times later — "Mrs. ... that was certainly a risky, difficult surgical procedure." But I never seemed to receive back from her what I had hoped she would say: some small appreciation for my concerted effort in going that extra mile for her son. But not being a neuroanatomist, she can't be expected to understand the complexities or risks involved in such an operation. Within her mind an operation is only an operation, and I, as the doctor, was merely doing my expected job. The only point of relevance in her mind was that I had cured her son — nothing more. My self-fulfillment necessarily had to come from the self-realization of a job well done. One of my closest friends, a true scholar in his own right, once gave to me a poem entitled: "The Guy in the Glass" (by Dale Wimbrow, 1934). That guy is the one we must all answer to when looking in the mirror each day. What does he expect?

~~~

One of the primary objectives throughout this book has been to use it as an educational vehicle for disseminating information that, sooner or later, may be important to all of us. Among other points already addressed, I feel that it is incumbent upon me, as a neurosurgeon, to share my observations and experiences regarding a handful of accident cases; and, in so doing, I hope to arouse "awareness" so that people may avoid harm to themselves or others. One can't begin to list all of the countless situations that individuals may encounter in life which might expose them to serious injury or death. But people seem to ever-so-
~~~

frequently forget that we live in a physical world, and, within the blink of an eye, a good day can turn into a very bad one. Included below is a small cross-sectional sample of head injury cases which one might anticipate encountering in a community neurosurgical practice. With the exception of the last patient, they fall within the realm of "avoidable" injuries, and are presented primarily as a caveat for those who engage in potentially dangerous activities.

Case #1: This man was a blue-collar worker in his late twenties on whom I had operated two years previously for an acute subdural hematoma after a serious fall. We have already cited a very high mortality rate associated with this condition, but he was one of the lucky 20-30% who recovered and returned to work. Because of associated brain contusions and concomitant scarring, he was left with residual posttraumatic epilepsy. However, his grand mal seizures were well controlled with medication. Because he had gone a year without any convulsions (while on his medicine), he took it upon himself to stop taking it altogether. In this particular instance he not only discontinued taking his essential medication, but, without thinking, continued the potentially dangerous activity of scaling telephone poles at his work. One day when working high in the air, he suffered a major grand mal convulsion causing him to fall far to the ground, again striking his head, and again resulting in an intracranial hemorrhage. I believe he was the only patient I ever attended upon whom I had operated on two separate occasions for independent injuries resulting in acute subdural hematomas. However, after this second incident he was not as fortunate, having been left with severe brain damage, and no longer able to work.

Comment: Anticonvulsant medications basically suppress the triggering of potential seizures and do not treat the underlying cause of epileptic activity. Patients may mistakenly think they are cured after a period of time in which they go seizure free, and may take it upon themselves to discontinue the medications without consulting their physicians — a dangerous practice.

Case #2—involved a ten-year-old female who was cleaning the hooves of her horse when the animal kicked her in the head. I can vividly recall the pediatrician calling me from the ER late one afternoon, urgently asking me to see this nice little girl with a badly depressed skull fracture. We operated that night, and she ultimately recovered unscathed from her injury. This was in sharp contrast to a more severe case my partner had operated upon early in the 1970s. That particular child had sustained a more massive blow with extensive brain damage. She persisted in a vegetative state for several years, later to expire.

Comment: Horses can be very unpredictable and potentially dangerous animals whether one is standing beside them or in the saddle. While adults are always vulnerable, children are even more so, simply because of their youth and lack of experience. It has been my experience that parents all too often entrust their children to engage in dangerous activities without proper instruction or repetitive words of caution.

Case#3: This incident involved a twelve-year-old boy who was brought in by ambulance after having fallen out of a tree house. Upon my initial examination, he was found to have fixed dilated pupils and no spontaneous respirations. Although temporarily placed on a ventilator, he was confirmed brain dead, and life-support systems were later terminated. This case was particularly tragic, simply because the little guy was just having fun doing what most boys like to do. His emotionally-charged medical management was compounded by the fact that I had known the family very well for years. Also, by having children of my own, I felt the agony of their unbearable loss — and think about it to this day. The following weekend I promptly dismantled my own children's tree-house, much to their dismay.

Further comment: I am not necessarily suggesting that the idea of tree-houses should be abandoned, but perhaps thought should be given to enclosing them and building them closer to the ground. In contradistinction to most adults who are cautious of their moves, the unwary young mind may easily become distracted when having fun, opening up the possibility of a disaster.

Case#4: In the early 1970s, the Ford Motor Company introduced a series of vehicles that were touted as being "quiet" to drive by excluding outside extraneous noise when the windows were closed. Climbing into such a comfortable car was a young mother leaving home for work one morning. After shutting the door and starting the engine, she waved "goodbye" to her husband who was standing on the front porch. As she began to back up, she noted that his waving had become more intense — indeed frantic! Rather than signaling her farewell, he was trying in vain to get her attention, but she could not hear him shouting. Unbeknownst to the mother, her 30-month-old toddler had managed to wander behind her car, which by now was in motion. The terrified father began running in desperation toward the vehicle. At that moment his wife sensed a "bump" before sharply hitting the brakes. To the parents' absolute horror, they found the whimpering child lying on the driveway directly in front of the rear tire. Seized with panic, they fetched him into their arms and hastily drove to the emergency room. After hearing this chilling story from these grieving people so overwhelmed by fear and guilt, I turned my attention to the little boy. Across the parietal eminence of his small head was inscribed a full set of tire tread marks, tattooed into the bruised scalp. A palpably depressed skull fracture was also evident. Paradoxically and seemingly inconsistent with this violent injury, the child was perfectly alert, showing no clinical signs of structural brain injury. The rather extensive skull fracture without associated evidence of cerebral damage was corroborated by a CT scan. Later in the operating room we elevated the depressed cranial bone without any complications. He remained perfectly normal during follow-up for one year, and because his EEG was normal at that time we discontinued his prophylactic anticonvulsant medication.

Comment further: Despite the gruesome nature of this "crush" injury, there was no loss of consciousness, simply because the kinetic energy forces of acceleration-deceleration ordinarily causing movement of the cerebrum (e.g., boxing, football, falls, and auto accidents) were absent. For the same reason, the child was spared the translational shearing of neurons or tearing of bridging veins that we normally associate with severe closed head injuries.

Case#5: This incident happened to a middle-aged man merely attending his work. He had just repaired a flat truck tire and, after having fitted it back on the rim, was beginning to inflate the tire with compressed air. For reasons unknown — perhaps mere distraction— he overinflated the tire, resulting in an explosion. The hurling metal tire rim caught him squarely across the forehead. After the EMTs wheeled him through the ER door, it was immediately evident that he had sustained a severe bifrontal compound depressed skull fracture. A CAT scan disclosed extensive lacerations of both frontal lobes of his brain as well. In the operating room, we debrided the wound, and elevated the depressed shards of bone. Postoperatively, his lengthy incomplete recovery was punctuated by clinical evidence of severe brain damage. Here lay an individual with little control of arms or legs who, drooling from the corners of his mouth and uttering little more than unintelligible sounds, remained helpless and bedridden.

While this man survived in little more than a vegetative state, I had experienced a similar case my first week in practice back in 1971. That unfortunate worker, however, expired within minutes after admission into the emergency room, the skull offering virtually no resistance to that forcefully driven tire rim.

Comment: Almost any responsible person who has been confronted with a flat tire is aware of the potential danger of over-inflation when using compressed air. Nonetheless, many fail to use a tire gauge or exercise the necessary caution when doing so. Pressing on the tire or simply kicking it are insufficient means of estimating the pressure. We should not need to be reminded by the trauma surgeon, who has witnessed these grim injuries, to remain aware of the potentially dangerous nature of this activity.

Case #6—is presented as a fair warning to the young male who often takes chances trying to impress the girls and his friends — another tempting motivation in search of a serious accident. This twenty-five year-old man was waterskiing down in the bay one Sunday afternoon. The boat pulling him was taking fast, wide, sweeps near the shore. This activity imparted a centripetal force which literally "whipped" the exhilarated young man through the shallow water. Because of a gross misjudgment by both the helmsman of the boat and the skier as well, the latter veered in dangerously close to the shore on the last pass. His body and head tragically slammed into a dock piling, killing him instantly.

Comment: This case can be summarized in but a few succinct words: a horrific tragedy resulting from bad judgment by both parties while "showing off."

Case#7: Celebration activity after graduation from high school often entails heavy drinking of alcoholic beverages by youths whose bodies are mature, but who lack the good judgment, experience and cautionary restraint that come with age. Late one Saturday evening following graduation, a group of heavily intoxicated youngsters were involved in a violent automobile crash. The critically head-injured student whom I was asked to see was, ironically, the son of a daredevil of international fame. My initial examination sadly confirmed that the lad was brain dead, the status in which the EMTs had found him at the scene of the accident. This implies a tremendous force applied to the head at the moment of impact. I vividly recall presenting this grave news to the divorced, grieving parents, both of whom by this time were in the waiting room. Understandably devastated, they wanted "anything and everything" done —cost being no issue — to bring back their son.

Comment: The lesson taught is that fatal injuries show no respect for either joyous occasions or people of fame. The frail human body must be protected from the forces of nature by caution and sound judgment. Teenagers often exercise neither, and it is up to the parents and teachers to warn them of life's dangers.

Case#8: Rather than being an example of bad judgment, the following case is representative of one with absolutely no judgment. This patient was seen by my partner when he was on weekend call. It seems that two (possibly more) men in a mobile home park south of town had been consuming large quantities of beer most of the evening, and began boasting of their marksmanship. It defies the imagination to hear that the foolish man in question agreed to have his cohort of similar mentality shoot a beer can off of his head from several feet away. Immediately one thinks of the legendary William Tell upon hearing of this asinine stunt. But the shooter, lacking the prowess of Tell, placed a fatal bullet directly between the eyes of his human pedestal. What an unnecessary tragedy this was by two men in a moment of drunken "macho pride"…or was it stupor?

Like most head injuries, the preceding cases were totally preventable, even though some occurred during innocent, well-intended activity. As is so often the case, the latter two were tainted by alcohol. Rarely, we encounter one, much like a bolt of lightning occurring out of the blue, such as the unique case described below.

Case#9: This adverse event happened to a little preadolescent boy who was in a boat in the Gulf fishing with his dad and several other adults. Suddenly and without any warning, a beast from the sea flopped into the boat, violently knocking the child down. He struck his head on some object in the boat and was rendered immediately unconscious. By the time he arrived at the hospital he was beginning to regain consciousness, and during the course of the night became fully alert. Further history, as gathered from the father, proved amazing. The "large fish" proved to be a manta ray, the father estimating its weight at somewhere around 300-pounds! It took several men to lift this monster fish off of the child and out of the boat. Ultimately the boy made a full recovery without any evidence of either brain or other bodily injury and was discharged from the hospital the following morning.

Comment: This case is not presented because I am fearful that one of our readers will have a manta ray fall on him, but rather to alert people to beware of potential unexpected dangers virtually anywhere and at any time. Our clinical practice throughout the years has collectively been replete with unusual cases.

~~~

Back in 1990 when my case of hepatitis B was confirmed by liver biopsy, and treated with alpha interferon, the current medical thinking at that time was conducive to my continuing to operate as a surgeon. However, sometime in 1991 a dentist in South Florida was found to have infected several of his patients with the HIV virus via contaminated needles used in his office. Because the hepatitis virus is considered much more contagious than the HIV agent, a dictum was advanced by the CDC stating that any medical provider harboring either virus should not engage in invasive surgical procedures; more implicitly, they should not enter a major body cavity during surgery. Although this announcement represented the antithesis of what had been standard medical opinion not twenty-four months earlier, it rightfully was designed to protect the public. For me personally, it was to radically change my life. At a time well into my career when probably performing at my best as a neurosurgeon, I was compelled to step down— at least until such time as I could clear the virus from my system. Clearly, it was the only thing to do in order to prevent spreading the illness to others. Frank and I had previously anticipated retiring at age 62, but certainly not prematurely at the age of 55. Moreover, during the course of my additional medical workup for the disease, my physicians discovered complications of the viral infection within my body: cirrhosis of the liver and concomitant esophageal varices. The latter triggered a very disquieting thought, for I immediately reflected back to those awful nights as a young intern when confronted with the desperately ill patients hemorrhaging from them. During the course of a phone call from my internist in which he disclosed this latest medical information, my obvious question was, "Jesse… how long do I have… ten years?" He paused for a moment and replied, "Yes… probably 10 years."

This seemingly never ending cascade of bad news finally brought me into a reality check. Major life-changing decisions were in order. Foremost was the realization that I might not ever again be able to perform surgery. When asked about this many years later, I can
~~~

truthfully say that I have missed those challenges that only neurosurgery could offer. Where my partners were concerned, I could have eased their burden by continuing to see patients in the office, but I couldn't have helped to relieve them of the ever-present surgical load and the untimely, stressful demands of the emergency room. They were in desperate need of more help!

The second immediate concern was one of a financial nature. Fortunately, several years previously our clinic group had enrolled in an excellent disability insurance program, which did provide me with adequate financial security until age 65. After that time my retirement would then kick in.

The remaining question I had to ask myself was what was I going to do for work? One realistic possibility entertained was to become a clinical neurologist, but that would have entailed going back into a residency program and essentially starting over. Keeping in mind the possibility of a prematurely shortened lifespan, I wasn't happy with the prospect of spending part of it back in school, especially since there were other avenues of life that I wanted to explore.

After having worked very hard for over 21 years in the private practice of neurosurgery, I decided to proceed forward with that second childhood dream: I would focus on my ranch as a cattle breeder. I well recall that day in his office when my accountant encouraged me to "merely switch occupations", which I was ultimately able to do. I tried to be optimistic and proceeded with almost the same fervor with which I had practiced medicine. With all of the land and equipment already at hand, I was on track to build a model cattle operation and enjoy every minute of it.

For anyone jolted by a life-changing illness, especially if accompanied by a loss of profession, he is suddenly confronted with an unexpected fork in the road. Foremost, one must remain composed in seeking out various alternatives. In a timely manner, a friend of mine quoted to me the words of a former East German military pilot after the tearing down of the Berlin wall. The pilot was asked what he was going to do now that the Germanies were reunified. The airman wisely replied, "A pilot is always looking forward." Sooner or later one's mind is good at sorting things out, and, like the pilot, I very quickly found myself looking persistently forward.

Foremost in my thinking was the possibility that I would eventually clear the hepatitis virus from my system, and that I should always remain prepared to return to my surgical practice. In order to maintain my state medical license, it would mean continuing to read medical journals and to attend national meetings, which I did for the better part of the ensuing ten years. Also, I needed to pursue some work along medical lines to keep me focused scientifically. I therefore sought out various medical activities in addition to working at the busy ranch.

I was soon to learn that the state of Florida needed focused, retired physicians to review the records of Medicaid patients in which there were suspected improprieties regarding provider services and billing. After having been accepted for the job, I drove over to the Medicaid office every couple of weeks, and loaded up my car with stacks of patients' charts for review. While this hardly measured up to the excitement of a neurosurgical practice, it did serve the important purpose of preserving my self-identity as a doctor.

If I may amplify on that last point: At some level everyone probably needs a "self-identity," and needs to maintain a positive self-esteem and a "healthy sense of worth." Out of concern, I have observed several of my retired physician friends who, after having lost their self-identity as practicing physicians, had fallen into the throws of a serious depression. As I have frequently expressed to them, there is a lot to learn, to see, and to do in this world, offering us numerous opportunities to become experts on any number of things. More than once I have retold the story of the East German pilot.

Another medical undertaking of mine concerned a temporary appointment as the chairman of a worker's compensation medical board, also involved in examining deceptive billing practices by providers throughout the state of Florida. Being chairman of the committee entailed my over-seeing the multiple cases collectively designated to the reviewing board members. Having at least two reviewers agree on any improprieties was mandatory before making any formal accusations against the provider. I vividly recall the first time that a fellow pulled up to the front door of my house in a van, and began unloading stacks of large boxes filled to the brim with patients' charts for my review. Only then did I realize what a daunting, time-consuming task this would be. After weeks of study and preparation by the six reviewing doctors, we met together at the formal board meeting, bringing each provider individually into the room, and presenting him with the alleged infractions. I regret to say that I was sadly disappointed in some of the flagrant abuses we encountered in this small minority of providers. Some of the accused were high- profile doctors, one even being the eminent author of a well-known authoritative textbook.

Another field of endeavor occasionally occupying my time over the ensuing twelve years was partaking in medical-legal work. For the most part the cases in which I was involved were old patients of mine, most of whom having been injured in motor vehicle accidents. Because of the late discovery of injury, the cases often ended up in court for compensation. Having been the patient's doctor, I was called in as an expert witness on behalf of my patient (the plaintiff).

Along the same lines, for a brief period of time I made myself available to review the merits of potential medical malpractice cases. In an isolated incident I was contacted by an old fraternity brother of mine from Northwestern who, after years as a practicing physician, decided to go back to law school and become a trial lawyer. He consulted me on two separate injury cases, neither of which had any merit as far as I was concerned. I could find absolutely no negligence on the part of the attending doctors. Despite Jim's persistence in trying to find medical fault, even going so far as flying a patient to Tallahassee for me to examine, I honestly told him he simply did not have a legitimate lawsuit in either case. With all due respect to my friend, and even though his clients were indeed injured it was not the result of medical negligence. In my opinion these would have been considered frivolous lawsuits. That was the last I ever heard from Jim.

But despite all of these various and sundry endeavors, my primary occupation and self-identity ultimately became one of a true cattleman— not to be mistaken for a "gentleman farmer" who sits by and gives directives to others — for I began to work very hard seven days a week, doing just about everything on the ranch.

~~~

Valencia had always wanted to meet Dr. Bucy, the man she had heard so much about as an inspiration and influence in my life. In the summer of 1992, my wife and I thus set out for Tryon, North Carolina, and drove up the side of the mountain to visit my dear mentor. It brought back fond memories — twenty years past — when my entire family stayed with the Bucys. With high anticipation, I sought to introduce her to this robust, vibrant, intellectually astute man who was internationally recognized as a giant in neurological surgery. As we pulled up into his driveway, and he strolled out to the car to greet us, I was aghast by the drastic change in his appearance. He had become very
~~~

gaunt, feeble and rather subdued, the picture of a man seriously ill with a debilitating disease rapidly depleting the substance of his body and the energy of his mind. As I gazed into his eyes, a part of me wept inside. We later sat in his living room, occasionally looking out of the large window to the bottom of the mountain below, while reminiscing over our mutual acquaintances and experiences of old. After visiting over tea for perhaps the better part of two hours, it was time to bid my teacher and friend farewell, realizing that I would probably never see him alive again. With the fondest of memories, I was about to close another long chapter in my life. As we silently drove down the hill, I was sadly leaving behind the man primarily responsible for my becoming a neurological surgeon.

Dr. Paul C. Bucy passed away in September, 1992, his name to be inscribed in the world's medical archives as one of the foremost neurosurgeons of our time.

~~~

In 1992 President Bill Clinton appointed his wife, Hillary Rodham Clinton, as chairman of the White House Task Force on Healthcare Reform. Many of us in the medical profession were alarmed by the sweeping changes being proposed, even for a system that was so crippled and in such need of repair. While sitting around the table at our annual Capital Medical Society Valentine's dinner in 1993, several doctors suggested that I write a paper which would propose interjecting physician input into the national debate on healthcare reform. After writing that paper, it was sent both to our United States senators and also to the Executive Vice President of the American Medical Association. Printed below is the article as published in the Capital Medical Society newsletter in Tallahassee in 1993.

Finding a Reasonable Solution in Healthcare Reform

While there has been great concern over rising healthcare costs during the last few years, it has escalated to perhaps the main topic of conversation in recent months. One senses a near frenzy emanating from the haste to present a broad plan to the people and to please everyone. However, to the dismay and concern of many, the medical profession thus far has been excluded from any participation in this area. While both federal and state officials are ignoring any physician input into the decision-making process because of alleged conflicts of interest, they are
~~~

depriving themselves of a valuable source of information in cost-saving measures.

The following paragraphs are not intended to attempt solving this gargantuan problem but merely to vividly show that there are obvious areas of extreme waste of monies in current-day medical practice. By touching on but a few areas and sharing my thoughts on their solutions, I would hope that my colleagues would be invited to contribute further input. To wage any type of effective war, all branches of the attack force must be involved, for to exclude anyone would merely guarantee defeat.

Briefly, by way of background, I am a neurological surgeon who, after twenty-one years of practice, had to retire from clinical medicine because of chronic illness. At a recent dinner of our medical society in which solutions to the current healthcare crisis were freely discussed, several of my colleagues asked that, because of my unique situation, I become involved. They agreed on some of my ideas and shared their own with me as well. You see, I have not only lived through an era of great medical advancement but have also observed great increases in neglectful spending as well. Because I am retired, I have nothing to gain other than the satisfaction of contributing to the solution of this monumental problem.

The federal and state changes currently are focused on: health access, cost containment, insurance reforms, health regulation and tort reform. My comments, based on personal experience and observation, will be primarily confined to cost containment matters but will touch on regulation and tort reform as well.

In the early 1970s we, in neurosurgery, had to rely solely on air encephalography and cerebral angiography, in most instances, for the localization of intracranial mass lesions. Because these were invasive procedures carrying significant risk, they were not performed indiscriminately but only after careful assessment of the patient's clinical condition and the findings. The number of such studies, and hence their cost, was thus dictated by the specialist who was in the best position to order them and were based upon his clinical judgment. There was no waste of financial resources on the studies as the indications were firm, and the person ordering them most qualified.

Then came the CAT and later the MRI scans which have revolutionized the diagnosis of intracranial lesions and have saved countless lives. However, the price tag for these procedures goes way beyond expectation. In a discussion with one of the leading local HMO directors, it was learned that imaging studies have had a major impact on cost in that managed-care setting. Contrary to the days when but a few angiograms were done in an institution, there has been an avalanche of scans performed. Because they are low risk, noninvasive studies— anyone can order the test. Let us now analyze this point.

People entering the emergency rooms around the country who have had trivial head injuries, uncomplicated headaches, metabolic or drug disturbances— to name a few— may get a scan. Very often they are not seen by a person with expertise in the neurological field, but rather by a screening physician who begins with an expensive scan.

CT scans have been anchored in many small communities without clinicians available to know how to properly order the test. For example, for years I received countless patients with low back pain referred to me from our outlying referral area with a plain CAT scan of the back. A plain lumbar CAT was of little to no localizing value to us. If the patient simply had a low back strain, the CAT was not indicated. If, on the other hand, the patient had the clinical findings of pathology; e.g., lumbar disc, tumor of the cord, etc., he needed contrast myelography with the CAT or nowadays an MRI. In either instance, the scan done prior to referral was wasted, and the examination later repeated by someone more knowledgeable of low back pain. Computerized brain scans are often ordered simply for expediency and for defensive medical reasons, when clinical observation and re-examination might have well sufficed. For example, an ER physician is reluctant to send home a patient with a headache after a minor head injury without a scan. We are talking about an alert patient who was not unconscious, and who had no abnormal findings. In a neighboring town a few years ago, such a patient was sent home, but was somehow lost to adequate follow-up, and later proven to have a chronic subdural hematoma. After lawsuits emerged, ER physicians and neurologists alike were forced to order scans on many with very minor head injuries (and there are a lot of them).

Without apparent consideration of cost, many radiologists will recommend duplicate studies; e.g., CAT on top of an MRI, when one test alone might have sufficed. Admittedly, there are situations where the studies complement one another and give additional information, but this is not always the case.

On occasion the radiotherapist will order follow-up serial scans on the irradiated patient without first consulting the primary neurologist who is managing the case, and who is in the pivotal position to recommend further treatment. Ordinarily, another scan is dictated by clinical change rather than merely to satisfy the curiosity of the therapist eager to visualize an early therapeutic effect of his radiation.

Another area of duplication of scans occurs when a patient obtains a less expensive scan from a lesser quality scanner in the community, and is then referred to a specialist whose standard of practice relies on higher quality imaging and quality control. Not infrequently, I have had to repeat outside MRIs done for low back pain in which axial slices were not cut through the lumbar disc in question or not through the conus medullaris to exclude a tumor.

There are other examples of inefficient ordering of these extremely valuable, yet expensive, studies, and the costs defy the imagination when multiplied nationwide.

A second area of financial drain with little return is the continued excessive treatment of hopeless conditions. As a senior consultant for Medicaid in our state, several such examples of expensive care have been brought to my attention. One such case involves a child with hydranencephaly (congenital absence of the cerebral hemispheres), whose total medical care the first year of life, having been paid by a private insurer, was $758,000. He is now three years of age, has but a tiny remnant of brain tissue even present, exists in a vegetative state and is totally ventilator dependent. He requires private duty nurses no less than 16 hours per day amidst a totally dysfunctional family. This child, with continued good care and yet absolutely no hope for <u>any</u> meaningful recovery, had an average cost to Medicaid of $197,737 annually during the second and third years of his life. It is because of such unreasonable cases that it becomes mandatory that society establish the guidelines as to the extent it is willing to pay for such conditions.

For years we struggled with the concept of brain death and educating the public to accept it. Now we have convinced both the legislatures and the people that it is fruitless to keep a brain-dead individual artificially alive. It would seem that this concept could be expanded with the help of wise but carrying members of the medical profession to include such cases as those alluded to above. Second opinions in these hopeless cases would be mandatory. Just as brain death cases are backed up by the statutes, so would the above.

Another controversial issue within the category of the brain injured is when to begin and to what extent should expensive rehabilitation be carried out. As an illustrative case, I mention the middle-aged brother of a prominent citizen in our community who sustained a violent head injury. After the acute phase had passed (perhaps three weeks), and it became evident that this man would survive, the family insisted that he be sent to an expensive rehabilitation center elsewhere in the state. Because he remained deeply comatose, I recommended strongly that we defer such therapy until such time that it became evident that he would improve to the point where he could utilize it. This is analogous to waiting for a child to attain a certain age before teaching him to walk; i.e., the brain must be ready. The man's family listened to many other health care workers (nurses, social workers, and therapists) who were neither versed in neural injury nor cost containment, and, against my advice, persuaded the family to have him transferred to the rehabilitation center. After several weeks of unsuccessful therapy, and a bill of $60,000, the man was returned, unimproved, to our community.

Rehabilitation of the brain and spine injured patient, be the cause trauma, stroke or other etiology, is of unquestionable value in appropriate cases. But the primary neurologist or neurosurgeon should make that decision, and not the patient's family.

As we look around us in the daily practice of medicine, the concerned thinking individual must ask serious questions about our healthcare delivery system: How long are we going to continue to support the conception, delivery and neonatal care of crack-cocaine babies? When is society going to impose birth control measures on these addicted women who repeatedly deliver dysfunctional babies and monstrous medical bills to America? To what extent is medicine obligated to save every baby presenting to a neonatal intensive care unit irrespective of size, extent of brain damage or irreparable, often grotesque congenital malformations? Are there limits as to the extent of <u>non-essential</u> care that medicine should deliver to the elderly? When should aggressive treatment such as blood element transfusions, expensive medications and intensive care strategies be stopped in those pre-terminally ill with fatal diseases such as AIDS and cancer? In a recent study it was found that in hopeless cancer cases, the cost per year of life gained in patients with solid tumors was $82,845 and it was $189,338 for those with hematologic cancers.

There are, of course, humane considerations here as well as financial. Furthermore, a blueprint for the solutions may be drawn from the private sector perhaps with the support and direction of the federal and state governments and with the full cooperation of those who write and uphold the laws.

Defensive medical practices have to some extent been discussed under excessive imaging studies. Contrary to what has been voiced by a few in this country, it does indeed exist and is quite significant. To best illustrate this point, I was contacted several years ago by a concerned neuroradiologist. He informed me that one of the local neurologists insisted that each time a myelogram (spinal dye test) was done on one of his patients (most of which were done for obvious herniated discs or back strain) that a full battery of chemical and bacteriologic studies be done on the cerebrospinal fluid. As absurd as this seemed, the neurologist made it clear that he did not want to leave any room for a lawsuit. I checked into the cost which, then in the early 1980's, was $300 extra added to the base cost of the dye test. If everyone shared his view, the added cost would be staggering, considering how many myelograms are done nationwide each day.

Furthermore, there is no question that defensive medical practices also drive up the costs within both hospitals and nursing homes. Astronomical bills are mounted up in the elderly until each has taken his last breath. For instance, it is frequently the case that a senescent individual, pre-terminal with cancer, might sustain a minor fall from a chair or bed. The nurses, out of either panic or out of administration policy designed to avoid a lawsuit by an unhappy family, will call the doctor. The doctor, despite his awareness that the patient's age and pre-terminal condition had long before dictated the patient's imminent death, now feels the pressure to order a multitude of x-rays to rule out hip, rib and long bone fractures, a CAT of the head and probably a neurosurgical consultation should the patient be the least bit confused. He must do this not to save a life ready to cease functioning prior to the fall, but rather to protect the institution, its personnel, and himself from the wrath of the family and its attorney.

In other cases where a terminal cancer patient runs a fever, he may receive a myriad of blood tests, consultations, and expensive intravenous antibiotics until the inevitable last breath is taken— all for the same reason. For, despite impending death, "everything must be done" to assure those present that the death was most certainly an act of God and not due to negligence.

Sometime in the future, perhaps in one year or perhaps in twenty, this point will finally be acknowledged by those who ultimately orchestrate control of the healthcare problem. Let sound clinical judgment dictate the course of events. If there are, indeed, true deficiencies in judgment or improprieties in care, then let those boards responsible for licensing nursing homes, hospitals and physicians investigate those improprieties.

In a recent McNeil and Leherer News Hour interview with HHS Secretary Shalala regarding medical costs, she claimed that curbs on rising physicians and hospital fees would slow down the rate of increase. Her explanation of the current rate of increase was "an economic incentive to order more tests," and her solution was to be more efficient in ordering them. I think this points out clearly the perception of the problem as viewed by an administrator rather than by someone practicing in the trenches of medicine. The points made thus far by this author refute the idea of primary personal financial gain by those ordering these tests by introducing many other complicated factors, defensive medicine being merely one of them.

There have been many proposed solutions to the escalating costs of medical care, and it might be well to touch on this subject as it is apropos to this paper. Frequently, there has been talk about cutting back on the education, hence, the availability of physician specialists, while concurrently endorsing an increase in general practitioners in managed care facilities. While we unquestionably need primary care physicians, who can more efficiently diagnose and treat any given complex medical problem than the specialist? I have seen a number patients who have been sheltered from the specialist because of budgetary constraints by an HMO; specifically, patients who had advanced neurological deficit from spine disease and who needed urgent surgery to relieve them of pain, reverse their deficit, and return them to work.

Another solution mentioned is capping insurance premiums. That will do nothing but create chaos under the current circumstances. If on the other hand, there can be a reduction in needless expenditures, and better utilization of funds available, caps might be of value.

While there are undoubtedly multiple possible solutions to the problems alluded to above, I would like to share some of my ideas: It would be particularly important to see physicians return to those principles taught in medical school and instilled by their preceptors regarding clinical judgment. After a careful history and assessment of the patient, most well-trained doctors have a good idea as to what the problem might be and can lay out a differential diagnosis. They may then order only those tests which are reasonable in confirming the diagnosis rather than to haphazardly order a shotgun array of studies merely to build a litigation shield. And rather than reduce the number of specialists, we should support a reasonable representation of them in the medical framework, for it is that clinical judgment of the specialist, in many instances, that leads to the correct diagnosis and treatment. On the other hand, when the generalist admits a patient to the hospital, I think it is medically wrong to initially consult half-a-dozen specialists covering several different body systems merely "so nothing is missed" (I have frequently seen this done), but rather to request assistance only for the solution of the problem that brought the patient in.

Once the specialist locks onto the problem, then he alone is in the best position to order the necessary ancillary tests. Indeed, the neurologist or neurosurgeon is in a much better position to say whether or not a CAT or MRI is indicated in any given case based upon his neurological training and his clinical judgment. The generalists might not like this approach, but recalling the earlier part of this article, it would vastly cut back on unnecessary scans. Years ago, the family physician would not have considered ordering a pneumoencephalogram, nor would a neurosurgeon today order a cardiac angiogram. The fact that the CAT is noninvasive and easy to access should not be a license for anyone to order the procedure in most instances.

In the case of spine pain, the patient who is followed by the family physician and who fails to improve, should then see a spine specialist. The latter will then decide whether the condition warrants an immediate scan if there is a neurological deficit or, to the contrary, if the patient can be treated conservatively and avoid that expensive radiological procedure. The author is the neurosurgical consultant to the Florida State Hospital in Chattahoochee, where we have, in effect, implemented this system. Rather than having the ward physicians order brain scans, the patients are first seen in the neurological clinic. It is at that checkpoint that the decision is made regarding imaging studies. There has subsequently been both a reduction in the number of scans ordered and in the cost to the state as well.

Each specialty could study this issue from its own perspective, and guidelines could be structured. For such a system to be successful it would require the cooperation and support of the legal profession and this is why: If in spite of the best clinical judgment of the ordering physician, an adverse result occurs because of the delay in ordering a scan, the case would first be reviewed by a panel of his specialty peers. If the panel finds that the specialist used prudent judgment, regardless of the outcome, he should not be held liable. If on the other hand there was a gross error in judgment— they would so state— and the doctor would be subject to litigation if that course were chosen by the patient. This system would protect the doctor practicing good clinical medicine and who is cost-conscious; it would also lead to considerable savings in healthcare dollars. As an example, we might again refer to the cases of trivial head injury in which scans are ordered without hesitation. If, in the judgment of the neurosurgeon, the patient might best be closely observed for any change (alert patient with no abnormal findings on examination) without a scan, then the system would back his judgment.

Citing yet another example: We might consider the chronically complaining, neurotic patient who has had headaches for years and has a normal neurological examination. Given the fact that the patient had a normal scan one year previously, the doctor may exercise the option of following the patient in the office for the development of any neurological abnormalities rather than ordering scans every six months. He has used appropriate judgment here at a substantial cost savings. Should this patient, despite this decision, spring up with an unsuspected tumor, the panel would still support the neurologist's clinical judgment.

On the other hand, if the scan was not ordered on a person not ordinarily plagued with headaches, and whose eye grounds harboring papilledema were not examined, the neurologist has not practiced good clinical medicine. If, for whatever reason, this case should be presented to the review panel they would necessarily judge against the clinician. Using this type of discretion in my neurological group alone would have saved thousands of dollars annually.

Each specialty would employ its own judgment guidelines and each would provide its own panel. These review bodies could be set up much the way the peer review panel is set up for Medicaid in the State of Florida, but in lieu of the Florida Medical Association the specialty societies would supply the reviewers. This concept would again distinguish "bad outcome" from "negligence" while lending support to the conscientious clinician trying to exercise sound medical judgment within the framework of cost consciousness. Cost savings would probably be in the billions of dollars. The AMA estimates $15.1 billion was spent on physician-ordered defensive medicine in 1989.

Once again, these decisions are made by the joint efforts of our governmental officials, the medical profession and society at large. A process to educate people must be enacted. The people now feel they have the right to demand what test is to be done or how long a loved one can remain alive in a vegetative state. In my practice I so often hear such statements as: "even if his chances are one in a million, I want to take that chance," or "just keep him alive, doctor, and we will hope for a miracle." People must now be cognizant of the odds of recovery and accept the restrictions imposed, so there are funds available for others. Again, we have educated them on brain death and have legal backing. Why can we not do this regarding other matters?

In summary, some of these issues are straightforward, while others represent radical departures in our thinking. However, all are reasonable. Before pouring billions of healthcare dollars into a system proposing coverage for all citizens, we must first analyze what is wrong with the current delivery system and where the money is going.

Good health is important to us all, but we must define the controls and limits of expenditure. Just because a patient bumps his head and the family "thinks a CAT should be done," or because a family demands that its 80-year-old grandpa should be kept on a ventilator— doesn't necessarily mean that either is indicated in the judgment of the attending physician in particular, or in the eyes of society in general. That money might be better spent repairing a young working father's hernia so that he can return to work and support his family.

Cost containment issues in health reform are going to force budgeting strategies at a lower level, and the changes will not be to everyone's liking. Hence, these will knowingly raise questions as to one's right to life-sustaining treatment, especially in the elderly, the terminally ill, the brain injured, and those progeny of drug addicts — to name but a few. We can only anticipate an escalation of discrimination suits in the wake of proposed change.

The efficient solutions enumerated here will not work without the support of our legal system. The trial lawyers will argue, as they have for years, that the injured patient has his right to a day in court. Indeed, that

> is true if he is hurt through negligence. But society must stand behind the doctor who may have had a bad result, even though the execution of his judgment was proper.
>
> Perhaps by implementing the proposed system, it would be appropriate to consider integrating a patient insurance compensation system into this paradigm to cover those injured, but not through negligence. The private malpractice insurers could continue to cover the doctors for true malpractice behavior as determined by the review panel.
>
> Again, this paper is not intended to solve the cost-containment subject. It is designed to demonstrate physician insight into the complexities of medical practice not recognized by those on the outside of the medical field. Valuable input into the answers in solving these problems must also come from doctors. Finally, we understand the reluctance of our federal and state leaders to allow physician input because of conflict-of-interest concerns. Granted, doctors to this point have thwarted the intrusion of government into the practice of medicine. They have been handcuffed with regulations, paperwork, and fee regulations. However, most all of them agree that a change in our system is necessary. Furthermore, many, by virtue of experience and wisdom, would be valuable contributors to healthcare reform. Just as the government asks the engineers in the aerospace industry to build celestial navigation systems for spacecraft, so should they ask the doctors to help build a sound healthcare system.
>
> Not only is there a potential pool of active, willing, concerned physicians that would like to participate in shaping healthcare reform, but there is also a reservoir of retired academic and private practitioners out there who would be neither encumbered by financial conflicts nor restricted by time constraints who would be invaluable in shaping up this reform. In any event, I hope this is done with deep forethought and not just in haste to get something before the American people.
>
> I liken this unrestricted spending on healthcare monies to a black hole in the cosmos, where the unlimited intense gravitational force not only can bend light waves but also is capable of devouring infinite quantities of spatial debris fed into it.

This article was enthusiastically endorsed by the local medical community. It was later forwarded to the editors of the Journal of the Florida Medical Association, and, in the spring of 1994, I received the FMA's First Place Award for Best Guest Editorial. Such an overwhelming acceptance of this endeavor by my state-wide peers was humbling, indeed. However, there is a downside to this story. The editor of our Capital Medical Society Newsletter, after asking my consent, chose to send the article under his own cover-letter to Ms. Clinton. Our attempts to get the attention of either Ms. Clinton or the two state senators fell upon deaf ears. Despite the support of the Florida

Medical Association —we were not given the time of day in Washington, D.C.

~~~

Now, in turning to a subject of interest to most sports enthusiasts, the fall of 1993 was an exciting time for football fans in Tallahassee. In addition to a superb defense, Florida State possessed an offensive machine which would efficiently march down the field time and time again under the direction of its talented quarterback, Charlie Ward. Known as the "fast-break offense," opponents found it difficult to stop and frequently were subjected to a rout. As a fan, it was fun to watch Ward as he spotted his receivers all over the gridiron. If none were open he would react, "quick as a cat," in running for the necessary yardage to obtain a first down. At season's end, Charlie Ward received the Heisman trophy as college football's most outstanding player for 1993. Also, after winning the ACC conference, the team was invited to play Nebraska in the Orange bowl to decide the national champion. On January 1, 1994, with Ward engineering the scoring drives, combined with a stout defense and Scott Bentley's four field goals, the Seminoles beat the Cornhuskers 18 to 16 to claim their first National Championship.

~~~

Early in 1995 Frank approached me concerning the Bryan Robinson Neuroscience Foundation. Since 1979 when Bryan had passed away, Frank had been president of the Board. Now he was retiring and was planning to move away from Tallahassee. After discussing future changes in the Robinson Foundation with the other board members who were prominent local citizens, he requested that Dr. David Robinson, Bryan's son and a local internist, Dr. Fred Vroom, one of our clinic's neurologists, and I sit down as newly appointed board members. We all graciously accepted and so began our tenure in continuing what Bryan and Frank had begun many years previously. While the Bryan Robinson Neurological Foundation was a distinct entity for many years, it later became conjoined with the Tallahassee Memorial Hospital Foundation as the B.W. Robinson Memorial Endowment for the Neurosciences. After its inception, the primary mission of the foundation had always been in the support of neurological nursing education at TMH and the procurement of advanced equipment for the hospital. Going forward in the late 90s the focus of the endowment turned to a program of awarding small research grants to promising neuroscience research fellows, primarily at the University of Florida at Gainesville and at Florida State University. To honor any given current year's grant recipients, an annual awards dinner is held at the hospital. In addition, outstanding recipients from the prior year (and their respective professors) are asked to update us on the current status of their acknowledged research and to enlighten us on their future scientific objectives. Throughout the years I have found reviewing these research projects not only to be both personally enlightening and intellectually stimulating but have also been inspired by the enthusiasm of all of the researchers and professors during their presentations. As board members we become participants in helping to support and encourage the work of some of the future neuroscientists of America. Much of this research, usually weighted in neuroanatomy and physiology, genetics and molecular biology, aims at the root causes of some of our most perplexing neurological conditions, such as Alzheimer's disease, ALS (Lou Gehrig's disease) and stroke, to name but a few. Having continued this endeavor well into my retirement years, I think all of the board members would agree with me that this has been a very worthwhile investment of time.

~~~

Despite my premature departure from the practice of neurosurgery, Valencia and I remained optimistic about the prospects for the future and enjoyed life to its fullest. While both of us worked long days— she in nursing and I at the ranch— we were always together on off-time, continuing to enjoy our animals, the outdoors, and traveling. We even briefly took up skiing when visiting my sons in Washington state, something I had always wanted to do but could never afford as a youngster growing up in Colorado.

But then in early 1995, after we had just become comfortably established in our newly constructed home, Valencia developed a persistent cough. For years I had tried unsuccessfully to get her to stop smoking and passed the cough off as nothing more than due to cigarette irritation. After several weeks of showing no improvement, we deemed it
~~~

advisable to obtain a chest x-ray and scheduled an appointment to see our family internist.

On a Friday, the day the chest film was to be taken, I was working at the farm, when later in the morning my stepson drove up. He said, "You need to call Dr. Bailey right away." My heart began to race as I hastily jumped into my truck and drove to a nearby neighbor's home to use his phone. The reason for my sudden alarm was simply because Dr. Bailey was not our primary internist but rather a lung specialist. With my ear pressed tightly to the phone, I heard him say, "Jim, things don't look good at all. Valencia has a lung tumor." Overwhelmed by life's darkest fear and nearly speechless, I vividly recall uttering… "Bud, what you are saying has just destroyed our lives." For the remainder of that weekend, I was so distraught and anorexic that I scarcely ate a morsel of food and seemed to walk around in a daze. Deep within myself, I helplessly felt a growing void. I was unable to deny my agonizing thoughts or to avoid the prospects of the painful medical truths with which we were confronted. While trying to disguise my deep concern, I was very cognizant of the dismal prognosis for surviving even one year with cancer of the lung, should that prove to be the definitive diagnosis. The following Wednesday a needle biopsy confirmed my worst expectation.

After the initial shock we, like other positive human beings with faith and courage, set out to conquer this horrible disease. As a first line of defense, the surgeons elected to perform a thoracotomy in hopeful anticipation of resecting that portion of the lung harboring the neoplasm. But during the exposure, the tumor was found to have spread to the regional lymph nodes, and the surgeons did nothing further than to close the incision. Postoperatively as Valencia was wheeled into her hospital room, still in a deep stupor, I embraced her, whereupon she uttered into my ear… "Honey, as I was waking up, I overheard the doctors in the operating room say that the lymph nodes were positive." There were no longer any prospects of withholding the grim prognosis from this very intelligent lady with an abundance of medical acumen.

Over the next few weeks my wife received a full course of irradiation therapy to the chest, but both she and I knew this would merely be palliative in slowing the tumor growth and would not eradicate it. Meanwhile, I had heard that there was ongoing experimental clinical research at the University of Texas regarding immunotherapy for cancer. We contacted the investigators there, and they sent us a protocol containing the criteria for admission into their study. But we were later hit with yet another crushing bit of adverse news: Valencia didn't qualify for the study, because of her poor immune response to the required intradermal injection of test antigens as administered locally by Dr. Bailey.

As a source of diversion from the treatment that summer, I took her first to see Thomas Jefferson's home in Charlottesville and then on to Washington, D.C. on what I used to call "The All-American Tour," years ago when taking my children there. We saw just about everything and spent days-on-end in the Smithsonian Institution alone. However, I began to notice that she was faltering and was losing her endurance when walking around all of those historic buildings and monuments.

After we returned to Tallahassee late in the summer we began looking at houses on the weekends. It was something light and fun for us to do as an escape from the reality of all that we were now facing. One day while perusing a real estate magazine, she spotted a rather large, gorgeous home with majestic white columns in the front, reminiscent of those designed by Thomas Jefferson both at his home at Monticello and at the University of Virginia. Having just returned from seeing those beautiful structures that summer, we were intrigued with the likeness to them of this home right here in Tallahassee. Valencia begged me to drive her over to look at the place one Sunday afternoon, and, after a tour, she fell immediately in love with it. Her heart was clearly set on having that home to call our own. While it was a house whose beauty almost anyone would have appreciated, I felt that it was far more than either we needed or could afford. But I must simply ask… how do you say "no" to someone whom you love so very much, and whom you desperately don't want to lose? I thought to myself… perhaps this magnificent home is just the medicine she needs! Possibly it will give her that positive host response necessary to fight off the cancer. That healing potion consists of distraction, happiness, and a strong motivation to live on — despite the formidable odds. We made the sellers an offer, and were able to obtain a mortgage to swing the deal. Valencia's smile, which could light up a room, again returned. During that process she and I again found happiness. To once again quote the East German pilot— we were "looking only forward."

Then several weeks later after returning home from a hard day at the farm, and while I embraced her at the door, she asked me to feel her neck. She thought there might be a "lump." As I palpated in the area above her clavicle, I was mortified to find a very hard, enlarged, sentinel lymph gland. As a physician familiar with cancer, it was unmistakable that this node was pathologic. The fear and desperation experienced months previously overwhelmed me once again. The cancer was no longer localized to the chest but had now escaped to involve her entire petite and fragile body. Things suddenly became hopeless. While trying not to outwardly telegraph my feelings — yet weeping inside— I held her tightly and kissed her cheek.

The next 6-8 weeks were hectic. We began chemotherapy with all of its side effects, and, with a sense of extreme urgency, I tried to concurrently prepare our new home for occupancy. Once she began the intravenous anti-cancer medications, she began to fail rapidly. It then became a race against time, not to save her life which was impossible at that point, but to buy precious time for her to enjoy her remaining months in the home of her dreams. During one of her chemotherapy sessions in which she was hospitalized, I had the nurses hang a large framed picture of our new home on the hospital wall by her bed. When people would enter the room, she would point to the picture, and, in her soft weakened voice, would proudly say, "My husband bought that house for me."

I had painters, electricians and wallpaper hangers stumbling all over each other while working under a rigid timetable. Finally, at the time of the move, I paid for two moving vans, working simultaneously, to get the job done in one day. Once having moved in, I then hired one of my best hospital operating room technicians, who also owned a cleaning service, to bring in his crew and clean things up to make it livable.

While purchasing and moving into this beautiful home was quite an achievement, it sadly didn't change the course of my wife's relentless illness. Eight weeks after we moved in, and shortly after celebrating her 41st birthday, she passed away. It was devastating beyond words. I had lost the one I had come to love so very, very much.

A suffocating loneliness and reactive depression consumed me for months to follow, draping over me like a pall. Neither the bright rays of sunshine nor the joy expressed by shoppers in the mall could any longer energize me. When seeing friends out in public, I would avoid them. In short— there was no reason for happiness, for I had seemingly lost all that mattered. I would gladly have traded all of my earthly possessions just to once again see her smile for but a moment. I visited her grave-site daily for no less than 22 months and found it difficult to get anything else accomplished. The loneliness of trying to manage all of those cattle in the vast open fields day after day without her at my side was almost more than I could tolerate, only to return to an equally lonely house at night. There was no escaping the loss of a major part of my very heart and soul.

I kept recalling that while sitting at Valencia's bedside during her last remaining days, I had read in his biography of Thomas Jefferson's reaction to his wife's premature death.

> To quote Jefferson, … "From 1793 to 1797 I remained closely at home, saw none but those who came there, and at length became very sensible of the ill effect it had upon my mind, and of its direct and irresistible tendency to render me unfit for society and uneasy when necessarily engaged in it"(26).

Recognizing the ill effects that his own melancholy was having upon him enabled Jefferson to eventually recover; he resumed his greatness while becoming the third president of the United States three years later in 1800.

Finding sources of comfort, such as my self-identification with Jefferson's experience, can embolden one to recover. Similarly, I found it very consoling in speaking with friends who had overcome their own emotionally-crippling losses. They served to aid my healing in a very positive way. This is not to say that we shall ever forget a departed loved one, but we must learn (although often with great difficulty) to live with the loss. As most of us know, grieving after the death of a loved one is a normal process and must be dealt with before recovery can begin. Despite recognizing this, and as a physician who had helped so many deal with their own grief, it was no easier for me. Nonetheless, the dark cloud eventually lifted, and the sun again began to shine.

Honoring her personal request, I established the Valencia B. Geissinger Endowment for Behavioral Health at Tallahassee Memorial Hospital in 1998. I have since felt that this was probably one of the better things I have ever done in my life, not only by contributing to the TMH Foundation, but also by perpetuating her name as a part of the medical center for many years thereafter.

Two of Valencia's children continued to live with me in the big house until their educations were complete. Her daughter, Angela, later married after finishing nursing school but will always remain a close member of my family. She is a woman possessing the virtues of the highest integrity, a strong work ethic, and a keen empathy for the feelings of others; qualities appreciated by both her peers at the workplace and her family at home. I have been extremely proud of her.

ELEVEN

A Fork in the Road

~~~

After having spent well over one quarter of a century in medicine after graduation from medical school, I was eventually able to reconcile the fact that I would pursue an alternative vocation.

During the early nineties, substantial progress was made in the development of our ranch operation. At the Pavo site we not only re-fenced the circumference of the entire 152 acres but also constructed important cross-fencing as well. This provided us with four large independent fields not only for purposes of rotational grazing but also allowed for the provision of isolated bull-cow breeding units. One quickly learns that standard wire fence, no matter how substantial, will fail to keep the powerful large herd sires from breaking through and fighting, hence, the rationale for reinforcing any common fence between two fields with high-voltage electric wire. As a source of power for the 7,000- volt electric fence, a neighbor let me tap into his electric grid in the loft of his barn and run the line over to my property.

A spacious three-pen corral was centrally located with access from all of the fields and was gated in such a manner that the cattle could be driven into it from any given pasture for purposes of separating and working them, or running them down a loading chute into a trailer. Also, large tanks within each of the pens served as independent water sources for the respective pastures.

When speaking of water, one project looms indelibly in my mind. Without any available help, I constructed a 1,200-foot pipeline from the well pump down a hill to the corral. Even though I rented a power trencher, it was another one of those brutal jobs carried out in the hot, humid, Southeast with insects and thick, sticker bushes fighting me every step of the way.
~~~

Despite years of hard work, my re-shaping of this Georgia landscape gave me a great sense of accomplishment, the newly renovated spread subsequently proving to be a very efficient, safe environment in which to carry out my cattle operation for years to come. I can not begin to describe the sense of pride I felt standing on a hill, overlooking my own expanse of pastureland containing its segregated units of beautiful cattle serenely grazing on the thick, nutritious grass.

Further south at the Monticello ranch, significant progress was made as well. By having the power company eventually bring in a line, we were not only able to operate two deep wells as independent water sources, but, like the Georgia farm, were able to isolate the various pastures with electric fencing. However, with the expansion of the herd it seemed as if there was an ever-increasing need for more equipment, the sum of which translating into much more work in any given week. For instance, instead of buying high-protein winter feed for the calves, we began grinding our own by combining cottonseed and corn; consequently, the need arose for a grinding mill, several wagons and another tractor. Admittedly, I have always enjoyed farm equipment, and, like woodworking tools, I always seemed to find an excuse to buy more of it.

I used to drive my F-150 pickup truck over to a cotton gin in Georgia and load my peanut wagon with up to nine tons of cotton seed. As I hauled it back one time, I experienced two of the wagon's tires simultaneously blowing out, causing a few moments of terror. Had not those blown tires been on opposite sides of the huge, heavy wagon, we surely would have turned over in the middle of the highway. The full wagon weighed over four times as much as the truck and was connected merely with a simple tongue and ball hitch.

A second smaller John Deere tractor was also purchased to help facilitate the haying operation. As previously mentioned, after adequate drying, the hay must be expeditiously raked and bailed to prevent spoilage when the afternoon showers arrive. While that may be the ideal situation, it seldom works out as expected. Not only might the weatherman be wrong in his forecast, but equipment has a nasty way of breaking down at the most inopportune times. I can't begin to count the times that, while in the middle of some type of field-work, I would sense the unmistakable odor of leaking hydraulic fluid. There are innumerable seals and hydraulic lines susceptible to leakage and rupture on all of these pieces of heavy equipment. Sometimes the problem can be repaired on the spot within hours, but more often it means a day or two. In the case of a mechanical breakdown after having already cut the hay, there were occasions in which I lost an entire cutting (translating into thousands of dollars) when the rain began to fall. Meanwhile, the tractor or baler sat idle in the shop awaiting repair.

When speaking of putting up hay, I am reminded of an interesting experience worth sharing. On a warm, sunny mid-summer afternoon, while in the midst of raking my dried hay, I spotted a healthy-sized Eastern diamondback rattlesnake crawling into one of the hay windrows. After marking the spot, I hurried to the barn to obtain a rake and from the truck my .44 magnum pistol. Wondering if the snake was still there I quickly returned to the site. Sure enough, as I raked away the hay the poisonous reptile came slithering out. While I waited patiently for that perfect shot, he sensed me and coiled up on an area of freshly cut grass, preparing to strike. One learns from experience that it is best to patiently kill the animal with a single well-placed bullet. The unpleasant alternative is missing with a hurried shot and having to chase him around haphazardly, as he continues to crawl and dangerously hide under the piles of hay. After I fired that shot with the powerful revolver, his head lay separated from the still-writhing body. As I curiously bent over to closely inspect what I thought was his inert head with open eyes— his fanged jaws suddenly sprang widely open with lightning speed! The force generated by the jaws against the ground both rotated and lifted his head toward me in a threatening move. The menacing head was not only alive, but deliberately attempted a last strike when it visually perceived danger. I have since recounted this eerie, unsettling, experience to others, one person relating to me that he was aware of a similar incident in which the unwary observer was actually envenomed.

~~~

Long after Valencia passed away, it seemed that I continued to work even harder at the ranch, becoming increasingly obsessed with making a "go of it." Because she was no longer at home to greet me at the end of the day, I had no incentive to embark on the 26- mile ride home in the evening and often worked until total darkness fell.
~~~

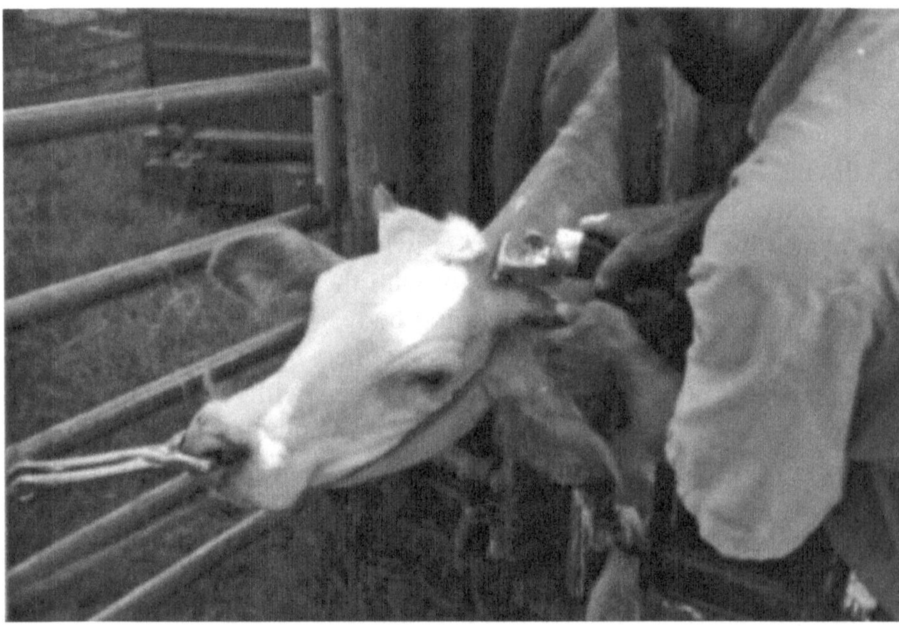

The Rancher

Preparing for a de-horning operation.

But despite all of the intense labor and expense, it seemed that I was consistently beset with bad luck. After a few years, I decided to have my herd evaluated by the BBU (Beefmaster Breeders Universal) inspector out of Texas. With the realization of having heavily invested in cows with sound genetics and bulls of a similar constitution, I could hardly wait for the inspector's conclusion. But both to my surprise and great dismay, he found all kinds of unsound characteristics within the progeny of my herd, and they graded out as mediocre. What I proudly had thought was an exemplary herd of Beefmaster cattle was nothing more than average in the eyes of that critical examiner.

Furthermore, there appeared to be some serious problems regarding my expensive bulls. One herd sire which I had purchased out of Texas, while visibly an attractive, muscular red bull, seemed to prefer eating grass all day as opposed to breeding with his group of open females. After his first sub-standard breeding season, I loaded him into the trailer and hauled him up to a reputable veterinarian in Moultrie, Georgia. After a physical examination and semen analysis, it was concluded that one of his testicles had been destroyed and was atrophied (most likely from having been kicked). What's more, the other gland was deficient in both the quantity and quality of the sperm it produced. I had to realize an expensive loss on that day he rambled out of my trailer at the stockyards. Bulls are good for one thing only, and it is financially not feasible to feed them all year if they fail to settle the cows. Recall that "fertility" is one of the Beefmaster Six Essentials.

Then there was my expensive, prized, herd sire jointly purchased with Fred Thompson several years previously at the big "Cow-Town Classic" sale in Dallas-Fort Worth. He was an enormous, showcase animal with feet reminiscent of a small elephant's in size, and testicles that rivaled tennis balls. One Saturday morning, while relaxing in Tallahassee from a tough week's work, I received a frantic phone call from my friend, Banner Lee, in Pavo. He said, "Jim, Crossmatch has a swollen infected sheath. It has been dragging on the ground in the dirt, and he has been stepping on it." For those readers unfamiliar with bulls, the business end of a breeding bull is not to be confused with a good-looking head and broad shoulders. In a somewhat desperate attempt to preserve this elegant-appearing animal's breeding potential, I took a day off from work and trucked him up to the College of Veterinary Medicine at Auburn University in Alabama. Because of his "pendulous sheath" they recommended the animal be circumcised. With all of that having been said and done, his deformity was nicely corrected by the veterinary surgeons, but he was never to regain his prowess as a herd sire. We eventually had to send him "down-the-line" to the meatpacking house just like the red bull.

Because the majority of the young bulls which I produced also possessed pendulous sheaths like their sire, Crossmatch, they failed to bring a premium dollar irrespective of where I sold them. Similarly, my two-year-old females, also lacking a trim underline, failed to bring a top price when taken to a prominent Beefmaster sale in Tifton, Georgia. After several calf crops, it became painfully evident that I was not getting a good return on my initial investment in these expensive animals.

There comes a time almost like a "point of no return" in the cattle business. Not only had I invested substantially in the land, equipment and animals but also in a great deal of time and effort in building up this small cattle breeding enterprise. I found myself at a cross-road, namely, at a point in time to re-evaluate my position in this business. While perhaps an unrealistic expectation, it was inherent in my personal makeup to persevere in meeting this new career challenge. After further consideration, my future goals in the Beefmaster business consisted of both expanding the size of my herd, and simultaneously striving even harder for breed improvement. I was determined to "breed out" any undesirable genetic traits in the future progeny of my cattle.

To this end, I first attended a national Beefmaster Breeders Symposium at Texas A&M University in College Station. It was a three-day well-attended educational event, and I came away very optimistic. Subsequently, while keeping both sound genetics and the Six Essentials in mind, I later upgraded my herd with additional high quality female base cows. Ultimately, I envisioned having four premium "bull breeding units" each of which was to consist of an exemplary herd sire and twenty five base cows.

One of the premium quality herd sires proposed was to be the son, through artificial insemination, of a nationally well-recognized, yet now deceased bull named "Mountain Man." Before his death, this bull's valuable semen had been extensively collected and preserved, to later be made available for purchase by Beefmaster breeders throughout the nation. The cattle literature supported his strong genetic traits by promoting his sons who had exceptional conformation themselves, and who consistently sired quality calves with high weaning weights. I flew out to San Antonio and drove to the ranch where the Mountain Man bull had lived, and where he had been immortalized with a monument. I purchased one of his branded, registered sons, whom I named Piton after the metal mountain-climbing spike.

To procure the other three highly-valued herd sires, I planned later that year to fly to San Angelo, Texas. That was the site of the Lasater Ranch, owned and operated by Lawrence Lasater, the son of the founder of the Beefmaster breed, Tom Lasater. It was October, 1996, when I flew out to the Lasater Ranch in great anticipation of their high-volume Beefmaster bull sale. To this cattleman it was an exhilarating experience renting a car at the airport and driving over to the large expanse of stock pens harboring an impressive collection of attractive bulls that were to be auctioned the following morning. Immediately after climbing out of the car, I was greeted by the very personable Mr. Lasater. I took great pleasure in shaking the hand of the man who carries the name synonymous with the Beefmaster breed. Laurie was not only a preeminent, well-respected cattleman but a fine person who could be rightfully proud of carrying-forth what his father had begun during the earlier part of the 20th century.

I well remember spending the entire Friday afternoon and early evening hours intensely studying the premier bulls to be auctioned off on Saturday morning. Time and again I would re-inspect those animals in which I was most interested, focusing on their overall conformation to the breed and their traits for reproductive efficiency. An informative catalog had been provided, outlining the pedigrees and the time-measured weight gains for each animal in the sale. Of paramount importance to me were the genetic backgrounds of this impressive group of prospective herd sires, which presented no potential inbreeding conflicts with any of my own base cows. Through a process of elimination I was eventually able to scale down my choices, often walking around alone within the pens while within arm's length of these behemoths. That by itself makes a strong statement as to the "disposition" of these gentle beasts. Considering there were hundreds of bulls on display, it wasn't a simple task picking out exactly what I wanted— but it certainly was fun! At the auction ring the next morning, I was very fortunate to have bid successfully on those three animals which I thought best suited for my herd, especially given the highly competitive nature of the auction. I could hardly wait to get them trucked back to Monticello to join Piton.

On Sunday morning after the sale, several of us were invited to take a grand tour of the Lasater ranch which in itself was an experience. One can only imagine driving for miles upon end through a great expanse of well-fenced pastureland with exemplary animals scattered about grazing. To this day I can envision those large groups of lengthy, voluminous females with perfect conformation, which had allowed them to drop and nurse the robust calves seen at their sides. Worthy of emphasis is that the very nature of this business is founded upon good genetics, and the ability for the females to produce large quantities of milk, accordingly raising sturdy heavy calves who will later command a premium price on the market.

The weekend came to a close with a delicious, farewell steak dinner in which we all enjoyed the camaraderie. This was certainly a very positive experience not only to observe a gold-standard cattle operation but also in associating with some very fine people as well — a memorable weekend in the cattle business.

~~~

Thus far I have written primarily about my vocations of neurosurgery and cattle ranching. Now I have a story which encompasses both.

A friend of mine, Hank Pollard, was the ranch foreman of a rather prominent cattle operation east of Monticello. He was the man who, twelve years previously, had first ignited my interest in the Beefmaster breed. Considered by many as one of the most knowledgeable cattleman in Florida, I would often confer with him regarding questions of herd management.

I hadn't seen Hank for quite some time after my retirement, when one day his wife called me at home on the phone. She sounded very concerned while relating to me that her husband had not been acting normally for several weeks. Although she couldn't precisely put her finger on the problem, she claimed that he just "wasn't mentally himself." In view of the fact that Hank had already recently seen his primary physician who could find nothing wrong with him, Janet asked if I would please examine her husband.

The following morning, I called him up out at the ranch where he was employed and asked if it would be convenient that morning for me to check him over. He hesitated for a moment before saying that he was quite busy, further adding that it was imperative that he work a large group of cattle in the holding pens in order to get them segregated. After a moment of silence he then replied that, once finished, he would then be happy to comply with his wife's request for an examination. Later in the
~~~

morning, I drove thirty- five miles over there from Tallahassee with medical instruments in hand, fully anticipating his work would be done by the time of my arrival. To the contrary, I found him struggling all alone, fervently trying to complete his work. He was so preoccupied with this rough, rowdy bunch of cows that he didn't even initially notice my presence. He was fussing with the large heavy gates, while at the same time trying to segregate a group of unruly animals storming around in every which direction. Being all too familiar with the frustration of one man trying to do the job of several, I approached the corral to offer my assistance. We then teamed up, and, working together, we eventually got the cattle appropriately separated out, much to Hank's relief.

After catching our breath and a drink of cool water, we strolled up to the ranch foreman's small office building, where I prepared to open up my small black bag. It had already become apparent to me while watching Hank work the cattle that he seemed sluggish and reacted slowly to the incessantly charging, obstreperous animals. Normally, one must be decisive and act quickly in diverting the cows through the cumbersome, swinging steel gates. Also I had noted his marginal agility in coordinating the gross movements of his extremities. This can be a dangerous occupation under the best of circumstances, and the cowman must be very facile in the use of his arms and legs to remain out of harm's way.

Once inside the ranch office, the most notable finding was the flatness of Hank's affect; namely, he had a loss of appropriate emotional response. Also quite apparent to me, he was both generally slow in his motor and verbal responses and had a tendency to gaze off into space with a vacant stare. On the other hand there was no evidence of any type of paralysis or visual disturbance. In relating to me his more recent medical history, he disclosed that several weeks previously he had severely "bumped" his head on the heavy steel squeeze-chute. Although neither headaches nor other subjective symptoms had been a particular problem, it was several days after that particular incident that his wife began to notice changes in his demeanor. Having known Hank for fifteen years, my findings represented a distinct change in him. Considering the timing of the relevant history of head trauma followed by the progressive nature of his symptoms, I felt strongly that he was probably harboring a chronic subdural hematoma. In fact, I was so certain of the diagnosis that I immediately called Jenny at the neurological clinic from my truck cell-phone, telling her that Hank was going to need surgery that afternoon. In the meantime he needed an emergency MRI scan, and the neurosurgeon on-call alerted that the patient was on his way to Tallahassee.

By that afternoon Hank was whisked into the operating room at TMH for removal of what proved to be an unusually large chronic subdural hematoma, the mass causing a dangerous shift of his brain. This enormous lesion had, indeed, posed an imminent threat to my friend's life. The liquefied clot was successfully evacuated, but Hank's postoperative course was a stormy one, marked by recurrent runs of grand mal convulsions. The violent seizures were eventually brought under control with medications, and his ultimate recovery complete.

Hank subsequently left the cattle business and began teaching at Florida A&M University, where he has since remained. Through the years I have spoken several times with my friend and his wife, who are both understandably very appreciative of what was done to diagnose and reverse the course of his serious illness. When recounting this story to both the Pollards and to others, I have often concluded by saying, "I'm probably the only neurosurgeon in existence who physically helped a rancher work his unruly cattle in a holding-pen minutes prior to diagnosing a dangerous intracranial mass." At the very least — it makes for a good cowboy story.

~~~

Before closing the book on CNS trauma, let me comment on the important subject of cerebral concussion, and how it relates to the overall spectrum of brain injury. The long-term ill-effects of having received multiple concussive blows to the head, recognized for years in the sport of boxing, are now being recognized with increasing frequency in football players.

As critical background anatomical information, there exists within the core of the brainstem an assembly of special "arousal" neurons that lead to higher brain centers, their influence ultimately "projecting" to the frontal lobes. This "reticular activating system," as it is called, is the brain's alerting system, and is of key importance in determining wakefulness and sleep. Early in the 20th century, neuroscientists demonstrated that if this multi-synaptic nerve pathway is surgically interrupted in experimental animals, they will remain in a persistent state of sleep.
~~~

If during a head injury the cranium is either set in motion when accelerated after a forceful blow or abruptly decelerated upon striking an object, the brain, being the consistency of gelatin, will actually become distorted within the skull. In so doing, the reticular system of neurons will be momentarily physiologically interrupted, and will "shut down." The ensuing state is one of disrupted cognitive brain activity or even a total loss of consciousness. After a variable period of time, these "stunned" neurons will resume functioning, whereupon the individual will again begin to recover. Bearing this concept clearly in mind, we used to think of concussion in purely physiological terms which, in the strictest sense of the word, does not in itself portend structural brain injury. We have subsequently learned, however, that there is often much more going on in the brain at the time of an impact than merely the "off-on" quality of consciousness. When examining the brains of persons who have repeatedly received concussive blows to the head, investigators have found microscopic evidence of permanently injured neurons.

To carry the analysis one step further, there is evidence that there are "lesser" degrees of concussion which may be manifested by such symptoms as headache, dizziness and disorientation. In point of fact it has been estimated that a complete loss of consciousness probably occurs in perhaps only 10% of the total concussed group. This then begs the very important question: Of the remaining 90% of individuals with "milder concussions," what is the incidence of permanent neuronal injury?

Because of this anatomically documented correlation between a succession of concussive blows to the head and permanent brain damage, the medical recommendation of abstaining from this contact sport after three concussions can now be appreciated. Furthermore, the total magnitude of cumulative injuries resulting in irreversible harm may not become apparent for many years thereafter.

Intense scientific and social interest is being generated to study this problem in football players in an effort to understand and, hopefully, eliminate the syndrome of "chronic traumatic encephalopathy." One area of clinical research being contemplated is to establish normal baseline cognitive data in athletes before competition, thus allowing post-injury evaluation in terms of degree and permanency. This information can be correlated retrospectively with the number and extent of concussive symptoms. These data in turn could be implemented in future areas of injury prevention. In addition, closer attention will be paid to the head-injured athlete on the playing field. He will no longer be able to decide for himself to reenter the game, and "play through" an injury to the head as he might have done with a bruised shoulder or a cramp in his thigh. It has been expressed by those knowledgeable on this subject that, in the years ahead, we are going to see major changes in the way the game of football is played.

A second critical point to be made concerns the relationship between concussion and subdural hemorrhage. In lecturing to the family practice resident doctors, I always tried to make the following point: If the forces causing brain movement during acceleration/deceleration are of such magnitude as to cause a concussion, those same forces can certainly cause shearing of bridging veins to the brain, leading to subdural hemorrhage. This is precisely why anyone who has had a concussion should be observed closely for any later headache and/or deterioration of function. One of the causes of the "talk and die" syndrome is to overlook the situation in which the victim initially loses consciousness from the blow to the head (concussion), later awakens to function, but over the course of time, he again deteriorates and dies from an intracranial hematoma.

This concept, while always important in any concussed individual, becomes particularly important in rural America, where time and distance to the nearest scanning facility and neurosurgeon may be problematic. Under those conditions during a Friday night football game in which a young player sustains a head injury, the coaches and family alike must maintain a keen sense of awareness as to possible sequelae beyond those of a simple concussion and allow time for medical intervention, lest it be too late.

After this discussion, some of the cases described in the book probably now become more meaningful. For instance, there was the toddler whose head was run over by the car; yet, he did not lose consciousness—simply because the cranium was pinned down, the brain being constrained from movement.

And then there was the cowboy, Hank Pollard, who struck his head a severe, decelerating blow on the steel cattle chute. While Hank didn't get into trouble with the slow, accumulation of subdural blood and fluid for several weeks (later being saved by a craniotomy); he could have easily ended up a "talk and die" victim.

~~~
~~~

Because the ranch was now a full-time occupation, the next several years were focused on trying to make an earnest "go" of it. In so doing, one quickly learns to develop "tough skin." By failing to describe some of the adversities facing the rancher, I would be remiss in presenting the reader with an accurate picture of farm life. In contrast to the hospital environment in which the surgeon is provided the luxury of anything that he might need, the rancher can only rely on himself in his struggle with nature's many forces.

Such a seemingly straight forward task as maintaining one's fences becomes ever so consuming. If neglected for even a short period of time, what initially appear to be merely small, nuisance weeds profusely grow into thick, towering, plants or even trees. The trees eventually become inextricably entwined within the wire of the fence, and, if ignored for just a few years, the fence will lose its structural integrity. Eventually, the entire mess must be laboriously bulldozed down, removed, and replaced by an entirely new enclosure. If the problem is never addressed, the branches of any ingrown trees begin to encroach on the periphery of the field, making it both cumbersome and dangerous to drive a tractor beneath them when cultivating or mowing. The alternative to "doing nothing" is to spray the fence rows annually with powerful, sometimes environmentally unfriendly, herbicides. Chemicals that may work for one year or two may become ineffective, after which resistant weeds then begin to grow. Despite herbicides that are increasingly more powerful, expensive, and toxic to the person applying them, there often emerge dense woody-stemmed, thorny plants that one can almost never eradicate. I have even gone so far as to try, unsuccessfully, to burn them out. Keeping in mind this annoying, ongoing problem, imagine its total magnitude when applied to literally "miles" of fence rows.

Because ranching essentially deals with biological systems, there exist many parallels with the practice of medicine. The well-recognized phenomenon of such systems becoming resistant to pesticides (analogous to bacterial resistance to antibiotics) is a serious problem for the rancher, not only with regard to weeds but to insects as well.

Years after having established my hayfield, I would often stand by the barn on the hill overlooking the field, mesmerized by the tall, blue-green Bermuda grass undulating with the early morning breeze sweeping through it. One can't begin to appreciate the investment of time, effort, and expense in preparing the soil, planting, and later fertilizing the grass to establish such a field. Then one summer day, early in my haying career, I noted that the hay had seemed to have lost its green luster.

Thinking no more of it, I left town for a medical meeting. Upon returning only one week later, the entire field had suddenly turned brown — as if wiped out by a hard winter frost. Close inspection revealed countless thousands of swarming small green worms, consuming every last viable blade of grass. I was to soon find out that these insects were the larvae of moths, and because of their propensity to march relentlessly forward and so consume an entire field within days they were called Army worms. The next time these pests first made their appearance evident on the freshly grown hay, I sprayed the field with a potent chemical known to kill them. After two seasons of fighting this recurring larva, I figured into my schedule a spraying routine early each July when the worms usually showed up. But with increasing frustration, the magnitude of the problem only escalated; after several subsequent seasons, I found myself spraying up to four times each summer. Needless to say, this was not only demanding of my time, but also generated increasing costs for both chemicals and diesel fuel. Simply stated, the Army worms were becoming resistant to the chemical and were virtually taking over my valuable hayfield. With each passing year, the grass became sparser and began to permanently lose its vigor.

Citing these pest encounters doesn't begin to even touch the scope of problems testing the mettle of the rancher. Times of extensive drought not only lead to insufficient summer forage for grazing but also to reduced hay production for ensuing winter feed as well. I can recall one prolonged dry summer in which several farmers in our area, despite having vast acreage, had to sell their animals simply because the grass wasn't growing.

Another on-going problem concerns the deterioration and/or breakdown of farm equipment. The hot, humid, day-time atmosphere of the late spring and early fall followed by declining nighttime temperatures promotes concomitant heavy condensation of moisture. This in turn rapidly corrodes and deteriorates expensive equipment. I recall one year having paid $3,000 for a brand-new disc hay mower which, after only twelve months (even under the cover of the barn), was so rusty that it looked like something out of a junkyard. I tried to re-paint and even spray it frequently with protective oil and diesel fuel, but rust in the South is like a cancer. It would recur despite my well-intended efforts. In time, heavy metal may decompose in shale-like flakes, and the equipment must be discarded. Replacing it causes great anguish when the profit margin of farming is predictably so slim to begin with.

Speaking of equipment, there are incessant mechanical breakdowns and the customary exorbitant expenses of having things fixed. In constantly fighting all of these and many other adverse elements, both natural and human-induced, the farmer is often lucky just to break even. It is almost impossible for the small-time operator to financially get ahead in any meaningful way.

I have just mentioned but a few of the many, recurring problems encountered on a ranch, but I found strength in meeting those challenges and tenaciously tried to overcome them. At the end of the day, when all is said and done, there exist many positive intangible rewards in ranching which might include: feelings of great accomplishment when overcoming the innumerable obstacles; a strong sense of pride in the beauty of one's ranch and animals, and finally— a very healthy lifestyle. While enjoying my alternative occupation to the fullest, and despite any adversities, I elected to pursue it throughout the nineties and beyond.

~~~
~~~

TWELVE

A New Beginning

~~~

After having worked alone very intensively day after day for weeks upon end at the farm, I began to feel like a serious recluse. Then after several months, something fortuitously happened which greatly helped me through the grieving process of having lost my wife. A long-time friend, Bob Doherty, who had been a college fraternity brother and later my roommate at Northwestern in the late fifties, decided to retire in Florida. Bob had taught Arabic at the U.S. Military Academy at West Point for many years, while at the same time bolstering up his résumé with twelve postgraduate college degrees from several preeminent universities in the area. After his latest academic achievement, a law degree, he and his wife, Anneliese, came to visit me in Tallahassee. Liking the area very much they decided to retire here and ended up buying my old house. After purchasing the larger home for Valencia, I had been encumbered with two mortgages, and the Dohertys relieved me of one of them. It was to both of our advantages since they were strongly attracted to our beautiful former home which was located in a quiet, gated community. Having these good friends nearby helped me immensely to recover from my personal loss, and for years to come we were to have many wonderful times together.

Once I began to see my way out of the gloom of having lost Valencia, I eventually began to seek female companionship. I had always been a person who preferred the stable relationship that only marriage could offer. Even as a youngster my first natural choice seemed to be one steady girlfriend with whom I could pal around in sharing my experiences. One day in the late nineties I was introduced to a very attractive lady with a gorgeous smile and magnetic personality named Elaine. After having exited an unhappy first marriage several years
~~~

previously, she was seeking a trustworthy companion with whom to settle down. At the time Elaine had three children, Lisi, Natalia, and George, from her prior marriage. After nearly two years of courtship, she and I boarded a plane for Lake Tahoe where we were happily married on January 4, 1999.

Among other things, Elaine seriously rekindled my interest in snow skiing. It was not only an adventuresome form of recreation which we could enjoy together, but it also offered other advantages as well. We began to visit my sons and their families on an annual basis out in the state of Washington and would ski as a family. My younger son, Roger, previously a member of his high school ski team, was also very helpful in my progress on the slopes. There were four ski resorts within three hours of my sons' homes in Spokane. Much more important than the skiing, however, was my re-connecting with my boys, and mending the emotional wounds which had resulted from the divorce from their mother twelve years previously.

Elaine and I have always enjoyed traveling together and sharing the unique and often unexpected experiences. In 1998, Dr. Roy Barineau, a humanities professor at Tallahassee Community College, organized the first of two successive yearly trips abroad to the cradle of western civilization. In reflecting back to my undergraduate college days at Northwestern, one of my favorite courses was the history of the ancient world. It was taught by Dr. Carl Roebuck who was one of those rare, innately gifted teachers who could bring what many would consider a very dry subject into the students' lives as a most interesting and colorful story. At last, long after my retirement, I now had an opportunity to re-live that epoch of time which Professor Roebuck had so elegantly introduced to us so many years ago.

Our travel group consisted primarily of educators, several of them retired, plus other prominent citizens in our community, including a member of the Florida House of Representatives. We soon found ourselves to be a very congenial, adventuresome group with similar academic interests and senses of humor. Elaine and I were honored to share with them the wondrous experiences provided by traveling to both Egypt and Greece.

With all things considered, the adventure to Egypt was probably the most fascinating trip I have ever taken. Within hours after awakening on the day after our arrival, we found ourselves atop a camel, viewing in the distant desert the pyramids of Giza silhouetted against the rising sun. These majestic structures were built during the Fourth Dynasty (circa

2,500 B.C.) and are the only remaining intact structures of the "Seven Wonders of the World." An hour later we stood in awe at the base of those stone monuments and were given the opportunity to enter. An acute anxiety attack, induced by claustrophobia, precluded Elaine's descending more than a few feet down the dimly lit, confining, shoulder-width decline. Not to abandon this unique experience, I proceeded downward with the rest of our group into the deep subterranean bowels of the pyramid of Mycerinus. With enhanced illumination by a battery-operated minor's headlamp worn by a member of our tour group, we crawled on hands and knees through the damp, morbidly silent and eerie chambers from that far distant past. One could just imagine the excitement, years ago, as the archaeologists uncovered the marvelous artifacts from these same dark, stone corridors.

Later that morning we were bused south of Cairo to Saqqara, the site of the great step pyramid of the Pharaoh, Djoser. That structure, built in the Third Dynasty (circa 2,658 B.C.), was allegedly the first known pyramid in Egypt. It was designed by the great architect, Imhotep, who was also later deified as a healer. Of medical significance, the Greeks later equated Imhotep with their own god, Asklepios, an important piece of history which we amplify upon later (35).

The next week was spent sailing south "up" the Nile, interrupted by brief stops at several places of great historic interest. One such place was Karnak which, in covering some 250 acres, is considered the most remarkable religious complex ever built on earth (4). Highlighted among its many magnificent, bold stone structures are temples, chapels, columns, statues, obelisks and even an avenue lined with human-headed sphinxes.

Later, after sailing further south to Aswan, we saw a quarry where the gargantuan obelisks of antiquity had been chiseled from stone faces by multitudes of workers. These granite structures of incomprehensible weight, capped by pyramidions similar in appearance to but much smaller than the Washington Monument, were then loaded onto vessels, and shipped 100 miles north on the Nile to later be erected at Luxor. The technological achievement of this consummate feat of engineering, like the construction of the great pyramids themselves, remains extremely difficult to comprehend for such an early period in history.

The last leg of our journey took us to Abu-Simbel, the temple of the great Pharaoh Ramses II. Highlighting the façade of this temple are four 65 foot seated colossal statues of Ramses himself. Back at the Cairo Museum, on the day prior to our departure from Egypt, we observed in awe the actual mummy of Ramses II. Allegedly, this "greatest of the pharaohs" was the Egyptian leader at the biblical time when Moses directed the exodus of the enslaved Hebrews from Egypt. In essence, we momentarily imagined ourselves back in a time capsule — a spectrum in time embraced at one end by the colossal structures illuminating the power and deeds of the great pharaoh's during life, and at the other by their mummified remains. Within that time span is one of mankind's longest and most fascinating stories.

The trip to Greece was an equally enlightening experience. After initially flying to Athens and becoming acquainted with the area, our Grecian experience was then divided into two components: several days on a guided bus tour of the Peloponnese, followed by a cruise of the Greek islands.

On the first day, after crossing the Isthmus of Corinth, we visited the ruins of Mycenae. This was considered the most famous city of prehistoric Greece and the capital of the mythological great king, Agamemnon (49). Outside of the citadel of Mycenae we visited what is thought to be the most imposing example of Mycenaean architecture, the Treasury of Atreus, also known as the Tomb of Agamemnon (22). Students of ancient history will recall that Agamemnon organized the expedition against Troy in the epic Trojan War.

Our excursion then took us to Olympia, in many ways a nostalgic site to visit. Not only did we see the ruins of the great temple of Zeus, another of the Seven Wonders of the World, but also the Olympic complex as well. While much of the large complex of buildings was built in the fifth century B.C., the stadium, as we saw it, had been constructed in the fourth century B.C. We entered the stadium through the historic vaulted passage, and, while sitting in the sunshine on the ancient graded earthen embankment (said to have provided seating for 45,000 spectators) — we could for a moment vicariously imagine viewing the splendor of those early games (21).

Later in the land journey, we stood at the historic battle site at Thermopylae where King Leonidas and his 300 Spartans temporarily held back the massive Persian army led by Xerxes in the year 480 B.C. That engagement has always been considered one of the great strategic battles of all antiquity and the epitome of bravery against overwhelming odds.

Seemingly everywhere in Greece, whether visited by land or by sea, were places of great historical importance, but none is more relevant to this book than Epidaurus. For here was the epicenter of our medical heritage: the Cult of Asklepios. According to Struckmann, over a period of 1,000 years this cult expanded on an international scale, Epidaurus being its center (23).

As history tells us, the mythical son of Apollo, Asklepios, was later recognized as a demi-god by the Oracle of Delphi. This stimulated the wide acceptance of his cult which had been ordained as one of healing. After the devastating plague (429 B.C.) during the reign of the great Pericles, the cult of Asklepios took on an even greater meaning. Asklepios then became recognized as a savior, and it is said that the Greeks associated him with the great physician-healer, Imhotep, of Egypt. Statues of Asklepios reveal him carrying a staff around which is wound a snake. The staff symbolically represents fertility and power, hence, the god's power over life and death. The snake not only can determine life or death, but, because it sheds its skin, it equates to healing and immortality. The caduceus that symbolizes medicine today maintains the staff and the snake. Furthermore, the ancient Greek physicians were called *Asklepiadai* and felt they were descendants of Asklepios. Hippocrates, long thought of as "The Father of Medicine," was considered the 18th in succession to Asklepios (23).

In reflecting back to those early days at Northwestern, when Professor Roebuck unfolded the interesting story of the ancient world, little did I realize at the time that someday I would visit, in person, the geographic locale where our medical heritage had its origin.

~~~

Several years had passed during which I had no steady help at the farm. From time to time I would latch on to some unemployed young fellow in Jefferson County to help me with some of the heavy work, but, for the most part, I did everything by myself. Upon remarrying I found a new companion in Elaine who was a good sport at helping with some of the tasks such as grinding feed and driving the small tractor during hay harvesting. But simply stated, it is very hard, hot work, and she freely admits not only to being anxious that she might get hurt but also to a morbid fear of stinging insects and poisonous snakes.

After struggling together for a year or two at the ranch, I was fortunate to find an eager, energetic young man to help me almost any time I needed him. Alex was a successful building contractor in Tallahassee who had started up and managed a thriving business by his
~~~

mid-twenties. During the course of a conversation while he was doing some renovations at our house, he expressed a genuine interest in helping me at the ranch. In turn I would be his mentor and teach him all I knew about the ranching business. He also envisioned having a small cattle operation of his own someday. I proceeded to schedule large two-man jobs in such a way that, after first getting his own men settled into work, Alex could then be at my side for days at a time if necessary. This is best illustrated by the "cattle drives" up to Georgia in the spring and back to Monticello in the fall. Sometimes it would take as many as six trailer loads over two days just to get the mama cows all moved. Moreover, it takes two people to cut them out (i.e., to separate specific animals) and load them onto the trailer. To the novice this may not seem like much, but many are the problems encountered. The lead cow, for instance, might turn around in the trailer and try to exit against the flow of the others coming down the loading chute, which is only 2 feet wide. Once the cow is "stuck" in the narrow chute, there suddenly occurs a bi-directional impasse. As many as a dozen cows may then have to be backed up into the loading pen before starting the process all over. Or sometimes a cow might either lie down in the chute or get hung up over the side of it trying to jump out. Suffice it to say, there are a number of large, imposing bodies dangerously banging around, resulting in a great deal of yelling, whip-wielding and manure-sloshing during this rowdy process — quite the antithesis of working in a quiet, clean operating room at the hospital.

Another facet of the cattle business concerns the veterinary work, which incidentally must be done on a timely basis throughout the year. This necessitates first getting the grazing animals collected in the distant field(s) and then herding them into the corral. I found this procedure most easily accomplished first by learning who the "lead" cows were and then enticing them to a tub of sweet-smelling feed placed on the tailgate of my truck. Soon to follow were the others, as Alex would rhythmically honk the horn, thereby creating a Pavlovian conditioned response as he drove up the fenced "trap" to the corral. In the meantime, I was out at the periphery of the field driving the ATV, encouraging the stray animals to coalesce with the rest of the herd to follow the truck. This technique proved quite reliable in herding the cattle, especially from the remote fields of the 152-acre Georgia ranch. Without question, this method was more efficient and much safer than riding a quarter horse as in past years.

Once captured in the pens of the corral, the animals could either be segregated for loading onto a trailer, or driven down the narrow wooden chute where they were individually immobilized in the large steel head-gate for branding, veterinary work, etc. Besides giving preventative vaccinations for a number of diseases, we also de-wormed them twice a year. Any observant traveler can spot, at a mere glance, cows standing by the roadway that have been neglected and not de-wormed by their owners. They are gaunt and "hollowed out," having both protruding ribs and bony hindquarters. Rather than investing a little time, effort and money in worming medicine, many farmers just push the grass on their scrawny animals hoping for them to gain weight. However, instead of packing more meat on the cows, it is the parasitic worms which derive the nutrition from the forage, the farmer becoming the ultimate loser at the stockyard.

Besides helping me with rounding the cattle up, Alex was invaluable in assisting me with de-horning and castrating the animals. Once locked in the head gate of the squeeze chute, the often frustrated and sometimes unruly cattle were firmly held captive for our work. Horns were nearly always removed from all of my animals, males and females alike, for they are potentially dangerous weapons that can inflict serious injury against both man and beast. The horns, depending upon how large, were cut off either with de-horning shears or a wire saw, similar to the Gigli saw used by the neurosurgeon to cut cranial bone flaps. The base was then cauterized with a hot iron to staunch the bleeding.

Earlier in the book I had stated that our purpose in raising purebred cattle was to raise seed stock for the commercial cattleman. In large part, the ultimate goal was to produce large, "meaty," fertile bulls which the commercial cattleman could use to upgrade his herd, thereby siring large calves. Succinctly stated, I was in the bull producing business. But, as previously acknowledged, not all of my young bulls were acceptable to be sold as breeding stock. Necessarily, I castrated the inferior males resulting in steers with tender meat to be sold at the stockyards.

In the years to follow Alex continued to faithfully assist me with all of these tasks, irrespective of the weather or other adverse circumstances. As the herd grew in size, so did the work. Moreover, as our time spent working together improved the efficiency of the ranch operation over the years, our friendship commensurately grew stronger.

~~~
~~~

THIRTEEN

From Surgeon to Artisan

~~~

With the passage of time I achieved my goal of four bull-breeding units, efficiently combining two farms with adequate grass and fencing. The ranch operation then became somewhat routine, leaving me more time during the year for other outside activities. This afforded the opportunity to begin thinking about another passion of mine — a well designed workshop and the longing to build fine furniture.

After obtaining my backup 75-HP John Deere tractor, a second barn was constructed in which to store and protect it. This smaller building was also later to serve as a suitable workshop. With a little effort, the wiring was upgraded to safely serve the requirements of the high-voltage machinery, and the plumbing revamped to supply me with inside water facilities. I could scarcely have wished for anything better than to focus on building furniture in my shop, while at the same time enjoying the presence of my large, but gentle, cows serenely grazing the thick grass adjacent to the open overhanging doors. I was comfortably ensconced in my new environment, even though I could no longer practice surgery.

To regress for a moment, I hadn't built any furniture since the late 1970s when I first purchased the farm. Between a busy surgical practice and utilization of any free time in building infrastructure at the farm, there was regrettably little time left for my family and virtually none for woodworking. Prior to starting the farm, I had built the mahogany gun cabinet discussed previously and a small cherry end-table in which I had turned the legs on my small shop lathe. However, perhaps the most elegant piece of furniture to date had been a "corner desk," also crafted out of mahogany. This was a self-designed piece of furniture with the legs and carcass jointed at 45° angles like an isosceles triangle and finished with an appealing dark red, antique stain. To my utter dismay,
~~~

my first wife had absconded with this treasured desk when she left Tallahassee with my young children in 1987. I had invested so much of myself and was so extremely proud of the piece that I longed to know where it was. But when asked about the desk ten years later, no one seemed to either know or, for that matter, even care what had happened to it. Even one of my curious physician friends later asked me, "Whatever happened to that unusual triangular desk that you built?"

In later revisiting my furniture-building hobby, the first project contemplated was an attempt at replicating that attractive little corner desk. Because I had neither the old desk nor the plans for it, I decided to redesign another. This time, however, I envisioned two closely-jointed rear legs instead of one, as had the original piece. Rather than using a plunge router or hand-drilling and chiseling the mortises of the legs, I decided to purchase a mortising machine. This is an apparatus that bores "square holes," which if done contiguously will result in a long deep mortise in each leg. This serves to house the male tenons of the aprons of the desk, thereby jointing the legs together. To eventually find such a machine, I stumbled by chance into a catalog of commercial woodworking machinery manufactured by Grizzly Industrial, Inc. I ordered the mortising machine from the company and used it as a pivotal piece of equipment to build my newly designed desk. Quite pleased with the final product, I engraved it underneath as a gift to my wife, Elaine. The finished desk, as one of my good friends, A. J., once said, was reminiscent of a "spinet" piano when viewed from the side and rear. In any event it was far too pleasing to the eye to be isolated away in a corner as originally intended and, to this day, stands proudly in our parlor. Because of the technical difficulty in cutting the inclined fold-down writing surface, all but one edge of which being machined at three independent angles, I had come to appreciate the immediate need for additional woodworking machinery. Also, at about that time, the motor of my 25 year-old, reliable Craftsman table saw finally burned out.

As a result there necessarily followed a period of time in which I began acquiring additional standing machinery for the shop. Because the mortising machine which I had purchased from Grizzly was so well constructed, I decided to look at their table saws, planers and other floor model power tools as well. I felt that by investing in these fine machines, I couldn't help but improve upon my work. While eagerly perusing through the brightly-colored illustrations of the thick Grizzly catalog, which so eloquently displayed its beautifully painted industrial woodworking machines, it reminded me of when I was a little boy in the

1940s looking at the equally appealing Lionel train catalogs. Those were the days when scaled-down steel toy trains, similar to the tools of the time, were also built to last forever—not even a close resemblance to the fragile plastic toys one usually finds on the shelves of stores today. Since I envisioned a long future of woodworking, I began purchasing the heavy, precision-ground, cast-iron machinery so reminiscent of my grandfather's high school workshop, the shop that had so captured my imagination when I was scarcely eight years old. In succeeding years and to the credit of Grizzly and other fine tool makers, I fortified my dream shop with a wonderful assortment of these exquisite tools. With few exceptions they were made outside the United States, yet were similar to those made in our country back in the pre-World War II era. Those in my generation can well appreciate the fine quality of tools and equipment manufactured in America at one time, and long for those days to return — improbable as it may now seem.

~~~

In 1998 tragedy again struck our neurological clinic. Dr. Mark Vogter, the young neurosurgeon who had joined Frank and me in 1988, suddenly passed away from a massive heart attack. The abrupt termination of his 40-year-old life was devastating to all of us. I had always said that, as a talented neurosurgeon, Mark was far ahead of his time. The entire community was sadly deprived of his expertise as a fine surgeon, and will forever miss him as a very popular man with a vivacious personality.

~~~

1999 was yet another big year for Florida State football fans. Chris Weinke became the university's second Heisman Trophy winner, and the Seminoles went on to beat Virginia Tech with its outstanding quarterback, Michael Vick, 46-29 in the Sugar Bowl game to win its second national championship. The team was also the first ever to be top-ranked in the AP poll from the preseason through the final vote after the bowl games. Also, as another remarkable accomplishment, from 1987-2000 the Florida State Seminoles put together 14 consecutive years of 10-win seasons and top-five finishes in the AP football poll, an unprecedented record to that point. For those of us local citizens who have identified with the team over the years, it had been a great ride with our splendid coach, Bobby Bowden.

~~~

The world as we had come to know it was about to change. At 8:46 A.M. on Tuesday, September 11, 2001, another event occurred which was to change the course of American history. Al-Qaeda, under the leadership of Osama bin Laden, was responsible for the hijacking of four airliners, two of which crashed into and totally decimated the Twin World Trade Center Towers in New York City, and a third caused major destruction to the Pentagon. A fourth plane crashed in a Pennsylvania field after the valiant passengers failed to subdue the hijackers. In all, there were 2,976 deaths and over 6,000 injuries of innocent people. As a result of both this act of terrorism and other subversive events, including the bombing of public buildings and mass shootings in schools and other public places, our lives have been changed forever. To protect the innocent from the rising tide of evil, our freedoms and personal privacy have seriously been violated. It has cost us dearly in many different ways. Not only is the very dignity of our citizenry undermined by the often impolite — if not blatantly obtrusive and curt — search and shakedown methods employed at the airports, but also in other public buildings as well. I recently entered a courthouse in a small fishing town on the Gulf Coast to pay my property tax, only to unexpectedly encounter a brutish woman with a badge and metal searching wand. Her aggressive attitude conjured up ambivalent feelings of humiliation and anger in this patriotic citizen, born at a time in our history in which most citizens could come and go as they pleased. I thought to myself while observing a young couple standing nearby, outwardly puzzled over my obvious disgust, that their young generation knows nothing other than a discomfiting level of government oppression. We all most certainly understand the need for increased security in these difficult times, but those behind that badge should be instructed in using some discretion by treating people with the dignity they deserve and not obtrusively acting like thugs themselves.

~~~

As we entered the new millennium there were destined to be significant changes in my life. Throughout the late 90s I had been heavily committed to ranching with little time remaining for woodworking. But now it had become increasingly more evident that the ranch was imposing an ever greater economic concern, despite my avid desire to succeed.

At one point in time, Elaine and I were running over 80 head of purebred females which, together with all bulls, calves and yearlings, constituted a herd totaling roughly 150 animals. If that wasn't enough, we even tried to breed Paso Fino horses, although on a minimum scale. The logistics of two people keeping all of these disparate groups of animals separated, watered and fed throughout the year, to say nothing of rounding them up for medical care or transport to Georgia, became problematic, indeed.

A frustrating incident occurred one day after we had just finished gathering up a large group of cattle and had segregated two subdivisions of cow/calf pairs. Each subunit consisting of roughly 25 animals was then diverted into each of two small adjacent fields as holding areas in preparation for transport to Georgia the next day. My Paso Fino stallion, who many times before had unobtrusively shared the same field with cattle, decided on that particular day to have some fun — ultimately at my expense. Without any warning he suddenly reared up on his hind legs while loudly snorting and pawing at the air, causing the startled cattle to frantically stampede. In a wild frenzy after being deathly frightened, they not only tore down a very well constructed barbed wire cross-fence fortified with a highly charged electrical wire, but proceeded to again mix with the group of cows from which they had just been painstakingly culled. As I set out to repair the damage and again separate out the animals, I began to seriously question at my age the wisdom of continuing the futility of this frustrating occupation. Rather than shooting the horse out of a fit of anger, I gave him away— saddles and all— to my sister-in-law, eliminating at least one of my immediate problems.

Another ever-present problem concerned marketing my cattle. The progeny of my more recently acquired Mountain Man son and the Lasater bulls were beautiful animals, so much so, that I couldn't find buyers who were willing to pay me what I thought they were worth. My county consisted of very hard-working farmers and ranchers of very modest means. They were simply interested in procuring straightforward bulls to get the breeding job done, not to be dazzled by my stately showcase animals — the heralded Six Essentials notwithstanding. Not that they didn't like the looks of my cattle, but only that they expected me to "give them away." My recourse was to ratchet up my marketing strategy by advertising in all of the prominent farm journals and bulletins in the Southeast. In addition, we widely distributed professional-grade business cards and photographs in strategic places of business and even posted elegant signs on a major highway. But the returns were meager, indeed. Simply stated, I was raising a rich man's cattle with little demand in a poor region of the South. This of course was in marked contrast to Mr. Lasater in San Angelo whose animals were in great demand by the owners of the large range herds out west. He could sell 50 bulls to a single commercial cattleman in Texas or California, where these premium herd sires served to fulfill the expectations of what they are bred to do — survive on harsh range conditions and produce hardy, robust calves.

Besides trying to market my cattle by "private treaty," I also took them to a number of different cattle sales throughout the years. One of the stockyards in Georgia, for example, had a highly advertised monthly "purebred" sale, which on occasion was exclusively reserved for Beefmaster cattle. Prior to one such sale, I enthusiastically hauled a load of my aging mama cows and a few bulls 90 miles up there, fully expecting to make some money. Soon after the beginning of the auction, however, it became painfully evident that things were not going well for the sellers. My wife has often recounted my walking out of that auction amphitheater with head hung low, bitterly dejected with my proceeds. The buyers paid me not even close to what purebred animals realistically should have brought, but rather the current price per pound of beef on the hoof. I might just as well have driven the animals up the road from our ranch to the local stockyard.

After so many years of hard work, much fortitude and uncompensated optimism, I finally began to reconcile the fact that I must reconsider the economics of the cattle business. Thereafter for several more years I began thinking more like a commercial cattleman rather than a breeder of seed stock. That is to say that ninety percent of my marketing was projected to be at the stockyards. Granted, I was able to continue selling a few prize bulls at a reasonably good price, but, for the most part, we castrated the males and sold them as steers. No longer was I to harbor the delusion of any general demand within my geographic area for animals from a prized, registered herd.

Several years later, a sobering event transpired which probably put the exclamation point on my remaining days as a cattleman. One evening as the sun was beginning to set, I received a disturbing phone call from the tenant who lived with his sick wife in a trailer on my Georgia farm. Stuttering with excitement he said, "Doc, someone has deliberately cut your fence, and your cows are standing ready to walk out onto the highway!" With fencing materials in hand, Elaine and I hastily jumped into the old Ford pickup and drove 45 miles up to the place — with old Mr. Griffin in the meantime holding the cows at bay. Upon examining the fence after my arrival, I verified that someone had indeed methodically cut five strands of barbed wire. I couldn't begin to conceive as to why someone would derive pleasure out of such a dangerous act of vandalism. Totally aside from the unnecessary work of repairing the fence and standing to lose some very valuable cattle was the potential of endangering the lives of any passersby on the busy highway. Colliding with a 1,500 pound beast(s) crossing the highway, while streaking along at 55-mph., is a recipe for disaster. The potential for damage and even loss of life was a very disquieting thought. Moreover, even if damages were minimal, I most likely would have faced an inevitable lawsuit. Although I was not directly culpable, a judge surely would have ruled against me in a court of law, evaporating my assets and drastically altering my life at a critical time near retirement. I could ill afford a chance that such an act of vandalism might recur and decided that warm summer evening, while repairing the fence, that I would exit the cattle business. All too often in our litigious society, one must go on the defensive to protect what he has worked so hard to accumulate throughout his life. It is shameful that our system, replete with predators seeking large judgments at the expense of others, doesn't often serve justice to the honest man trying to do the right thing. I recently heard this theme echoed on television, that is to say, small businesses throughout our land are frequently being threatened with often unjust and frivolous, expensive lawsuits by those seeking windfall punitive damages.

All things considered, I felt that it was the appropriate time to begin reducing the size of my herd and eventually selling out. Thus, when Alex and I finally hauled that last load of cattle to the Thomasville stockyards, I had no regrets in doing so. Paradoxically, I had no misgivings in having spent 20 years of my life actively engaged in the cattle business, for I had lived out my second childhood dream, one which I wouldn't have traded for anything. By having educated myself in almost all aspects of ranching, I had added another dimension to an already interesting life. It also afforded me the opportunity to meet a great many genuinely good, down-to-earth people, many of whom remain some of my best and lasting friends.

~~~

Fortuitously, it was at about the time of the wire-cutting incident in Pavo that I received a call from Mr. Werner Wilson, a spokesman for the Jefferson County school Board, inquiring whether I would be interested in selling part of my Monticello farm. It seemed that the state of Florida was offering $17 million to Jefferson County to construct a badly needed new high school. Posing some urgency to the matter were time constraints on both purchasing a suitable piece of property and finalizing a construction bid for the project; the unviable alternative was for the county to forfeit the money. Despite my being sympathetic to their plight, my initial response was a resounding "no." After all, an abundance of my life's energy had been invested into seeing that raw land developed into a beautiful ranch with its gorgeous, fenced, green fields and thriving exotic cattle. It was a memory I never wanted to relinquish. Not willing to settle for "no" as an answer, Mr. Wilson and his associate, Mr. Ulmer Miller, were persistent in meeting with me on subsequent occasions in an effort to swing a deal on the property. After further consideration, I recall a pivotal day later in the negotiation process in which the three of us were walking through the dense underbrush in the wooded area of the farm. At that particular time we came to an agreement on a price which averaged the value of the choice elevated regions of the property with the lesser value of the low wetlands. During the discussion, these amiable, low-key gentlemen, whom I always considered to be of the very highest moral order, further elaborated that the school board was interested in a parcel of land sizable enough to house the buildings and athletic fields not only for the high school but for future elementary and middle schools as well. After several more days of dialogue, our small group reached an agreement on a substantial parcel of the property. The entire school board subsequently came out and walked over the prospective land. From the onset, my farm was one of three potentially viable sites to build the schools, one of the other two belonging to the highly visible television news and sports mogul, Ted Turner. After further lengthy discussions among board
~~~

members and the county commission, the Geissinger property was ultimately chosen, much to the dismay of several very angry neighbors.

As a result of this transaction, within a matter of a few months I had disposed of all of my cattle and well over half of the Monticello property. After the sale, there remained the two farm buildings and 80-acres of land, the latter eventually being leased out to a young rancher and his family who lived down the road.

Having sold all of the land behind the barn and shop, it became immediately apparent that I faced another serious problem. There was some urgency in vacating the woodworking tools from my shop, for they presented an invitation for thievery and vandalism. Furthermore, since I no longer had any animals requiring my daily attention, it was foolish for me to waste both the fuel and time in driving from Tallahassee to the farm workshop in Monticello. Without delay I contacted Charles Reichert, the man who had constructed my original farm buildings and arranged to have him duplicate the workshop behind my Tallahassee home. I could now envision walking 50-feet to turn on a bandsaw rather than driving 50-miles a day to do so.

~~~

During this transition in my daily life from rancher to woodworker, there were also changes occurring elsewhere regarding my family. My two sons, both residing in the Pacific Northwest, were raising their own families and providing me with wonderful grandchildren. Jeff, my older son, had two beautiful, very sweet daughters, Autumn and Georgia, and a proud boy, Harrison. Roger, my younger son, was blessed with three cute daughters, Karrisa, Kelsie, and Kali. Jeff and Roger, much like their dad, have enjoyed a lifetime of both working with their hands and pursuing most outdoor sports, including hunting, fishing and skiing. I am proud of these young men, who are not only good fathers but also fine, productive, honest citizens. A father can ask no more of his sons. Unfortunately, distance has precluded my spending any lasting time with them. At one point Elaine and I purchased a gorgeous piece of property in Idaho, thinking that we could build a house there, but that possibility became infeasible in terms of money, time and distance.

On the home front my elder daughter, Kim, and her husband, Alvaro, a sheriff's deputy in Tampa, provided me with yet another prized granddaughter, Alina. I am proud to state that prior to her starting her
~~~

own family, Kim had not only earned a BA college degree, but later, after having become a registered nurse, proceeded to obtain a BS degree in nursing as well. In following the medical footsteps of her father, she then worked for several years as a neurological intensive-care nurse at the well-recognized Tampa General Hospital. Kim has, to some extent, kept me abreast of some of the current trends in neurological surgery as practiced in a university-teaching setting. My family in Florida, distance not being a factor, has been an ongoing source of love and inspiration during my later retirement years.

While speaking of exemplary families, I shall take this opportunity to briefly introduce that of my wife, Elaine. Her mother, Carmen, who lives alone in Miami, is best described as a kind soul, and indeed a pleasure with whom to associate. Elaine's youngest sister, Mini, who resides remotely from the others in South Carolina, possesses the same affable demeanor as her mother. Two other sisters, Rosita and Evelyn, are very successful business women who live in South Florida, Evelyn being my personal accountant. Many years ago I first became well acquainted with Elaine's youngest brother, Gilbert, when he visited us in Tallahassee. I showed him how to tag a newborn calf and how to shoot skeet with a 12-gauge shotgun. Her two other brothers, Ray and José, I consider close friends, both being of the highest integrity and persons with whom I can freely share life's many experiences.

~~~

Several months after the farm sale, Mr. Reichert fulfilled my high expectations when he completed the construction of my elegant new workshop. The thick cement slab, poured upon the deep underlying steel-reinforced cement footings, was built to support several tons of weight. The slab was also extended beyond the main building to function as the floor for a "lean-to," a convenient structure for sheltering other equipment such as my tractor-mower. Inside the shop, a one-ton mobile, overhead hoist was mounted on a steel transverse beam to allow placement and unloading of heavy equipment. Eventually, after the electrician had installed all of the lighting and required circuitry for my power- driven equipment, I was ready to have everything moved from Monticello to Tallahassee.

Over the course of time, I would often revisit those colorful pages of the Grizzly tool catalog and would purchase additional machinery for the
~~~

shop— implements that I felt were necessary if I were to continue to refine myself in emulation of my grandfather.

As already discussed, my initially-built furniture, for the most part, was usually self-designed, as opposed to using plans from a book. I would first conceive of the basic need for a special piece and then proceed to sketch it out on paper, keeping the proper proportions in mind. Utilizing the appropriate geometry and mathematics, the plans were then finalized with a careful consideration for both strength and beauty. During the actual fabrication process, there were often additions and deletions to the base plans in arriving at the final product. By making such changes, I could produce furniture, such as the gun cabinet, unavailable in most stores. Citing it as the benchmark example, others have told me that they have yet to see another as well constructed, functional or pleasing to the eye. Most store-bought cases serve to hold the guns, but lack the aesthetic appeal of having been hand-made and so personally designed. Throughout the years I've been asked by other hunters to build them fire-arms cabinets, indicating that there are indeed individuals who both appreciate quality workmanship and are willing to pay for it. In my own mind, the greatest compliment I can be paid is not that any given piece of my furniture is necessarily functional or even beautiful, but rather that it was constructed with the same pride and quality as the craftsmen of years past. I, along with my fellow woodworkers, am endeavoring to keep alive an old and ever-fading art form.

People often express to me an interest in perhaps getting into working with wood, but don't know where to begin. It is a self-education process, much like ranching, beginning first with undeterred motivation and fortified by an unyielding persistence during times of frustration. When getting started it is easy to become discouraged after a less than perfect first result. As I have done in previous chapters pertaining to other topics, I now offer a few tips that might be helpful to those interested readers.

To regress a bit, my approach to woodworking has always been a heuristic one, much like the study of medicine. It begins with a basic understanding of the nature of wood: its anatomy, characteristics of grain and strength, how it is machined, its finishing qualities, and its ability to exchange moisture while undergoing dimensional change under fluctuating environmental conditions. All of these factors have a bearing on what kind of wood should be utilized for a particular piece of furniture and the type of joinery employed.

And not to be forgotten are the machines themselves. Whether it is a hand tool purchased in a local hardware store or a 1,000-pound monster ultimately trucked to the shop from some distant source, it is foolish to assume that, once installed, all one has to do is to use it! The serious craftsman must always first learn how to best use each device. There exists a continuum between maximum safe efficiency and pushing a tool dangerously beyond its limits of intended use. Furthermore, these machines must frequently be cleaned, calibrated, sharpened and— in the moisture-laden Southeast — protected from the scourge of rust. I once visited a local woodworker who had recently purchased a brand-new, industrial drill press from the Grizzly Company. Although scarcely a few months old, it had been relegated to the corner of his garage and looked like something from a World War II salvage yard. Its cast-iron surfaces, no longer bright and reflective, were disgustingly brown and deeply pitted from the rust of neglect.

So often when they first enter my shop, visitors will ask me why my equipment looks like new despite this terribly humid atmosphere. Several years ago I read somewhere how to prevent rust build-up. Because this is such a critical issue and often such an extremely discouraging one, I will briefly describe my technique.

As a first line of defense, I initially remove any current rust from the surface by first applying a coat of non-silicone based, wood-surfacing paste wax. Once dry, simply add a few dashes of mineral spirits and then scour it with a green 3M pad. If, after wiping it off and allowing it to dry, there is still rust present; I repeat the process. Once the rust has been removed, another final protective coat of wax is applied, and this time the surface is buffed with a dry, clean, soft rag. Finally, and of the utmost importance, each and <u>every</u> evening throughout the year, before leaving the shop, I cover the machine's cast iron surface with an unwrinkled, heavy cotton bath towel to absorb any condensing nocturnal moisture. By rigidly following this protocol, I have weathered entire seasons without rust eating up my valued equipment.

The field of woodworking has often been described as a…"journey without an end." There is no limit as to what one can learn en route to building his own "masterpiece," irrespective of its size, complexity, or the type of wood used. We have all begun by building what many consider mundane items, but to the beginner even the most "trivial" final product can become a thing of beauty, an uplifting accomplishment for which he can be justly proud.

After many years I have been very fortunate to have latched on to what has been referred to as an "armada" of power tools, representing nearly every size, color and shape. While over the course of time I had eventually learned to use them sufficiently well to build several acceptable pieces of furniture, I had always felt that there existed a serious void in my expertise regarding the use of hand tools. To take a hand plane to a beautiful walnut or cherry tabletop required much more courage than I, who had tackled any number of challenging surgical operations, could ever muster up. To the contrary— I yearned to become proficient in utilizing those basic hand tools that our forefathers had used so many years ago. I thus decided to learn the technique of building Windsor chairs, not only for the purpose of learning to fabricate something quite elegant, but also to overcome the fear of ruining a piece of furniture with grain tear-out in the process. To attain this goal, I enrolled in an introductory course in constructing sack-back Windsor chairs, taught by the world-renowned chairmaker and teacher, Mike Dunbar, the founder of the Windsor Institute in Hampton, New Hampshire.

For those readers unfamiliar with these chairs, they originated in England during the early 18th century and later rapidly gained popularity in our colonies. In its basic form, the chair consists of a thick plank with the legs, arm supports and the spindles supporting the steam-bent arm crest and curved back socketed into it. It is entirely constructed with hand tools. As a prerequisite for the course, much like the young doctor procuring his first black bag and the instruments to fill it, I had to purchase an assortment of unusual tools. For the most part these tools, many of which most people have never heard of, had to be custom-made and/or forged in far-off places in New England and later shipped to me in Tallahassee. Moreover, to comply with the explicit written instructions of Mr. Dunbar, I had to hand-sharpen them all with various increasing grits of sandpaper to produce an "invisibly sharp edge." I should have known at that point what was in store for me a few weeks later at "The Windsor Institute."

After journeying far north from Florida to New Hampshire and having settled down in a rooming house after purchasing some groceries, I was ready to begin the class the following day. The first class began on Monday at 8:30 A.M. when we were given a lecture by Mr. Dunbar on the history of Windsor chairs. We were then taken into the shop where protocols for each of the ensuing five days were passed out. The general scheme to be followed by the students was first to observe as the master or one of his skilled assistants began constructing a chair. In so doing they showed us how to use those intriguing, unique tools, as they engaged in the construction of a particular phase of the sack-back. The students would then return to their workbenches and replicate that phase of construction in building their own chairs. This protocol was to be repeated time and again each day and throughout the week until each of us had completed his sack-back chair.

During that first morning, we had to carefully hand-plane and steam-bend the arm rail, carve out the bow of the back with both the drawknife and spokeshave, and then follow by steam-bending it as well. Later in the afternoon, while using the same implements, we cut from raw blank pieces of red oak the seven spindles of varying lengths and tapering diameters for the back of the chair. Being the oldest in the class of perhaps one dozen students, I found myself at times struggling to keep up as I learned how to use these unfamiliar tools, while attempting to get the job done without shattering or splitting out the wood. And so went the week— constantly running on a treadmill much like the early days of college and medical school. I awakened almost routinely at 2 AM. each day disturbed by the idea of not only trying to remain caught up in my work, but truly wondering if I could make it through the week and complete it without seriously bungling up the chair. But like any task involving learning something new while under time constraints (which can be painful), I somehow managed to remain tenacious in building that interesting little chair. By week's end I had not only overcome the challenge of mastering how to construct a unique item of furniture in the same manner as our ancestors had done, but I had something tangible as a reward for my efforts— an intriguing, beautiful artifact that will be enjoyed by many for the ages.

Once I had arrived home in Tallahassee, I set forth to construct my own steam box for bending the necessary components of oak in preparation of taking my personal chair building skills to yet another level. I then searched the forest of my farm until I found a straight-grained, white oak tree which might be suitable for a chair. After felling the tree and dragging it out of the woods with my tractor (while cutting a hole in the fence to do so), the log was quarter-sawn at a local mill and then taken to my shop in preparation for a chair. After its completion, the bow for the back, the arm rail, and all of the long spindles in that second chair were from my farm; this added special interest and value to that particular piece.

Over the next three years, I periodically returned to the Windsor Institute to learn the art of building more complex and even more eye-appealing Windsor chairs. These experiences not only enhanced my skills as a wood craftsman but enabled me to meet new friends with a common interest. And just as I had years previously exchanged medical information with others at national neurosurgical meetings, I now had expert colleagues in woodworking with whom to share unusual or perplexing problems. Like the others attending Mike Dunbar's advanced chair-building courses, I eventually came to think of myself as a "chairmaker." The workmanship of these elegant, 18th-century chairs has subsequently been shared with others in our region, not only with occasional tours of my shop and home, but with formal exhibits as well. I considered it a privilege and honor to have been asked a few years ago to give such a tour to the Tallahassee Woodworkers Society, a distinguished group of skilled woodworkers from the greater Tallahassee area. In addition, after I built a complete set of sack-back chairs, one of them was exhibited in Thomasville, Georgia, at its "Cultural Center." Subsequent to that event, on August 24, 2007, I also entered a sack-back Windsor chair at the Physicians Art Show at the Westin Diplomat Hotel in Hollywood, Florida, in association with the annual Florida Medical Association meeting. I was humbled to receive first-place in the wood division of that event.

Over a period of time I have built an even dozen chairs, 10 of them Windsors of varying design, but each unique by its hand-crafted nature. The latter were all numbered, signed, and heat-branded. Among them was a writing-arm chair (reminiscent of the school-desk chairs used by the children during World War II), which I specifically made for my scholarly, long-time friend from Northwestern, Bob Doherty; it commemorated our association of over fifty years. The last Windsor to date (#10) was a Nantucket Fan-back chair built for my wife, Elaine. It is a large black chair with custom-carved rosettes in the ears of the curved upper-back crest.

I shall be forever grateful to Mike Dunbar and his group of distinguished assistants who served as my instructors. I enthusiastically recommend the Windsor Institute to any craftsman interested in this particular phase of woodworking.

One eventually comes to realize that it is the combined skills of using both power machines and hand tools that truly embodies the craft of woodworking. This cannot be better illustrated than when discussing the planing of a board. The knives of a power thickness planer, irrespective of their sharpness or the tool's precise calibration, will invariably leave "planer marks" in their wake on the freshly planed surface. If left uncorrected, this aberration can become painfully evident when a finish is later applied. A well-tuned hand plane and a wood scraper will deftly remove these blemishes, even without sandpaper. Parenthetically, I have become obsessed with fine, pre-World War II, Stanley hand planes and have begun collecting them. After purchasing an old refurbished, #4 Stanley Bed Rock smoothing plane from a collector in California, I found that I could remove a mere "whisker" of wood from a recently thickness-planed board. Thus, I now employ it as a surface finishing tool on virtually every such piece. Much like some of our old surgical instruments, I find such eloquent tools indispensable for fine work. I've often told my woodworking friends that I like that #4 so much, I feel like "taking it to bed with me."

After several years of a chairmaker's mindset, I began to genuinely question whether my skills might be up to making anything else of significance. With some trepidation I later began building other articles of interest. As my first "period" piece of furniture, I built a Queen Anne porringer-top tea table (circa 1750) with hand-carved cabriole legs. I obtained the plans for this beautiful table from the *Fine Woodworking* magazine, the author of the article being Dan Faia. Several years earlier Dan had been one of my talented instructors at the Windsor Institute when I built that first sack-back Windsor chair.

A more recent article of furniture constructed was a "Huntboard" (sideboard) designed by Garrett Hack, at the time one of America's most talented and visible woodworkers. Arguably it is one of the most difficult — yet attractive — pieces added to my collection to date. It also incorporates a study of "wood-movement" in its construction. More aptly stated, each of its major individual components is fabricated to allow expansion or contraction during its exchange of moisture with the atmosphere, thus obviating any fracturing of the wood. Visually, it stands as a relatively long and narrow, yet tall, piece which is made of quarter-sawn straight-grained cherry. It is handsomely supported on thin, hand-planed, tapered legs which contain decorative inlay bandings of holly and ebony. The centered, aesthetically pleasing front three drawers, each proportionally decreasing in height, are embraced on either side by small cabinet doors containing panels of flame birch. Interestingly, the latter present an illusion of movement when the observer changes eye elevation. The birch panels are tastefully bordered with ebony, while all

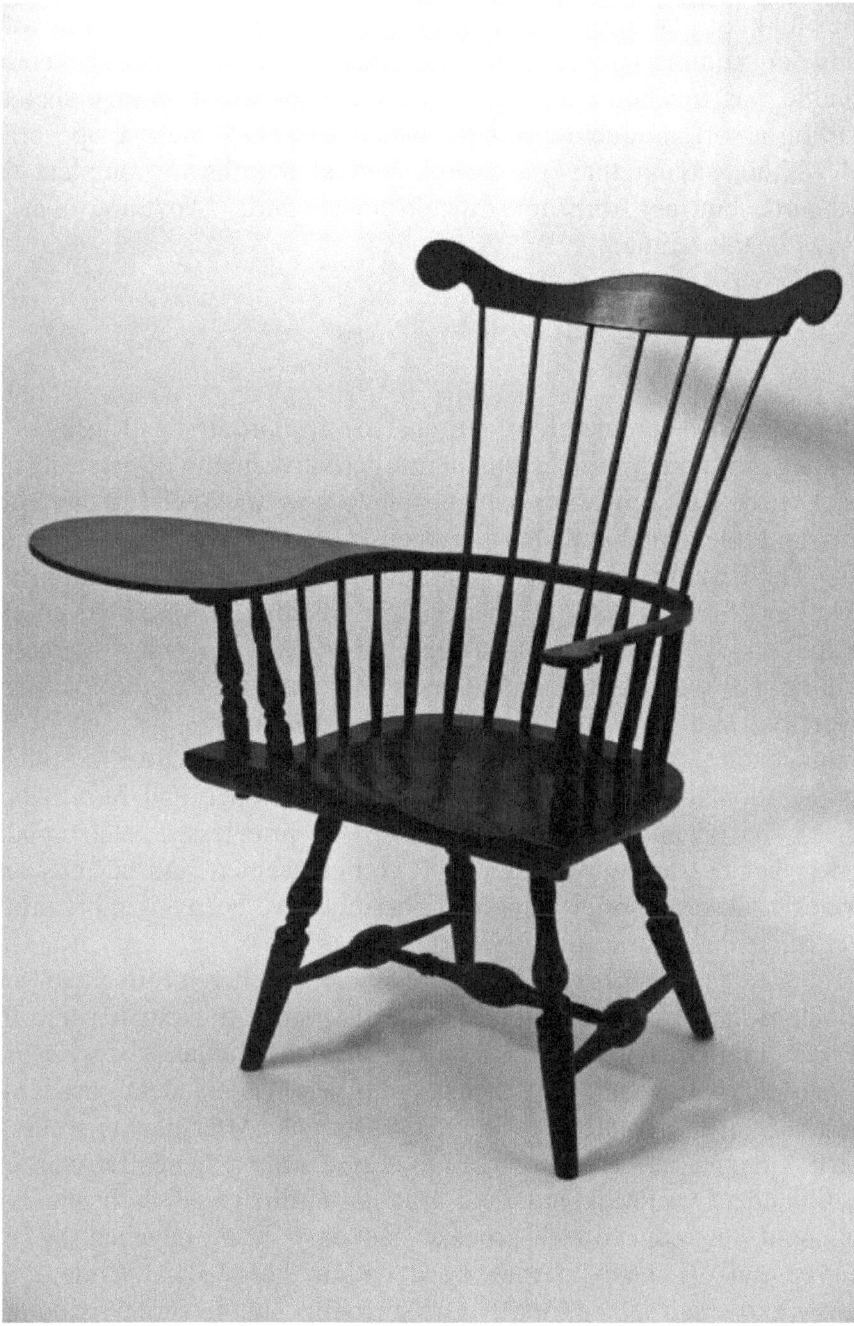

The Chairmaker

Windsor "Writing-arm" chair — crafted by the author for his long-time friend.

of the pull knobs are hand-turned of the same material. The top of exotic bloodwood contrasts nicely with the body of the cabinet. The entire ensemble was finished with eight coats of hand-buffed, orange shellac, imparting a soft antique appearance which lends striking eye appeal. It goes without saying that it took me several months to complete the Huntboard, but as Abraham Lincoln once said, "Anything that is worthwhile takes time."

~~~

While I had prematurely terminated my professional life as a neurosurgeon, and was later pursuing alternative paths of interest, my wife, Elaine, had simultaneously begun to sow the seeds of her own professional development. Having been so involved raising her family during her first marriage, the opportunity for a college education had eluded her. Soon after we exchanged our wedding vows, however, she enrolled in the Tallahassee Community College, soon thereafter obtaining her AA degree. After then matriculating to Florida State University, she first received her BA degree in the school of communication, followed later with both an MPA degree in public administration and an MIS degree in library science and information studies. The beaming smile on her face was priceless as she proudly stood in her cap and gown after each commencement. As her husband and most ardent supporter, I couldn't possibly have been any more proud of her achievements.

The medical school at Florida State University, heretofore a two-year curriculum in the basic sciences, in recent years had expanded into the four-year Florida State University College of Medicine. My wife first became employed at the medical college as student academic coordinator at the Tallahassee Regional Campus. After having received her MPA degree she was promoted to administrator, thereafter working directly under Dean Mel Hartsfield. Her extraordinary scholarly standing throughout the educational process has only been matched by the intensity and efficiency of her work within the Medical College, as recently expressed to me by the dean himself. Her self-motivation and exemplary achievement at the middle-age of life should serve as an inspiration to others.
~~~

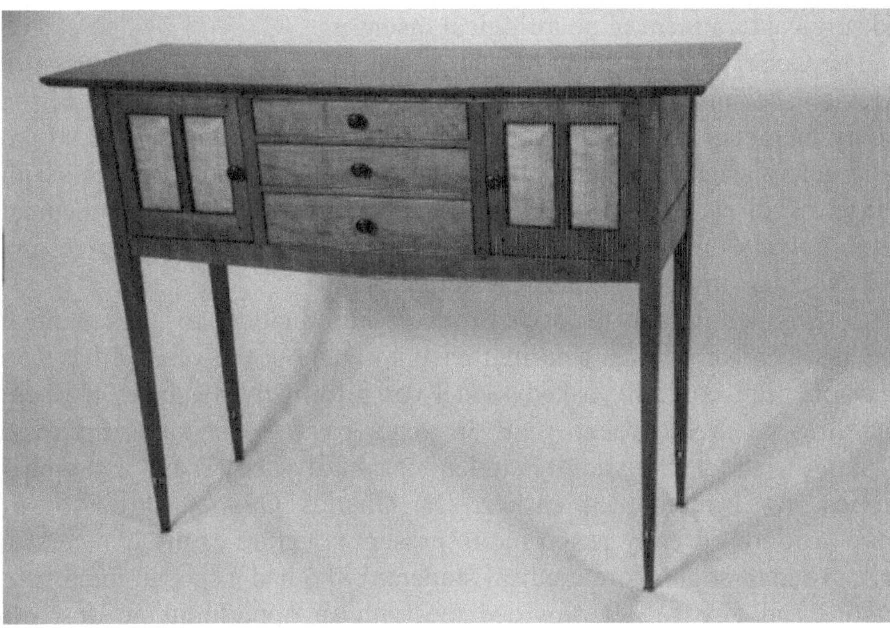

The Artisan

Elaine's affiliation with the medical school has also served to reunite me with the medical community. As previously mentioned, I had basically isolated myself both at my farm and in the workshop over the years, probably serving as a subconscious subterfuge from my forced departure from the practice of medicine. It had been painful to prematurely relinquish the field of neurosurgery, ending so abruptly a life-long goal. Let there be no mistake: retirement after so many years of hard work is kind to the body, but I shall always miss the fascination of medical science, more specifically, the challenges in both the diagnosis and surgical treatment of neurological disorders.

The College of Medicine has, however, afforded me the opportunity to revisit medicine in several different ways. For instance, many of the faculty members are old colleagues of mine, contemporaries with whom for so many years I shared the front lines in treating those befallen with injury and disease. We not only reminisce about old mutual medical cases, but discuss the changes occurring both in medical practice and medical education during this new millennium.

Equally important has been my re-introduction to the medical students themselves. On a formal basis throughout the years, I have on occasion been cordially asked to deliver informative lectures to them regarding my field of expertise. In years past, the sessions involved speaking to the neuroanatomy students primarily about head and spinal injuries. As I mentioned earlier, Dr. Charles Ouimet, professor of neuroanatomy, recently asked me to present a lecture of my choice to a large group of sophomore medical students, who had a special interest in neurological disease. It provided me with an opportunity to dust off some of my old 2x2 slides, root around looking for an antiquated projector, and to resurrect my affinity for neurosurgery. I tried to expose them to clinical topics not ordinarily emphasized as part of their standard curriculum. Some of those topics covered included the diagnosis and surgical treatment of interesting pituitary tumors, intracranial aneurysms and cases of trigeminal neuralgia, all of which seemed to capture their interest. This was attested to not only by their questions after the presentation, but by the later feedback as relayed to me by Dr. Ouimet.

I should like to recall another special event transpiring several years ago when Elaine volunteered to have the regional medical campus Christmas party at our home. Not only were the medical students attending, but the various deans of the College of Medicine and many of the faculty members and administrative staff as well. During a "fire-side chat" with a few of the students, I discussed the surgery of a number of intracranial conditions, pointing out on a human dry skull the various standard approaches used by the neurosurgeon.

That experience caused me to briefly reflect back on my own life as a neurosurgical resident at Chicago Wesley Memorial Hospital, sitting at those white tablecloth dinners with eminent professors of neurosurgery from around the world and listening with fascination to their experiences in the early days of our specialty. I would like to hope that my personal reflections on neurosurgery during the latter half of the 20th century, in conjunction with those of my colleagues, will continue to serve as a source of inspiration to others; namely, reflections that will stimulate future generations of physicians and neuroscientists to cross new frontiers in the diagnosis and treatment of disorders deemed impossible during our lifetime. Awaiting the investigators of tomorrow are solutions to the treatments of such prevalent pathological conditions as cerebrovascular disease, spinal cord and traumatic brain injury. Far from being solved as well are the perplexing problems of the aging brain and of other entities that destroy the human intellect, whether they are the cause of the prevalent dementia bearing Alzheimer's name or the more uncommon dementia of the prion-based Creutzfeldt-Jacob disease. Finally, there remains the solution to the treatment of the dreaded malignant gliomas that snuff out the lives of so many during their productive years. The mere prospect of subduing these complex and atrocious maladies of mankind, causing so much pain and suffering to both the patient and his loved ones, should be strong motivation to any student entertaining the neurological fields of science and medicine.

My association with both the medical students and the post-graduate students, whose research has passed before us on the neuroscience foundation board, has served as a primary impetus in my deciding to write this memoir. While being able to strongly identify with these young people in their quest for scientific knowledge, and at the same time reflecting back on my own past, I have been encouraged to share my own life's experiences with these future generations.

~~~
~~~

FOURTEEN

Viewing a System Gone Awry

~~~

In 2009 healthcare reform was the centerpiece of newly-elected President Barack Obama's agenda. The $2.3 trillion a year (and rising) medical bill for the nation was staggering, yet many citizens lacked sufficient coverage or had none at all. Congress had been struggling to address the discrepancies of health coverage within the current system, while attempting to cobble together ways of paying for it. As a surgeon who has witnessed a number of disconcerting changes in our healthcare system over the last two decades I, like so many others, have agonized over the fact that the President and the Congress did not at the onset begin their analysis of the problem by asking the important question: Just why is it that our system is so very costly and inefficient?

Several years ago a movie entitled "*The Doctor*," starring William Hurt, was released. It portrayed a prominent surgeon who unexpectedly found himself in the unfamiliar role of a seriously ill patient, giving him an entirely different perspective on the practice of medicine. He ironically now found himself not only the "patient's advocate" but a victim of the system in which he had practiced. I have been retired now for several years and have had a similar experience, not as a patient with a serious disease, but as a surgeon who is witnessing today's practice of medicine while positioned outside of the medical arena. Perhaps I can share some of the problems I have observed from my vantage point.

Always keeping in mind that we are a capitalistic society which must also care for the disadvantaged and needy, any meaningful, affordable reform will be difficult at best to achieve, but with a concerted effort we can certainly improve.

Some time ago at a dinner party I asked one of the young surgeons in town how his practice was going. Fully expecting him to discuss
~~~

challenging medical cases, as we had done routinely for the previous 25 years, I was surprised to have him so quickly reply by telling me "how much money he was putting on the books." At the time I thought his intent was to indirectly inform me as to how many patients he was seeing, implying the good service he was providing for the community. However, each time I saw him his response was always the same. I finally began to glean a certain boastfulness concerning his medical success— measured solely in economic terms.

Soon thereafter another incident occurred, this time involving my wife. Elaine had been bothered for years with both an inflamed tendon in her right wrist and what we call a "tennis elbow," also on the right side. On several occasions each area had been successfully injected with cortisone, totally relieving the pain. Although the injections in the wrist were well-tolerated, those into the tightly bound tissues of the elbow were excruciatingly painful. As the months passed, the wrist discomfort became refractory to the repeated injections, and the pain disabling enough to preclude her even using a pencil. We thus sought out a highly recommended surgeon who was confident that by surgically exploring her wrist and cleaning out the tendon sheath he could rid her of the pain. Because she had also begun to concurrently experience a recrudescence of the elbow pain, I asked whether, while she was under the anesthesia, he could spare her the intense pain of a future cortisone shot by injecting the elbow at the same sitting. He didn't hesitate in saying that he would be happy to do so. The paper work in hand, we were then off to the business office to settle the finances. Because we were under our insurance deductible, I had the business people print me out a statement for the actual cost of this relatively minor surgery, which was projected to be $1,200. There would, of course, be additional independent charges for the outpatient surgical facility and the anesthesiologist.

The operative procedures went well, and Elaine was happily alleviated of both sources of her arm pain. Two weeks later, however, when I received the surgical bill there was not one, but two distinctly coded surgical charges, each for $1,200. My immediate response was that this was a billing error. After all, the cost of a vial of cortisone couldn't possibly have exceeded $30, and there was no increased use of operating room space, anesthesia or more than three minutes of the surgeon's time for the elbow injection. I hand-carried the bill to the surgeon during Elaine's postoperative visit. After stating my concern over the charge, he replied that he would "look into it." Then, not having heard from either the doctor or the business office for several weeks, I wrote a personal letter describing the problem to the owner-director of the clinic — a physician who had been a colleague of mine (and I thought a friend) for many years. I mailed the letter directly to his home, anticipating that it would have otherwise been intercepted by an office clerk who might well have ignored it. Because my letter was never returned to me, it was evident that he had received it; yet, there was never any attempt to rectify the double charge, nor even an explanatory courtesy letter. While this ended up being an unexpected and uncalled for out-of-pocket expense, the real disappointment was the way we had been mistreated. The system was simply geared to squeeze every penny out of the patient, any moral high ground notwithstanding.

Several other pertinent points concerning the practice of medicine today are illustrated in the following case history. It occurred when I was away from home visiting a long-time physician friend. He related to me some of the problems he had recently encountered when trying to get medical relief from chronic back pain. Upon entering the office of the consulting spine surgeon in his community, he was first greeted by a nurse practitioner who obtained his history in an unconventional manner by having him answer a series of written questions on a "deck of cards." This was followed by a cursory check of his leg reflexes and nothing more. Following that brief encounter, the surgeon himself entered the room, and, in a brazenly curt tone, asked Gerald if he had any leg pain. After Gerald denied any pain radiating into the lower extremities, and in the absence of performing an examination himself, the insensitive surgeon abruptly replied, "I can't do anything for you." Gerald was then charged $360 and scooted off to a pain clinic without having received either a decent examination or the least explanation as to the source of his pain. I could tell that my friend was not only disturbed having been denied the respect of an M.D., but also, and worse, not even given that basic courtesy every patient should be granted. As a point of emphasis, this kind man had been a prominent, well-respected, older-generation, family physician in his community for many years, and the manner in which he was disrespectfully treated was deplorable. What's more, things were about to become even worse for Gerald, who not only voluntarily vented his frustration to me but showed me all of his medical bills as well.

The medical doctor working in the physician-owned pain clinic proposed destroying the nerves deep within Gerald's back, which he felt were the cause of the pain. The true underlying etiology of the patient's pain was lumbar spondylosis, as ascertained by my personal examination and review of the CT scans and the radiologist's reports. The treating doctor proposed that he would first inject the nerves with a local anesthetic, and only if that temporarily eliminated the pain would he then proceed to destroy the nerves. The method to be used was to employ a radiofrequency current delivered through electrodes placed near the facet joints of the lumbar spine. Gerald agreed, whereupon the anesthetic agent was injected. Any pain relief was marginal to none, but the therapist recommended destroying the nerves on one side anyway. After a great deal of maneuvering with expensive imaging equipment in the fancy facility, a number of RF lesions were made. When asked if he felt any pain relief, Gerald replied that he didn't notice any difference whatsoever. The therapist then insisted the patient return in a week for re-evaluation. Out of obligation, but with much trepidation, my friend returned, again emphasizing to the physician that there had been no remission of his back pain. But much to Gerald's surprise, the therapist replied… "Let's do the other side anyway." He went on to elaborate that on the initial visit Gerald had agreed to submit to a bilateral procedure. After resisting further attempts at coercion, my disgusted friend exited the pain clinic, never to return. He was presented thereafter with a bill to the tune of several thousand dollars!

This particular pain operation was first described in the mid-1970s, and initially captured the neurosurgical community's interest. However, further reports were less enthusiastic, suggesting that any favorable therapeutic results were marginal at best, probably in large part being due to the placebo effect. My partner and I, who were ordinarily quick to employ new effective procedures, were never impressed with the published data; and so we decided not to engage in the operation. One point that everyone did universally agree upon in those days was that a test injection of a local anesthetic must prove unequivocally effective before proceeding further. Such a protocol was certainly not followed with my friend, Gerald.

At this juncture I think it appropriate to highlight another related point that warrants mention. Throughout the years innovative medical instrument and device-makers have provided physicians and surgeons with highly refined equipment with which to do our jobs better. I always enjoyed the exhibits at neurosurgical meetings, and usually later managed to talk our hospital into buying some useful apparatus. But customarily, after purchasing these innovative devices such as the radiofrequency (RF) generator, laser or ultrasound machines, there was necessarily an increase in the cost of the surgical procedure. This then begs the critical question: Where do we draw the line on holding down the costs for new technology?

As a glaring example, there have been recent legitimate questions raised by knowledgeable experts concerning the cost-effectiveness of some of the newer spinal operations which, during the extensive methods of fixation, may employ the use of commercially-processed fusing substances and advanced metallic hardware costing thousands of dollars. Although there are firmly established criteria for some of these operations such as spinal fractures or instability, they are frequently done in patients with degenerative disc disease (spondylosis) — common in our aging population. The heavy cost borne by Medicare has recently been highlighted in the *Wall Street Journal* (6). Thirty years ago Frank and I had excellent results after performing cervical vertebral-body replacements using simple, straight-forward, reinforcing stainless steel plates and screws, after first using the patient's own bone as a graft. Late follow-up postoperative films showed excellent fusion and stability of the spine. Furthermore, those operations were performed at a fraction of today's cost, even factoring in medical inflation.

Last year I discussed this "cost-effectiveness" point with a former president of the Florida Medical Association. He related to me that he had just heard of a spinal operation performed by an orthopedic surgeon which entailed one afternoon's work and for which the surgeon's fee alone was $50,000!

Relevant to our discussion were matters substantiated by Dr. Atul Gawande in his highly acclaimed article concerning healthcare costs, published in the *New Yorker* (9). This is an erudite, well documented essay comparing medical costs and outcome in two border towns in South Texas. The 2006 Medicare expenditure per enrollee was $7,504 in El Paso County. In the town of McAllen, 800 miles southeast and of similar demographics, Medicare spent $15,000 per enrollee or twice that of El Paso. One of the doctors interviewed in McAllen admitted that he had often seen financial considerations drive the decisions doctors made for their patients. This appeared to be the general theme practiced in the town; namely, more tests, more imaging procedures, more surgical procedures— in essence, more of everything. An example cited was the typical woman presenting with a first-time episode of gallbladder pain due to a stone. A viable alternative treatment option would include recommendations for appropriate medications, a fat-free diet, reassurance and office follow-up. Dr. Gawande was told that when confronted with such a patient, most McAllen surgeons would proceed with surgery instead. Doing so would of course provide them with an immediate reimbursement from Medicare in contradistinction to a more conservative and less lucrative approach utilizing sound clinical judgment and office follow-up.

But interestingly, "more is not necessarily better"—a point not fully recognized even by some hospital administrators. Medicare ranks hospitals on 25 metrics of care, and on 23 of them McAllen's five largest hospitals performed worse, on average, than El Paso's. In the case of the Mayo Clinic, considered the paragon of medical care where the "patient comes first," the cost per enrollee in 2006 was $6,688 — even less than El Paso's. Because the physicians at Mayo may be salaried, any financial incentives to drive up costs are inherently eliminated.

Dr. Gawande discloses many pertinent and interesting facts as he explains these discrepancies in reimbursement, all of which are relevant to any discussion concerning the cost of medical care. His article should be required reading for all of those involved in writing healthcare legislation.

Each of the cases cited above serves to illustrate a specific point: The gallbladder surgery, by its very nature, dictated both greater and immediate reimbursement than medical treatment; the efficacy of the expensive RF treatment for the back pain remains highly open to question, and, at the very least, the procedure was not done according to protocol; the unreasonable fee charged by the orthopedic surgeon can in no way be justified; and finally, the entire scenario concerning the far excessive billing for the supplementary elbow injection during the surgical operation on the wrist was unscrupulous. As corroborated by Dr. Gawande in his article— medicine to a large extent is now being economically driven rather than patient-driven.

After learning of these and several other similar incidents involving different patients, I had lunch with a high-profile local physician. I told him about some of these encounters, and asked him what was happening to the practice of medicine today. If I may directly quote him: "The doctors have been forced by the 'system' to change the way they practice medicine." At the time I disagreed with him, believing it was nothing short of greed.

We have looked at just one aspect of what Dr. Gawande calls the "cost conundrum" (9). Now, take a look, if you will, at something else—factors affecting the workforce. My good friend Ron, who is a prominent retired dentist, had recently asked that I get him and his wife lined up with a family physician. His previous HMO had gone out of business, and upon entering their elderly years they badly needed a doctor. I gave him the names of perhaps six good physicians, all of whom I had helped to train in our TMH family practice residency program. In each instance, after initially speaking to the office clerks and using me as a reference, Ron was openly greeted — until he told them that his insurance was Medicare. With that having been said, he was informed every time that the doctor no longer had any open "new-patient" slots.

Upon relating this story to yet another of my older friends, who was a family physician himself, he told me of a similar recent personal experience. His granddaughter had just given birth to a baby, but the parents were unable to find a pediatrician for the newborn. Every doctor's office contacted told them that— "they were no longer taking any new patients."

Based upon these two incidents, I began wondering whether I was missing something. I had always been taught that, as medical doctors, it was our duty to always look after the sick and infirm. In all my years of medical practice I don't recall our office ever having turned a patient away, very certainly including even those without any insurance at all, and even despite those busy times when we were double- or even triple-booked in our daily patient slots.

Concerned, I began to scrutinize more closely what was occurring. With all due respect, it appeared that many family physicians were both over-worked and underpaid. I well recall years ago the annual negotiations with the directors of our local HMOs in meetings that were often fraught with disdain, as their representatives tried to ratchet down our neurosurgical fees. Frank and I tried to be reasonable during the negotiation process, but it seemed that we invariably lost ground. The reimbursement fees struggled to, at best, remain the same, despite the inflationary costs of our own overhead expenses.

Another such example occurred after my retirement, when some of us had invested in a diagnostic imaging center as a part of our retirement income. It was the same dilemma: Despite a huge capital investment in marvelous, state-of-the-art equipment, our reimbursement rates by both the local HMO and Medicare were hardly enough to keep the company afloat. Some of us later sold out.

As a result, there has unfortunately been a change in the way some doctors view their patients. A few of them are beginning to "cherry pick" their patients by opening up their daily calendars to only those with higher reimbursing insurance as opposed to Medicare or Medicaid. Alternatively, given the fact that the practice of medicine has become more business-oriented, like any business with declining reimbursement, physicians have reverted to increased volume turnover. The strategy is to herd more patients through an office-based practice in any given day (many of them never actually even seeing the physician) in order to increase the revenue stream. But the deleterious byproducts in so doing are a weakening of the time-honored doctor-patient relationship and not infrequently— a compromise of the treatment. More specifically, quick patient turnover begets scanty review of laboratory data, imaging reports, and past physical findings in the patient's chart. One example will suffice: A retired physician friend of mine recently disclosed to me that his wife had had an ovary removed three years previously, but nobody had bothered to read the pathology report until recently— it revealed cancer!

One day, while inconspicuously sitting in my pickup truck at a parking lot, I overheard a group of perhaps five blue-collar workers discussing their recent doctor encounters. They were scathing in their assessment of modern-day medicine, describing it as an impersonal, bitterly brief, assembly-line approach. This was not the kind of medicine practiced during my generation, when the "art and science" were integral to the practice.

Another example clearly illustrates the resentment that many patients are beginning to have regarding the impersonal way in which they are treated in physicians' offices. A local businessman in town recently told me of an experience in which, while waiting in the examining room of a medical office, a nurse practitioner entered to examine him. After refusing the exam and after a brief exchange of words, he finally said, "I'll just sit here and wait for the doctor; I'm paying to see him."

Besides trying to increase volume and using ancillary personnel to help do so, some doctors are even turning to alternative sources of income. Years ago, I had heard of an incident involving a student at one of the medical schools. He reported an office encounter with a family physician who was allegedly his preceptor. Apparently, the student found himself frequently standing idly around in the office while the doctor, rather than teaching the student, was involved in paperwork regarding a research study conducted by a pharmaceutical company. Outwardly disgruntled, he told the student, "You can't make any money in medicine anymore. You need some supplementary means of supporting yourself."

Sadly, it would appear that with decreasing reimbursement rates from most third-party payers, and, in some cases, locked-in capitation fees by the HMOs, many doctors have resorted to devising other means of enhancing their incomes in order to maintain a respectable living— at that after having to pay soaring office overhead expenses (rent, office personnel, malpractice insurance, etc.).

Dr. Thomas Russell, Executive Director of the American College of Surgeons (2009), recently stated, "Numerous economists, statisticians, politicians and others have sought to develop models that limit spending while continuing to ensure that Medicare beneficiaries have access to appropriate services. Yet we still find ourselves with a reimbursement system that is financially unsustainable and that is likely contributing to workforce shortages" (33).

~~~

Turning now to another extremely important, yet largely ignored subject relevant to health costs, consider the following case history: Late one August during a football dinner party, a civil engineer friend of mine called me aside, obviously distressed, to relate to me the following incident. His daughter, a local college student on summer break, had been involved in a single-car accident. Having just left her home, and despite carefully driving in a rainstorm on a paved road, her car suddenly careened into a ditch causing it to roll over. Seemingly unhurt, she called her dad who arrived at the scene at about the same time as the police and EMTs. Merle wanted to take his daughter home in view of the fact that she had no complaints at the time— appearing virtually unscathed from the accident. The police officers present told him that they thought it would be advisable for the ambulance to take her to the hospital just to "check things out." Being the conscientious man that he is, Merle consented to have them load his daughter into the ambulance. Later, after having spent several hours in the emergency department, she was released home with full assurance that she was fine. Two weeks later Merle received a startling bill from the hospital for nearly $14,000 and another from the local radiology group for $1,000. Because his daughter was out of school for the summer and not covered with health insurance, he was fearful at the time that this would be an out-of-pocket expense. Trying to console him regarding the medical charges, I asked him to fax me the bills. Besides the ambulance and emergency room fees, his
~~~

daughter was charged separately for CT scans of the abdomen, chest, pelvis, cervical spine and head. That is, indeed, a lot of imaging and concomitant radiation exposure for someone who was fine at the scene of the accident, and "wanted to go home."

This case represents a prime example of "defensive medicine" in its truest sense. In all of my years of practice — and we saw many cases with very severe, extensive body trauma — I would have a difficult time recalling an instance in which every body region was scanned. In those days we took the time to first examine the patient, and only then x-ray or scan the specific regions of concern.

Let us reconstruct what probably really happened with Merle's daughter. First, the police—not wanting to be held responsible for any liability — recommended she go to the hospital, even though she had no complaints at the time. Second, the ambulance was already there— and somebody had to pay for it! Merle wanted to drive his daughter home. He could have just as easily driven her to the ER if that was the recommendation. Third, the ER doc, already inundated with patients, quickly assessed her by asking if she hurt anywhere. Rather than run the risk of being sued should he miss something, despite a sound history, physical examination and limited pertinent CT imaging, he found it both more expeditious and safer to hustle her off to the x-ray department for head-to-toe CT scanning. This case is best illustrative of both the practice of defensive medicine and over-utilization of resources, in contradistinction to sound clinical judgment, observation, time, and perhaps, at the most, some mild pain medication. It gives us strong reason to pause for a moment: a $15,000 bill to someone without any initial complaints, and who frankly was not injured at all!

In the *Wall Street Journal* (2009, December 26) there was a summary article on the key congressional elements to-date on the proposed healthcare reform bills within the House and Senate respectively. Is it not surprising that tort reform was not even mentioned in that table. Yet the cost of defensive medicine alone is estimated at over $200 billion annually. If the cost of health reform is really the issue, why isn't this addressed? We all know the answer to that question. I have yet to become engaged in this or related discussions with a group of knowledgeable persons (not just doctors), but what they admit that the trial lawyers in our country have nothing short of a hammerlock on our society. The reader will recall that in past chapters I wrote of the following events: 1).The local newspaper's refusal (after consulting with the local attorneys) to publish our medical society's 1975 article on the medical liability crisis; 2). a legislature-approved, non-binding, state mediation panel concerning personal medical injury that was later declared "unconstitutional" by the Florida Supreme Court; and finally, 3). the indifferent responses by Hillary Rodham Clinton and both U.S. senators to my 1993 paper on healthcare reform (endorsed by the Florida Medical Association). Incidentally, the contents of that paper would be equally applicable today— 17 years later.

Students of American history are well aware that in the latter half of the 18th century, the young nation's fate was in the hands of a small group of versatile, often affluent men, many of whom were merchants, landowners and lawyers. Although most were educated, articulate and generally outspoken, they collectively seemed to possess a clear altruistic vision for our country, and have since been referred to as the "Power Elite" (29). Many would argue that today our nation is also controlled by a powerful, vocal, collectively wealthy group, consisting largely of a subset of members within the legal profession. Because they both comprise the majority of the legislative bodies writing the laws and also preside over the courts, they determine how business is done— usually to their advantage. In contrast to our forefathers, the current power-elite group nurtures, as its prerogative, self-serving interests that tend to erode, for their own benefit, our society rather than to enhance it. Few would argue that in reality our system, rather than being a true democracy, constitutes a professional class rule or an oligarchy.

Let me give just two examples clearly pointing out how the judicial system is tainted in favor of the plaintiff in Florida. The first entails an article recently published in the newsletter of the Capital Medical Society in which the annual report of the American Tort Reform Foundation (ATRF) was summarized. The ATRF ranks six areas of the country which have developed reputations for litigation abuses; that is specifically, "where judges apply laws and court procedures in an unfair and unbalanced manner generally against defendants in civil lawsuits." South Florida was ranked #1 in the 2009 report. Citing unreasonable jury awards, it was stated that since November 2007 there have been five separate medical malpractice trials with verdicts in excess of $30 million awarded to the plaintiffs (45).

The second example involves one of the statutes in Florida. My legal consultant has updated me on the details of a statute on the Florida books, about which few of our citizens are aware— "Comparative Fault." Although in 2006 there was a modification of the final pecuniary distributions concerning the previous Principle of Joint and Several

Liabilities, it still obtains that any awards in a personal injury suit are based upon the "court's estimate of the percentage of guilt".

Citing an example, I was asked to render a medical opinion in a case of documented, flagrant recklessness on the part of the plaintiff himself, who unfortunately was seriously injured in an accident. Even though the defendant was found only 10% at fault (and even that could have been contested), he had to pay out a $1 million award in what was a $10 million law suit. This comparative-fault rule is nothing but an invitation to frivolous lawsuits, and renders Florida a virtual paradise for trial lawyers. They are almost guaranteed a contingency fee in taking any case, whatsoever— even those of questionable merit. In contradistinction to Florida, Illinois, for example, has what is known as the "Not More Than Principle." In Illinois, if a defendant is not more than 49% responsible for the plaintiff's injury, he pays nothing. This law, few would argue, is more just for those unfairly accused of causing injury, and poses a strong argument for national tort reform. For years I have watched the doctors of our state plead their case regarding meaningful tort reform, but their efforts have largely been in vain.

Before continuing, I must emphasize that virtually no one would dispute that true negligence resulting in personal injury should be compensated, and most would agree that the person so injured is entitled to his day in court. Doctors who have consistently been found negligent should be appropriately dealt with through their medical specialty groups and state licensing bodies. Those bodies should have the power to see the doctor either rehabilitated or removed from his current practice, and not exonerated through clever, expensive, legal counsel.

In deference to those unfortunate patients who sustain injury from medical accidents (as opposed to acts of true negligence), there should be some means within our system of compensating them. In the past, one solution mentioned by others has been some type of "no-fault" insurance, similar to that seen in motor vehicle coverage. But the question of true negligence is not the issue here and is not to be confused with a bad outcome.

In defense of the honorable physician who has spent his or her entire life in the study of medicine, and while practicing in full accordance with the prevailing standards of the community, if a patient sustains a bad outcome (not incurred by the result of negligence), the doctor should not be assaulted financially and emotionally by the unhappy plaintiff's attorney. Because of just such an incident here in town, a very scholarly physician friend of mine was driven into retirement nearly 20 years prematurely, and has yet to recover from that degrading experience.

Of relevance, in my unpublished newspaper article of 1975 denouncing the lawyers who cried out that it was only the incompetent doctors who were getting sued, I pointed out that the targets of many large suits were the professors of surgery at the university centers. After all, they all are the ones bold enough to operate upon cases that the rest of us fear to touch. They are often the most skilled of the lot.

Aside from litigation for a bad outcome, there is another aspect of concern regarding lawsuits — the mere anticipation of one! Some of the younger surgeons in our area are comfortable in earning a living by picking only the "low-hanging fruit"; i.e., the straightforward and safest surgical procedures. Others, for instance the younger neurosurgeons in town, will simply avoid the more dangerous operations. In a defensive posture they refuse to treat intracranial aneurysms; without exception, every such case is now referred out to some distant university center. Individually, they have told me that venturing into this dangerous work is nothing short of an invitation to a lawsuit, should a negative result occur. No one knowledgeable in the treatment of this condition can argue with their logic.

Similarly, a few years ago many of the hospital emergency rooms in South Florida, because of the highly litigious climate and fears of a lawsuit, were having difficulty in getting neurosurgical coverage. Cases demanding such care were necessarily referred distantly to Miami. Earlier in the book I emphasized several entities that need immediate treatment if a fatal issue is to be avoided. What happens to the older child with rapidly increasing intracranial pressure from shunt-dependent hydrocephalus while riding in an ambulance, fighting traffic, en route from the Palm Beach area to Miami?

The reader will also recall the incident many years ago in which, over the phone, I steered a young general surgeon residing miles away through a craniectomy on a child in order to save his life from a rapidly expanding epidural hemorrhage. Today it would be a rare doctor who would venture out of his specialty in such treatment lest the consequences of potential liability, in the wake of a bad outcome, descend crushingly upon him.

Furthermore, as an indirect result of the legal oppression causing surgeons to eschew certain services, some patients, seeking those same essential services, may find themselves traveling far away from their communities to obtain them. This can be inconvenient, at times very costly, and even dangerous by delaying urgent care. Recently one of the professors at the medical school expressed concern to me that she had a crippled child, whom she had to intermittently drive 600 miles round trip to Birmingham in order to obtain specialty care. She had looked into a group locally which allegedly performed that specific type of corrective surgery, but they had refused to take her child as a patient. Although I didn't say anything to her I could only assume that, in all likelihood, they did not want to accept the liability risk relative to the child's complex problem.

Reading the preceding paragraphs demands the question: Why should surgeons with highly specialized skills and training be intimidated from providing relevant needed care to patients within their communities? In the early chapters of this book I described the intense and lengthy study required to become a neurological surgeon. But the education process does not stop with passage of the final board examination and certification. Reading the newsletter of the American Board of Neurological Surgery (2008), I see there is discussion concerning Maintenance of Certification. This not only evaluates the neurosurgeon's professional standing, life-long learning, self-assessment and cognitive knowledge, but also evidence of performance in practice. The latter requires the participant to track his proficiency and the outcome from a number of different categories, comparing his results with those of his peers. The public should be fully aware and take comfort over the ends to which most board-certified surgeons, irrespective of their specialty, are trained and the highest standards of practice to which they are held. The surgeon's overall knowledge and skill should not immediately be judged by a negative outcome; certainly, not when each and every day there is an inherent risk in virtually every operation he performs, granted, some more than others. In the particular case of the neurosurgeon, why should the sword of Damocles hang over him each time he enters the operating room to rid the patient of some often complicated hideous, danger lurking within the intracranial cavity or spinal canal? Similarly, why should the destitute patient, indirectly affected by the mere threat of that same sword, sometimes have no recourse but to travel several hundred miles for treatment? These are all reasons why we need tort reform, not only to free the doctor to carry out the duties for which he has been expertly trained, but to reduce the incessant "fear" of a lawsuit, thus allowing him to better serve the community. This can in itself reduce the burgeoning costs of defensive medicine.

For years physicians nationwide have been trying to obtain some type of federal protection from malpractice suits. In Florida we are up against such an imposing collective group of lawyer-legislators that every attempt at reform is stymied. For instance Texas was able to place a $250,000 cap on punitive damages; but only after much wrangling in 2003 were we lucky to get $500,000— and even that has been challenged. Physicians in practice must tip-toe through the process of vocalizing for reform, not individually wanting to become too visible, lest they might incur the wrath of their local attorneys. Even the AMA has been ineffective nationally, while the results of any state reforms are merely table scraps. After what I have witnessed during my medical career, I am going on record as predicting that the legal oligarchy of our day will forever determine the drumbeat to which we all march. That is— unless there is generated enough incentive and public support to unseat them. Although it would take a wide and concerted effort, the public is generally dissatisfied enough with the "Big Business of the Law" that changes could quite conceivably be achieved. Under the coordinated leadership of both the business sector of our country and the medical establishment (e.g., the state medical societies, and the voices of the influential, national medical specialty organizations), such change could both financially and politically be instigated. We do have a system in place in this great nation that will allow us to elect lawmakers who recognize the importance of meaningful tort reform in reducing medical and other costs of doing business. Those involved both in business and healthcare delivery can then be unshackled from the bonds of legal oppression resulting from those costly, time-consuming, demoralizing lawsuits involving so much that is so short of true negligence. It would seem to me that it is time for the citizens of this country to step forth in supporting this change. The doctors alone have been unable to do it.

~~~

Respecting other aspects of healthcare reform, I would like to emphasize again the objectivity of my observations as a retired, non-practicing physician. Like my colleagues who practiced medicine during the latter half of the 20th century, I have borne witness to significant change, as reflected in the preceding pages. This is not to vituperate any specific individual, group or facility, but rather to point out problems within our region, some rather thought-provoking, that I think echo those
~~~

voiced nationally. Only by acknowledging any improprieties or areas of waste and inefficiency can we then more rationally analyze and rectify them.

Thus far in this chapter I have endeavored to point out instances of unreasonable costs, modes of treatment of dubious value, poor communication among physicians and offices, overutilization of scans and other tests, misplaced or lost medical reports, etc. What's more, there is plenty of blame to go around. Anyone who has spent a night in the hospital can attest to what most consider excessive costs. And finally, we might ask, how does the patient himself figure into all of this? Let me cite a recent experience in that regard.

I was called by a friend to examine his son, a highly educated professional man, who was having a number of disconcerting symptoms in his arms, legs and spine. He was convinced that he was being overtaken by some horrible disease of the central nervous system. A thorough history and careful neurological examination, done by me on two separate occasions, failed to reveal any evidence of organic disease. To the contrary, he was under an enormous amount of stress at work which had created inordinate anxiety. My recommendation, after counseling him on the stress, was that we follow him closely with serial examinations. Like so many other patients in today's world, he went on-line on his computer, and began searching out exotic illnesses that might best fit his symptoms. Because his constellation of unrelated symptoms did not bespeak an organic disease, I again tried to reassure him after still a third visit. The next day I received a call from his father who reported that Blair said he had insurance that would cover the cost of an MRI scan, and that he would like to have one done. Suffice it to say, people today have wide access to medical information, but lack the medical expertise obtained only through medical school and experience to make rational sense out of what they have read. Yet they feel justified in requesting tests costing thousands of dollars, simply because "The insurance company will pay for it." In dealing with such patients, as I mentioned in my 1993 FMA article, the doctor must feel confident in taking a firm stand regarding ancillary tests and imaging studies based on his provisional diagnosis, just as I did with the young man discussed above. He must then carefully record all of his findings and his recommendations. The doctor's rationale in using good clinical judgment in accordance with standard practice should be supported by his knowledgeable peers, and not maligned by the lawyers as an act of negligence should his medical opinion prove incorrect. Just because a patient walks into the office and wants a scan doesn't mean that it is necessarily indicated. Nor should the doctor feel compelled to comply with the patient's wishes merely for the sake of practicing "defensive medicine." Incidentally, in the case of the young man discussed above in whom we did not pursue the expensive, unwarranted MRI, he finally began to listen to me. His psychosomatic symptoms have since entirely abated, and he has nicely compensated in learning how to handle his work-related stress.

While there are a number of interrelated complex problems associated with our current healthcare delivery system, they are by no means insoluble. In addition to tort reform, I shall touch below on some of the current thinking on other facets of cost containment.

In the earlier chapter regarding the1993 FMA-endorsed paper in which reference was made to various areas of wasteful spending, I touched briefly in citing several relevant examples concerning the highly charged subject of rationing medical resources under specific circumstances. I do not stand alone in believing that the concept of "spare no expense under any circumstances" is no longer tenable. The bench-mark example remains the brain dead patient, in which both the law and society have come to recognize the futility of indefinitely maintaining such an individual in an expensive intensive-care unit on life-support systems. But there are other similar medical circumstances that are currently less well defined or accepted. While some of these may be contrary to the Hippocratic doctrine, if organized medicine and the public don't accept this concept of reasonable rationing, then the government most likely will. This was corroborated in an article reflecting the views of Dr. Ezekiel Emanuel, a bioethicist and health adviser to President Barack Obama. That article clearly raises the question that not everyone may be entitled to "unlimited" care (28). This alone can be a significant factor in reducing the cost of healthcare.

Let us next look at the hospitals in the cost equation. There was a recent news clip on CNN reflecting the general concern over exorbitant hospital costs. An example given was the charge of $140 for a single Tylenol tablet. The hospitals argue that they must inflate such costs in order to cover uncompensated indigent care. But unfortunately the rest of us ultimately pay that cost ourselves through ever-increasing insurance premiums. And what about the poor man in the hospital whose insurance falls short of covering such a formidable, cumulative set of charges? Why should he go bankrupt under pressing conditions of a dreadful illness, refractory to treatment?

An enlightening article published in the *Wall Street Journal* reflected that lowering hospital costs is indeed possible — at least in India. In 2001, Dr. Devi Shetty, a cardiac surgeon who trained at Guy's Hospital in London, conceived of building a dedicated hospital for cardiac surgery in Bangalore. It is difficult to comprehend that this flagship heart hospital charges an average of only $2,000 per open heart case, as opposed to between $20,000 and $100,000 in the U.S., depending of course upon the complexity of the surgical procedure. The 1,000-bed facility employs 42 cardiac surgeons, and performs 3,174 cardiac operations per year, more than twice that of the Cleveland Clinic in the U.S. The secret to their success in bringing down costs is volume, and while doing so, they continue to utilize cutting-edge techniques and equipment. In describing his model, Dr. Shetty says… "What healthcare needs is process innovation, not product innovation." He is able to cut costs, for instance, by buying medical equipment directly from suppliers rather than sellers. They are even able to purchase indispensable equipment at reduced cost from large companies, such as General Electric, "because they are such good customers." For those who argue that quantity usually sacrifices quality, their mortality rate of 1.4% within 30 days of a coronary-artery bypass graft is better than the average of 1.9% rate in the U.S. This understandably is because each cardiac surgeon specializes in specific procedures, proficiently performing those operations many times per week.

Of equal interest to the high quality of the heart surgery performed is the sound way that the hospital is financially managed, including the insurance plan offered to the low-income working class. It might be important for us to take a closer look at this paradigm (1).

While hospital cost-cutting can be accomplished in India, it might be more problematic in the U.S. simply because of our highly competitive, <u>market-driven</u> system consisting of so many different players— both suppliers and consumers. Anyone standing on the sidelines throughout the country, when observing large hospital expenditures for any number of things, can only surmise that they must enjoy significant profits far in excess of any compensatory patient charges to offset indigent care. Like everyone else in these difficult times, it seems that they should be held accountable for what many feel are uncontrolled, carte blanche charges. As indicated recently in the *Wall Street Journal*, perhaps third-party payers will begin pressuring hospitals into curbing costs by controlling reimbursements (20).

At this juncture, allow me to share a few additional concepts cited by Dr. Russell concerning the current medical thinking on healthcare reform.

The market-based philosophy, much like that seen in large corporations, has been adopted by the healthcare sector, and is largely responsible for driving it as a "big business." Because this implies that "bigger is better," it is taken by the patients to mean that the more that is done in the way of medical tests and procedures, the better the care. Those paying for these tests provide physicians with incentives to meet this expensive "consumer demand." Quite otherwise, in order to reduce escalating medical costs, we must change to a value-driven system, that is to say, what can be done differently to provide equally effective, yet, more efficient and less costly care? Dr. Russell speaks of better use of information technology to maintain records and handle basic communications. This would vastly improve inter-physician efficiency and obviate unnecessary replication of costly laboratory and imaging studies. He also emphasizes the use of evidence-based medicine guidelines (32). The latter aims to apply the best available evidence gained from the scientific method to medical decision-making. This corroborates an important point I have tried to emphasize repeatedly by citing examples — the cost and comparative effectiveness of new treatment modalities should be determined by the statistical method. Furthermore, EBM seeks to assess the evidence of the risks and benefits of treatment.

The reader will recall in an earlier chapter the large random study in 1985, which statistically invalidated the extracranial-intracranial bypass operation for the routine prevention of stroke in certain cases of intracranial arterial occlusive disease. That study alone unquestionably saved hundreds of millions of dollars in future healthcare costs. Again showing how times have changed, a similar study was recently performed comparing the effectiveness of stent insertions in cardiac patients with chest pain as compared to drug therapy. This study, termed "Courage," reported in the *New England Journal of Medicine* (2007), showed no difference in the two modes of treatment. Yet many cardiologists, patients and device-makers haven't paid notice to the recommended guidelines from that study, namely, to initially try the patient on drugs. The expensive stenting procedure rate is now higher than ever. In an article in the *Wall Street Journal* (2010 February 11), there is a lengthy discussion as to why "Courage" has been ignored. The procedure economically favors its practioners, and the patient sees it as an "immediate cure" with the insurance company bearing the cost (48). It is indeed perplexing that 25 years ago during my generation there was enough integrity in our system that, despite the enormous worldwide investment of time and money in the cranial bypass procedure, it was abandoned in favor of less expensive drug therapy; yet, the "Courage" study of today has failed to impact the $15 billion annual bill on stent placements.

Sooner or later it seems inevitable that potentially expensive treatments are probably all going to be subjected to such "cost-comparative-effectiveness" analyses, and everyone is going to be forced to abide by the results. That is to say: Medicare and the insurance companies will only pay for the least expensive, yet equally effective modes of treatment.

Guidelines such as these would produce some standardization of care, coordinate care among physicians, and use resources more efficiently, while at the same time eliminating errors (32). There are currently in place throughout the country value-based provider networks implementing these concepts such as the Mayo Clinic, Cleveland Clinic and Kaiser-Permanente, to name a few. Some concern might reside in the fact that these networks, paragons of efficiency, encompass but a small geographic portion of the total expanse of health delivery. One might reasonably ask, "How do we deliver care for those living in smaller towns, far-removed from these large networks?"

The answer may partly lie in Dr. Gawande's *New Yorker* article, in which he refers to Grand Junction, Colorado, where some of Medicare's highest quality-of-care scores are achieved. The doctors there agreed among themselves to a system that paid them a similar fee whether they saw Medicare or private-insurance patients, thus reducing the incentive to "cherry-pick" the patients. The doctors also exercise peer review, and have committees overseeing costs and quality-of-care issues. Unnecessary surgery is frowned upon as are unusual complication rates. In other words, there is real accountability in that medical community. As a result, the problems in Grand Junction have gone down, quality has gone up, and costs have ended up lower than most places in the United States. This city of 120,000 citizens proves that with everyone working together quality reform is possible on a small scale (9).

It seems to make sense that as these value-based systems increase in numbers, the market will increasingly flow toward them, forcing others to change their way of doing business. Costs will fall. Referring again to Dr. Thomas Russell, I would like to quote his closing statement which resonates loudly in today's healthcare environment, "...We must instill the principles that set professionals apart from profiteers" (32).

In closing this chapter it is enlightening to record where our leaders are taking us at this point in time. Because of what we have all recently witnessed in Congress regarding healthcare reform, it might be well to look at what has happened in Massachusetts. In 2006 Governor Mitt Romney signed into law a plan mandating that most residents either have health insurance or have a fine imposed. The results of that plan have recently been well-summarized in the *Wall Street Journal* with a few of the salient points being listed below. While the number of uninsured citizens in Massachusetts has indeed dropped to three percent, 68% of the newly insured receive coverage that is either heavily or completely subsidized by the taxpayers of the state. Insurance premiums have necessarily escalated, with a family of four paying $13,788 annually, the per capita spending being 27% higher than the national average. Furthermore, commensurate with the increased load of patients there has been a relative shortage of doctors, and many of those are no longer accepting new patients. To make matters even worse, there are some people who "game" the system, buying required insurance only at the time of critical illness or surgery, obtaining their routine care elsewhere. This not only reduces the insurance pool but also translates into increasing emergency room visits (which jumped 7% in 24 months), thereby fiscally threatening some hospitals which have seen a reduction in their reimbursements for uncompensated care (44). Despite the obvious unexpected shortcomings and failures of the Massachusetts model, the U.S. Congress passed, and President Obama proceeded to sign into law on March 23, 2010 a very similar national healthcare plan.

No one can argue against the need for extension of coverage to the uninsured of our country or the mandates placed on insurance companies to neither deny nor eliminate protection for those who are ill or have pre-existing conditions. The argument lies squarely on the Machiavellian manner in which this legislation had been crafted and passed. It is easy for those without knowledge of the underpinnings of healthcare delivery to simply impose declarations and mandates and, thereafter, cleverly improvise ways (e.g., to the detriment of decreasing reimbursement for the doctors) for the taxpayers to foot the bill. But why did they not first look at repairing the flaws in our current system? To have first appointed a versatile committee of clear-minded professionals qualified to analyze, in-depth, the outlandish costs (defensive medicine just to name one) and other wastes before imposing more debt on our country clearly would have made more sense.

Many experts feel that, even now, meaningful changes in healthcare reform can be achieved, but only with honest bipartisan resolve, diligent study, and forethought. This can only be accomplished by utilizing resourceful, indispensable input from objective, knowledgeable, healthcare professionals and business leaders throughout the country. Such a committee was quickly assembled "after the fact" to analyze the details of the 2010 BP oil-spill in the Gulf of Mexico. One might then reasonably pose the question: Why not, with a concerted effort, organize a task force for an in-depth analysis of this complex healthcare issue that is affecting virtually everyone?

FIFTEEN

After the Journey—A Time for Relaxation and Reflection

~~~

It is hard for some to believe that I had spent 34 years in the Tallahassee area, and had never taken the time to set foot on magnificent St. George Island. Even my children had spent numerous days there on the beautiful white sandy beaches under the clear, blue Florida skies when on spring break from school. I must give full credit to Elaine who first introduced me to that scenic barrier island 100 miles to the southwest of Tallahassee. It is a virtual paradise, nestled in the Gulf of Mexico, where people enjoy their beautiful homes surrounded by the blue-green water, totally isolated from the chaos associated with the frustrating traffic and fast-food stores to which most of us are accustomed. Although we would never own a dwelling on this long, narrow island, I was intrigued by the shallow Apalachicola bay and the prospect of one day owning a small fishing boat.

When people retire they are generally expected to try their hand in at least some fishing; thus, I have never felt that I needed to apologize for time spent in indulging in that great pastime. Several years after selling the cattle, I had the opportunity of finally purchasing a used, welded-aluminum G3 boat as an introduction to the popular sport of saltwater fishing. My friend Ron, the retired dentist, owned a "pop-up" camper which he would set up at the state park on St. George Island, often fishing for weeks at a time during the summers. Reflecting back on my childhood days of camping and trout fishing in Colorado, I soon became motivated with the prospect of rekindling those interests along the Gulf of Mexico. Once having begun, we not only fished in the bay at St. George but also in the one at St. Joe Peninsula State Park, 50 miles to the west. After later purchasing my own fold-down camper, Ron and I
~~~

regularly began spending 4 to 6 weeks each summer enjoying our retirement at these gorgeous Florida state parks. Weather permitting, the days were spent boating and fishing, while the camaraderie of the evenings was frequently enjoyed in the camper over a delicious meal of freshly caught fish. Although at times it can be uncomfortably hot under the intense Florida sun, fishing far out in the bay provides a distraction from the heat and has a soothing effect on the mind. Novel sensations are aroused when one is quietly isolated from humanity on such a large body of water. The calm is interrupted only by the rhythmic slapping of the waves against the hull, synchronous with the constant to and fro motion of the vessel. And when least expected, a large gull might dive into the water nearby to snatch a fish, or a frolicking porpoise might happen along to gain attention. Manatees, large groups of stingrays and other interesting creatures appear at the most unlikely times, each serving to remind the vulnerable fishermen that he is but a mere guest in their vast, mysterious, dark-blue domain. And while enjoying the quiet and solitude, the silence may suddenly be broken when one is seized with the excitement of a large striking fish. The sensation one experiences as it then runs with the line while diving to greater depths, your rod straining and bending nearly in half, provides a great adventure for any outdoor sportsman. After the strike when beginning to reel it in, your excitement soon becomes tempered as you try to anticipate the nature of the fish you have on your line. After the drama has unfolded, one's efforts should at the very least be rewarded with a picture for the family album. Regarding such a picture, I would like to quote a priceless comment by my 12-year-old grandson, Harrison, when speaking to one of his little friends —"Most grandpas sit on the porch all day, but mine catches sharks."

As my enthusiasm for boats grew, Elaine and I later purchased a larger boat which is rigged with all of the latest and necessary electronic equipment, ample live-well capacity and storage space that qualify it as an excellent bay fishing boat. As one might expect of a neurologist, we had the name "Limbic Joy" painted in yellow on the boat's blue hull. Our vessel is usually launched at the mouth of the St. Marks River and powered into the Gulf of Mexico. When venturing out over the dark blue waters of the Gulf, often devoid of any signs of humanity as far as the eye can see, one enjoys a quiet serenity found few places on earth.

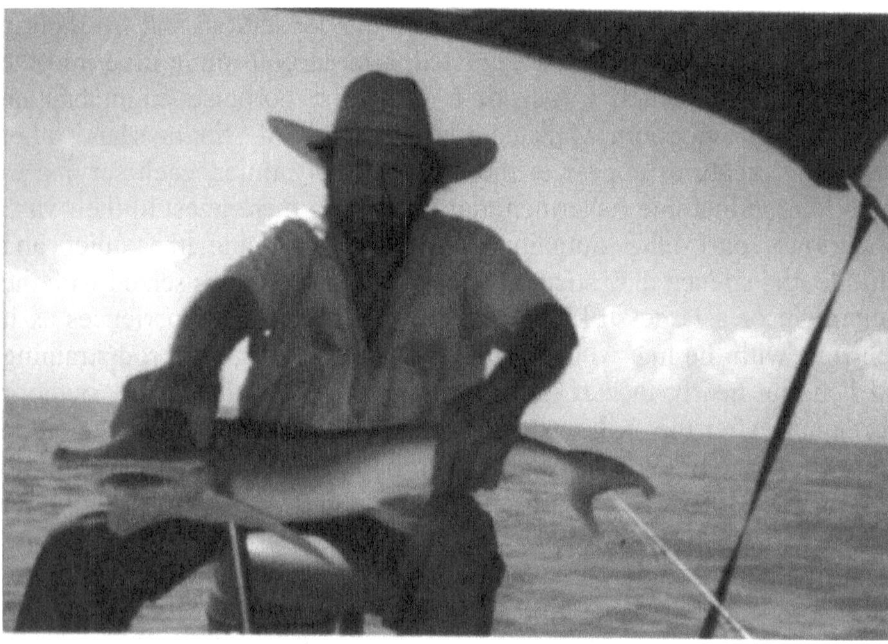

The Fisherman

Another source of pleasure during my later years has been that of corresponding, if not personally associating, with my previous professional friends from time to time. While generally considered a loner by nature, I still derive a great sense of enjoyment in attending medical functions, often recounting past experiences with old colleagues. I have always felt that those hard-working, conscientious physicians (most of the highest moral and professional caliber) formed the stable foundation of our exceptional medical community. It was, indeed, my privilege to have practiced medicine with them for so many years.

While there are far too many close personal friends to recognize here, I cannot omit our small "football group." Throughout the football season we alternate, as hosts, in providing the meals when enjoying the weekly televised Seminole games. Included among these special people is my old friend, Bob Doherty, whom I have known for 56 years and his delightful wife, Anneliese, who takes very good care of him. He and I go far back to the days at Northwestern when, as fraternity brothers and roommates, we battled through physics together. Then there is my good friend, Frank Melichar, now a retired neuroradiologist and his wife, Fran. I am indebted to Frank for his years of professional assistance in both providing his interventional work and also the interpretation of the detailed radiographs and computed images necessary for our neurosurgical success. Frank also helped me initially get started in the cattle business, an avocation in which he and Fran had excelled. Finally, there is Ron Kobetitsch whom I have frequently mentioned. He, like the others, is a true and loyal friend and my close companion during the boating/fishing adventures. Ron's wife, Gisela, who is both a thoughtful and generous person, completes our group's "circle of friends." During the "off season" we have also enjoyed movie-night get-togethers. As members of the same generation we reminisce over many of the old classic movies. The likes of Johnny Weissmuller, Boris Karloff and Lon Chaney Jr. conjure up memories of those Saturday morning matinees during the war when we were kids.

After having paid tribute to many of my friends and acquaintances throughout the book, I must now turn to my all important family. Time and distance have precluded my spending much personal time with my sons and grandchildren in the Pacific Northwest, but we do communicate from time to time. And speaking for all of my children and their children, both near and far, we have developed an emotional closeness that will remain forever in our memories. In my remaining years, I hope to see more of each and every one of them and perhaps leave with them an image with which they can positively identify, and which will, for them in their own lives, forever serve as a source of inspiration.

And finally there is my wife, Elaine. It wasn't easy for her to step into my life where the loss of Valencia had left such a deep void in my heart. But over the course of time Elaine and I have become very close. For a marriage to endure and become a solid, lasting bond, there necessarily has to be mutual respect, understanding, and the ability not only to communicate but even vent one's feelings during times of adversity and despair. This we have been able to do, and as a result our covenant is very strong. I have come to love and cherish her very much and couldn't begin to do without her.

~~~

If I may now reflect on an entirely different subject: When I drove my truck down to the coast last year to pick up our new boat, the owner of the marine store curiously informed me that an old patient of mine, owning a business in that small coastal town, wished to see me. Described as a large, burly, lumbering fellow with a bushy, red beard; he had apparently received word that I had recently purchased a boat. I eventually looked him up, and as he later stood towering over me it was hard to imagine that this was the same Archer MacCluster whom I had known as a little child. His case was discussed in detail in an earlier chapter. I first saw Archer as a baby in 1972 when he was referred to me as a case of obstructive hydrocephalus. After having placed a diversionary VP shunt in him, the next several years proved to be rocky in that he had required several shunt revisions. Keeping in mind all of the child's medical adversity, I still remember his parents who so stoically stood by little Archer with such deep love and concern. Despite the numerous hospitalizations and surgical procedures, he survived with his condition to achieve adulthood. While still grieving from the recent loss of his loving parents, Archer has now taken over the family wholesale fish business, managing it quite successfully, I might add.

After that touching experience last year, it seemed only appropriate to begin winding down my book on a neurosurgical note. While I have been busy ranching, building furniture and fishing for the last several years, my pediatric patients have, in the meantime, been growing into responsible adults. I therefore decided to look up three more of them, selecting each as representing a distinct pediatric neurosurgical entity.
~~~

What I am about to record I believe reflects the sentiment of most pediatric neurosurgeons. Those trying times spent in residency training were by no means wasted, as later realized when revisiting those patients who are no longer tiny babies or small children.

The second patient in this group presented to me in 1987 with a misshapen head. His case of craniosynostosis, termed scaphocephaly, was the result of a pre-mature fusion of the midline (sagittal) suture of the skull. Left untreated the head would have become elongated front-to-back, and when viewed from the front, it would appear both flattened from side to side and "keel-shaped" at the top. Most adults can recall at some time during their early childhood years in school such a child with an unusual head shape, and how the other children were quick to single them out. As described earlier, in order to surgically cure this toddler of his cosmetic deformity, we created artificial sutures in the skull along each side of the midline. This would allow future lateral expansion of the head commensurate with unrestricted brain growth.

Today Claude is now 23 years old, has been graduated from high school and has completed some college work. The reconstructive cranial surgery has provided him with a normal and cosmetically pleasing head shape as attested to by his relatives. He is currently working at the front desk of a local hotel.

Case #3 first appeared in 1972, when I was asked by a concerned local pediatrician to evaluate a six-month-old baby boy with an enlarging head. Because computed tomography was yet to be developed, I had to perform air ventriculography on him. The infant proved to have a large cyst within the posterior fossa of his head, and concomitant obstructive hydrocephalus. This rare condition, known as the Dandy-Walker syndrome, required independent shunting procedures to decompress both the cyst and the lateral ventricles respectively. The baby did very well after the operation, continued to thrive, and was followed in the clinic right on through his school years. I last saw him as an adolescent shortly before I retired, a time at which he appeared of normal intelligence and personality. Recently, during the process of writing my memoirs, I came across an old letter from Alvin which he had mailed to me soon after my retirement. I had stuck it in Doctor Walter Dandy's (the surgeon who first described this condition) historic book entitled, *The Brain*. In the letter, young Alvin was very kind in praising me for giving him a normal life. He went on to say … "I hope that one day in the future we will pass by each other on the street and you will look at me and be proud of the fact that I was a patient of yours. I hope to be a shining example of the great work you have done as a doctor."

How thoughtful and considerate for this young man to have written these kind words to his doctor; it was very much appreciated, indeed. Upon rediscovering that letter, I decided to contact Alvin, but he was nowhere to be found in our area. After a computer search, we finally tracked him down in Atlanta. I have since both spoken with him on the telephone and have acquired his picture. At 38 years of age I find the same nice-looking, affable person that I had recollected him to be as a youngster. Now he is a responsible, successful, married man, and I am indeed proud of him — as he had hoped in his letter 18 years ago.

Case #4, the last patient in this group, came under my care in 1979, two hours after her birth and weighing 7-pounds. She was born with spina bifida and a lumbosacral myelomeningocele. This was repaired immediately after birth, followed eight days later with a shunt for hydrocephalus. This anomalous condition is known as the Arnold-Chiari II malformation. She appeared to progress satisfactorily after the surgery, but as with Alvin I lost track of Lisa when I stepped down from practice in 1992. Sixteen years after my retirement, I happened to run into her mother in a small store in the coastal town of Apalachicola, Florida, and indicated to her that I would like to see my former little patient sometime.

Years later I called the patient's home, fully anticipating that I would first speak with her mother. To my pleasant surprise, I suddenly found myself conversing with a very intelligent, vivacious young lady, who was none other than Lisa herself. After subsequently being invited over to their home, I had a pleasant visit with the family. Lisa, now a very pretty young lady, is able to stand and walk, functions that I could not have begun to predict early that morning 31 years ago when dissecting those minute spinal nerves within the meningocele sack openly presenting itself on her tiny back. As I was leaving their home I silently recalled how Marshall and I had struggled together way back in 1970 at the Children's Memorial Hospital in Chicago as the only two junior residents holding down the neurosurgical service. The long days passed very slowly during those arduous six months in which we operated upon literally hundreds of babies and took night call every other night. As I stood at the doorway, with her mother looking on and Lisa smiling at me with such deeply felt appreciation; I gently touched my patient's head while thinking… "To have had just one baby turn out as well as this would have made all of that hard work during my surgical training worthwhile."

Prior to 1952 there was no effective treatment for hydrocephalus. The first valve-regulated shunt was developed that year by Nulsen, Spitz and Holter. Thirty years later, in 1982, the five-year survival rate for shunted cases of hydrocephalus was reported at 90% (34). We have just presented three cases here who are alive and functioning very well at 38, 38, and 31 years, respectively.

Recently, when reflecting back on our professional lives, my radiologist friend, Frank, asked me whether I would follow the same professional pathway if I had to do things over. I answered his question positively by relating to him my great sense of satisfaction in having recently contacted each of the above surviving patients— all operated upon as babies so many years ago— finding them now, decades later, such grateful productive citizens. His response was, "Jim, what you have done for them— no one can ever take away from you"

As a physician there is no greater reward than looking back on patients such as these, and enjoying the sense of accomplishment that goes with healing the crippled body. After all— that is the very reason most of us chose medicine in the first place. At the onset I had envisioned emulating my friend Jim's father, the Denver chest surgeon, who removed the mechanical pencil from the child's heart back in 1950.

In reflecting back on my life I have enjoyed, with few exceptions, learning new material from the early years of high school forward, always anticipating being a doctor like my grandfather. Because there was no self-doubt that I would attain that goal, I never felt that I was wasting time either when studying, or later when grinding away tirelessly as a resident in the hospital, just trying to survive through the night. After commencing with the study of neuroanatomy, neurology and surgery—eventually combining them— I knew that I had finally found my place in medicine. Like my resident colleagues, I became fascinated first with all of the intricacies of the nervous system and later the surgical means by which difficult conditions could be treated. Moreover, when matriculating through this process, the last thing any of us discussed was that of future income. To the contrary, we were passionate about what we had yet to learn and the future challenges confronting us in treating complex lesions— often positioned in seemingly impossible places within the nervous system.

Parenthetically, it was somewhat amusing to me to read one of the submitted critiques of Dr. Gawande's New Yorker article regarding the cost conundrum in medicine. The critic posed the question, which in essence asked— "Do you really think that you can get quality people to laboriously sustain the rigors of a residency if they are looking at an institutionally fixed, albeit reasonable, future salary as a surgeon?" Therein lies the very problem today as I see it! As previously written, in my day most of us felt that money should not be the primary driver, but rather to seek the rewarding sustenance of accumulating the knowledge necessary to become a top-flight surgeon. Referring again to the essence of what my insurance friend said so many years ago— "Doc, when you enjoy what you are doing and are proficient at it, the money will come naturally." Furthermore, I can't imagine practicing neurosurgery (even with a set salary) at an institution like the Mayo Clinic and not being happy with my chosen specialty.

What has just been said is not meant to de-emphasize the importance of a well deserved, decent income, but rather to clarify our priorities and purpose as physicians, past and present. The doctor must indeed be justly remunerated, for he is the very lifeblood of the entire healthcare system. It would seem prudent that a reasonable and reliably stable schedule of Medicare reimbursement is a good place to begin, since Medicare is the anchor above which all other payers seem tied. I use the word "stable" simply because we have seen repetitive, damaging Medicare cuts to doctors over the last several years. What they are paid for some of their services is so trivial that it is no wonder that they are no longer accepting Medicare patients. Many have difficulty paying their overhead expenses, to say nothing of ending up with anything resembling a well-deserved, decent income commensurate with their long education. Furthermore, the end result of poorly compensated provider-care could be very harmful to our entire society. Among other ills, out of the pure necessity of maintaining a physician workforce, it could lead to the lowering of our standards, thus allowing lesser qualified candidates to enter the field of medicine to care for future generations.

~~~

A few hours before writing this concluding section, I visited the home of one of my old friends, who had been a family physician for 50
~~~

years. As this unpretentious, introspective, elderly gentleman looked across the table at me through his spectacles, he began to reflect on his many years of dedication to his patients. With a sense of nostalgia, he asked me whether I thought that the way medicine is currently being practiced would ever revert back to the days of old. He and I began to deprecate on certain facets of medical practice today and agreed to deplore today's seemingly insensitive, mercenary, factory-like approach. Howard recalled his own days in medical training when, like mine, the subject of money was never even discussed. What's more, he had not even been taught how to set up and run a medical office. Of foremost importance, he was instilled with a "sense of responsibility" to his patients, and never wavered from being "on-call" 24 hours a day for the first 17 years of his practice. Being aware of my remote association with the medical school, he asked whether I could try getting through to the young students by addressing some of the problems associated with the practice of medicine today. Although I might not be afforded that particular opportunity, I did assure him that it was a major message in my book.

When we speak of today's problems in medical practice, just exactly what do we mean? Besides the economics of medicine, what else has changed from the days in which Howard and I both practiced? Throughout the book I have touched on many of the intangibles that are absent in today's medical community. Physicians used to respect the opinions of both their mentors and their colleagues. We were humbled by what we "didn't know" and stood ready to "pick the brains" of others whose wisdom and knowledge from years of experience far exceeded our own. The exchange of important information ranging from individual patients to entire medical topics, whether discussed in the hospital parking lot or in a formal daily x-ray conference, was commonplace. Today I have seen many who possess feelings of omniscience, resulting in their practicing medicine in relative isolation. They simply aren't curious as to what others might have to say, even those with many years of experience. When major, if not controversial, questions arose regarding diagnosis or treatment, we often adhered to the old adage that … "Two minds are, indeed, better than one…" and were wary of anyone who consistently felt that he had all of the answers.

This loss of respect and dissociation from one's peers may lead to a loss of camaraderie and later even to resentment. Previously we discussed the physician who became ill and couldn't even get his own partners to take night call for him unless he paid them handsomely.

Given these facts, it follows that there is a loss of respect for the patient as well. Nowadays, a nurse practitioner may be sent into the room on the first visit to gather the history and perform the initial examination. And not infrequently, the physician is nowhere to be seen until the day that he suddenly appears to perform the remunerative, invasive procedure. I believe the word "rapport" has been dropped from today's medical dictionary. In our day it was customary for none other than the physician to perform the initial history and physical examination, gaining both the confidence of the sometimes anxious patient and setting forth a provisional diagnosis.

For many there seems to have been a loss of professionalism over the last two decades, where individual providers or groups have preempted diligent service to others in favor of their own concerns. It is not just the love of money either. When we were in practice we, like most other physicians in our community, felt duly responsible both for our own individual patients and to the community as a whole. The last thing Frank and I would do in the evening, despite a very long day, would be to return phone calls to patients who had called our answering service after our office had closed. No matter how late it was, we would see them that night in the emergency room if necessary; or if the problem could wait, we would schedule to see them in the office the following day. In today's world, some doctor's offices are open only four days a week. Others have messages on their answering machines directing long-standing, loyal patients to the emergency room at the hospital during off-hours or on weekends, where they are seen, usually after a very long wait, by the emergency room physician. And should the patient need admission to the hospital at an inconvenient time, he may then be followed by a "hospitalist" (whose salary interestingly is incurred by the hospital), rather than by his own personal physician-group as was customary in days past. The "hospitalist," while not having the patient's office record at his disposal, must then rely on snippets of past history pieced together from either an unknowledgeable family member or a patient often too ill to accurately deliver it. Unfamiliar with underlying allergies, medications or past illnesses, the uninformed physician may embark upon a lengthy, time-consuming (possibly misdirected and dangerous), very expensive path toward the diagnosis, while relying solely upon laboratory work and imaging studies. Moreover, should the patient require inpatient surgery, he may not even see the surgeon postoperatively until weeks later during an office follow-up visit.

The "art and science" of medicine seem to have been largely lost today and have often been replaced by a cold, impersonal, sometimes rude, business transaction. Furthermore, when followed in the hospital by a total stranger without access to the office record, there may be a discontinuity of care— uncomfortably different from the way medicine was practiced in the past.

What I have described concerning the environment of today's practice of medicine may be disputed by some and might even incur the wrath of others in practice. Nonetheless, it undeniably reflects the observation and opinions of many retired physicians and current patients alike.

The negative medical encounters described in the last two chapters should not be misconstrued by the reader as representing the norm. However, because these incidents are seen with an alarming increase in frequency and represent such a marked departure from the way in which medicine was practiced during the author's generation, I find it very important to address them. The great majority of physicians who continue to place the patient "first" most assuredly deserve the full confidence and trust of those who are ill in times of need.

In my preface to this book, I mentioned the demographics of the "Lucky Few" generation. There are two other very important points made in Elwood Carlson's book that I would now like to point out, for they may be relevant in explaining the impersonal, revenue-based attitudes of today's physicians. First, it was documented that during the last two generations there has been a growing loss of "social trust" compared to what existed during the early generations of the 20th century. Today half of the members of Generation X (Born from 1965 to 1982) feel that others are "looking out for themselves first," and, at times, may be "trying to take advantage of you." This can be a negative force among physicians and might very well strain the doctor-patient relationship. Second, in his introduction to Carlson's book, Richard Easterlin emphasizes that as economic growth increases from one generation to the next, material aspirations increase commensurately. Each successive generation is raised on conditions of greater affluence (5). When my generation came along we felt that we "had to pay our dues" before driving expensive new cars or having cottages at the beach. Today there is a pervading sense of entitlement for immediate gratification. This cultural shift in thinking over the generations may in large part answer Howard's question regarding how medicine is practiced today, and whether it will ever revert back to the days of old.

Perhaps future students of medicine will reverse the pendulum back the other way.

I can only speak for the surgical specialties, which are seeking solutions to these problems of concern, and can only assume that others are addressing them as well. The subject of professionalism is currently being addressed by the American College of Surgeons. When this subject was discussed in the ACS Bulletin, Dr. Martin Luther King Jr. was quoted… "An individual has not started living until he can rise above the narrow confines of his individualistic concerns to the broader concerns of all humanity…" (30).

Citing another person's quote from that same ACS Bulletin … "As professionals, society permits us a monopoly on a body of knowledge. In return, our community logically mandates that we use our skills altruistically, and charges us with the responsibility of self-regulation…."

~~~
~~~

In Conclusion

~~~

During the course of this book, as a third generation neurosurgeon removed from Cushing, I have attempted to share my life's experiences in such a way as to leave somewhat of a footprint for those who might choose to follow. As the title of the book indicates, through my reflections as a member of the post-war generation, I have exercised my prerogative in giving my perspective on a number of different topics, including how medicine today is both practiced and how it is perceived by much of the public. I have also tried to identify local problems— in all probability a microcosm of our national healthcare system— and strongly feel, like many others, that they can be rectified. When viewing the inexorably rising cost of healthcare, we are witnessing yet another unsustainable "bubble," not unlike that of the burgeoning stock market or the housing boom of the last decade. While forced to feed these escalating healthcare costs, middle-class Americans are anguishing as they witness increasing deductions from their paychecks so their employers (local and state governments included) can cover the ever-increasing insurance premiums. There is no relief in sight, and any meaningful future household financial planning becomes impossible. If we continue to follow the current course, only the affluent will be able to afford medical care.

Conspicuous by its absence has been my personal opinion regarding advice to any prospective student contemplating neurosurgery in today's uncertain medical environment. Just the week before writing this last chapter, I was told that the college-bound son of one of Tallahassee's most visible professionals heeded his father's advice: "Not to enter medicine in today's climate." I would have to strongly take issue with that position for several reasons. First, it would seem unfair for us to dissuade any worthy, interested, motivated individual away from the field of medicine just because we, ourselves, are unhappy with the current system. Second, in consonance with what I have already written,
~~~

money should not be the primary driving force in that decision, as doctors will always continue to make a comfortable living. Finally, it is simply an absolute that we, as a society, are obligated to provide good doctors to oversee the health of our citizens. Simply stated: Healthcare is a necessity for those who need it and rewarding for those who deliver it.

Now if I might say a few words specifically about neurological surgery. Dr. Maurice Van Allen, who was one of my mentors in medical neurology at the University of Iowa, was board-certified not only as a neurologist but also as a neurosurgeon. One day when showing me how to perform my first myelogram, with eyes intently focused upon me, he solemnly said, "Jim, I know you are preparing for your future as a neurosurgeon, but you must understand that neurosurgery is awfully hard work!" Unfazed by his admonition at the time, I fully came to appreciate it years later and feel compelled to restate it here.

When two neurosurgeons, not associated with a university teaching hospital overflowing with house staff to assist with the work, endeavor to cover a hospital serving multiple counties, the workload at times is extremely demanding. There is an incessant river of patients which never ceases to flow. It is not unusual for the neurosurgeon to emerge from the operating room after an eight-hour, very taxing operation, not only to find himself confronted with several new patients in the emergency room but also a list of return phone calls to anxious physicians in outlying referral areas as well. In the meantime there are late rounds to be made in the NSCU and new consultations throughout the hospital waiting to be evaluated. And if that isn't enough, he could easily be summoned at 3 A.M. later in the night to repair a difficult myelomeningocele in a newborn in an effort to prevent meningitis and to preserve neurological function in the lower extremities. And so the work goes— like the flowing river— day after day, year in and year out. Dr. Van Allen was, indeed, both correct and wise in his advice to the naïve, young neurology resident.

With that having been said, it is now prudent to look upon our specialty in another context, one of academic fascination and personal challenge. Recalling that first major head case as a senior resident at the VA hospital in which, after performing a craniotomy, I trephined into the floor of the patient's skull to expose and remove his optic nerve tumor, I never ceased to lose my zeal for such challenges. To intently review the anatomy and plan the strategy of a difficult operation the night before and then to transform it into success in the operating room the next morning engenders the ultimate sense of satisfaction. It is the consummate ability of utilizing one's intellect, training and inherent skills in following the path of precision to surgical success that defines neurological surgery. To observe a patient who, prior to treatment, was comatose and critically ill, now again beginning to think, smile and execute a handshake of gratitude is the ultimate reward of being a neurosurgeon. Indeed, it is a just reward for the surgeon who has labored for so many years both as a student in the classroom and as a resident in the operating room.

Yes, even with all of the problems facing medicine today, I can endorse, without reservation, my chosen field of surgery to those who might aspire to engage in it.

In addressing the bright, prospective medical students of tomorrow, I exhort you to emulate the way medicine has been practiced in the past, namely, by embracing the philosophy and ideals of the venerable Sir William Osler to whom we have frequently referred.

Only by viewing the ill patient as a human being seeking our treatment at a time of need, rather than as a source of revenue and at times an inconvenience, can the doctors of today re-capture the patient's trust and respect — a relationship enjoyed by those of us from "The Lucky Few" generation.

In closing, I would like to leave the reader with this quote from Robert Louis Stevenson:

> "There are men and classes of man that stand above the common herd: the soldier, the sailor, and the shepherd not infrequently; the artist rarely; rarelier still, the clergyman; the physician almost as a rule. He is the flower (such as it is) of our civilization; and when that stage of man is done with, and only to be marveled at in history, he will be thought to have shared as little as any in the defects of the period, and most notably exhibited the virtues of the race. Generosity he has, such as is possible to those who practice an art, never to those who drive a trade; discretion, tested by a hundred secrets; tact, tried in a thousand embarrassments; and what are more important, Heraclean cheerfulness and courage. So that he brings air and cheer into the sick room, and often enough, though not so often as he wishes, brings healing." (15).

Glossary

~~~

AANS — American Association of Neurological Surgeons (formerly: The Harvey Cushing Society).

ACS — American College of Surgeons.

Anastomosis — An operative union between two structures.

Aneurysm — Circumscribed dilatation of an artery usually due to an acquired or congenital weakness in its wall.

Anterior — Denoting the front surface of the body; often used to indicate the position of one structure relative to another.

Aphasia — Impaired or absent comprehension or production of speech.

Arachnoid mater — A delicate fibrous membrane forming the middle of the three coverings of the central nervous system.

Arteriovenous malformation (AVM) —An abnormal connection between arteries and veins, usually devoid of intervening capillaries, and often resulting in an abnormal cluster of vessels.

Atlas — The first cervical vertebra.

Axis — The second cervical vertebra.

Axon — The single process of a nerve cell that normally conducts nerve impulses away from the cell body.

Babinski sign — An abnormal reflex when stroking the bottom of the foot, indicative of damage to the pyramidal tract cells of the cerebral cortex.

Capitation — A system of medical reimbursement wherein the provider is paid an annual fee per covered patient by an insurer.

Cerebellum — The large posterior brain mass lying dorsal to the brainstem within the posterior fossa.
~~~

Cervical spine — Relating to the neck.

Choroid plexus — A proliferative vascular fringe of pia mater within the ventricles of the brain which produces cerebrospinal fluid.

Circle of Willis — A cerebral arterial circle at the base of the brain.

CNS— Congress of Neurological Surgeons; also, Central nervous system.

Cognitive — Generic term embracing the mental activities associated with thinking, learning and memory.

Contrecoup injury of brain — Occurring beneath the skull but opposite to the area of impact.

Contusion — A mechanical injury (usually caused by a blow) resulting in hemorrhage beneath unbroken tissue

Corpus callosum —The great commissural plate of nerve fibers interconnecting the cortical hemispheres.

Craniectomy — Excision of a portion of the skull without replacement of the bone.

Craniosynostosis — Premature ossification of the skull and obliteration of the sutures.

Craniotomy— Opening the skull.

CSF — Cerebrospinal fluid.

Dendrite — The part of a nerve cell that carries impulses toward the cell body.

Diencephalon — The caudal portion of the forebrain consisting of the thalamus and hypothalamus, located between and deep to the cerebral hemispheres.

Dorsal — Pertaining to the back or posterior.

Dura mater — Tough fibrous membrane forming the outer covering of the central nervous system.

Epidural — External to the dura mater.

Efferent — Conducting fluid outward from an organ.

EMG (Electromyogram) — A means of recording electrical activity in muscles and nerves.

Foramen magnum — Large opening through the skull base through which the spinal cord is contiguous with the medulla oblongata.

Foramen of Monro — The slit-like aperture connecting the lateral with the third ventricle.

Fourth ventricle — A rhomboid-shaped chamber within the posterior fossa receiving spinal fluid from the third ventricle above through the Aqueduct of Sylvius; its floor being the brainstem ventrally and its roof formed by the cerebellum dorsally. Spinal fluid flows from this chamber into the subarachnoid space over the surface of the brain to be absorbed into the venous system.

Friable — Tendency to crumble into small pieces or powder.

Hydranencephaly — Absence of the cerebral hemispheres.

Hydrocephalus — A condition marked by an excessive accumulation of cerebral spinal fluid resulting in dilatation of the cerebral ventricles and raised intracranial pressure; may also result in enlargement of the cranium and atrophy of the brain.

Hypoxia — Insufficient levels of oxygen in the arterial blood or tissues.

Ilium — The broad, flaring portion of the hip bone, later becoming fused with the ischium and the pubis.

Infarction — The sudden insufficiency of arterial or venous blood supply in any organ resulting in a macroscopic area of necrosis.

Laminectomy — Denotes removal of the posterior arch of the vertebra.

Lateral — On the side or farther from the median or midsagittal plane.

Lateral ventricles — The two CSF-producing chambers within the cerebral hemispheres.

Medial — Relating to the middle or nearer to the midsagittal plane.

Medulla oblongata — The most caudal subdivision of the brainstem, immediately continuous with the spinal cord.

Myelography — Radiography of the spinal cord and nerve roots after the injection of a contrast medium into the spinal subarachnoid space.

Myelomeningocele — Protrusion of the membranes of the spinal cord through a defect in the spinal column, resulting in a fluid filled sac containing neural elements.

Necrosis — Pathologic death of one or more cells, of a portion of tissue or organ resulting from irreversible damage.

NSCU — Neurological special care unit.

Odontoid — The vertical process of the second cervical vertebra (axis).

Papilledema — Swelling of the optic disc, often due to increased intracranial pressure.

Paresis — Partial paralysis.

Pneumoencephalogram (PEG) — Radiographic visualization of the cerebral ventricles and subarachnoid space by the use of injected air into the subarachnoid space usually by lumbar puncture.

Posterior — Denoting the back surface of the body; often used to indicate the position of one structure relative to another.

Posterior fossa — The internal base of the skull where the cerebellum and brainstem rest.

Reticular Activating System — A diffusely organized neural apparatus through the central region of the brainstem that plays a central role in behavioral alertness.

Seizure (Epilepsy, Convulsion) — A disorder characterized by paroxysmal brain dysfunction due to excessive neuronal discharge.

Spondylosis — Often applied nonspecifically to any lesion of the spine of a degenerative (arthritis) nature.

Stereotactic — A precise method of identifying non-visualized anatomic structures by use of three dimensional coordinates.

Subdural—Beneath the dura mater.

Sylvian aqueduct — The CSF conduit between the third and fourth ventricles of the brain.

Sylvian fissure — The lateral sulcus of the brain demarcating the temporal lobe from the frontal and parietal lobes and containing the branches of the middle cerebral artery.

Synapse — The functional membrane-to-membrane contact of the nerve cell with another nerve cell.

Teratoma — A neoplasm composed of multiple different tissues not normally found in the organ in which it arises.

Third ventricle — The narrow, vertically oriented chamber in the mid-plane of the diencephalon deep between the cerebral hemispheres. It receives CSF from the lateral ventricles through the foramina of Monro and discharges it into the fourth ventricle through the Sylvian aqueduct.

Thrombophlebitis — Venous inflammation with thrombus (clot) formation.

Trigeminal neuralgia (tic douloureux) — Severe, paroxysmal bursts of pain in one or more branches of the trigeminal nerve.

Translational — Motion in which all particles of a body move with the same velocity along parallel paths.

Trephine (trephination or trepanation) — To remove a disk of bone — usually pertaining to the use of a hand brace and bit.

Ultrasonography — The location of deep structures by measuring the reflection of ultrasonic wave.

Venous sinus (dural) — Endothelial-lined venous channels in the dura mater.

Ventral — Pertaining to the belly or the undersurface of a structure.

Ventriculography — Radiographic demonstration of the cerebral ventricles by the direct injection of air or other contrast material into the ventricles.

Ventriculoperitoneal shunt (VP) — Operative procedure in which CSF is diverted from the cerebral ventricles into the peritoneal cavity for absorption.

References

~~~

1. Anand, G. (2009, November 21-22). The Henry Ford of heart surgery. Wall Street Journal, p. A-1, 12.

2. Bliss, M. (2005). Harvey Cushing: A life in surgery. New York, NY: Oxford University Press.

3. Brant – Zawadzki, M., & Norman, D. (1987). Magnetic resonance imaging of the central nervous system. New York, NY: Raven Press.

4. Bunson, M. (1991). A dictionary of ancient Egypt. New York, NY: Oxford University Press.

5. Carlson, E. (2008). The lucky few. Springer Science + Business Media B.V.: Springer.com.

6. Carreyrou, J., & McGinty, T. (2010, December 20). Top spine surgeons reap royalties, Medicare bounty. Wall Street Journal, p. A- 1, 20.

7. Davis, F., & Geissinger, J. (1975, April).Establishing a private practice in neurological surgery: preparations, problems and pitfalls. Surgical Neurology, 3 (4), 225-228.

8. DeKruif, P. (1996). Microbe hunters. Orlando, Fl: Harcourt Inc.

9. Gawande, A. (2009, June 1). The cost conundrum. The New Yorker. Retrieved July10, 2009, from http://www.newyorker.com/reporting/2009/06/01/090601fa-fact-gawande?currentPage=all

10. Geissinger, J. D., & Bucy, P. C. (1971, February). Astrocytomas of the cerebellum in children — long-term study. Archives of Neurology, 24, 125-135.
~~~

11. Geissinger, J., & Davis, F. (1976, November). Cervical disc disease and other causes of upper extremity pain. The Journal of the Florida Medical Association, 63, 872-875.

12. Geissinger, J., Kohler, W., Robinson, B., & Davis, F. (1978, July). Arachnoid cysts of the middle cranial fossa: Surgical considerations. Surgical Neurology, 9 (7), 27-33.

13. Geissinger, J., Zapata, C., & Deeb, L. (1985). Cushing's Disease— A cause of delayed growth and development. Surgical Neurology, 23, 636-640.

14. Gikas, P. (1972). Mechanisms of injury in automobile crashes. Clinical neurosurgery, 19, (pp. 175-190). Baltimore, Md: Williams and Wilkins.

15. Hinohara, S., & Niki, H. (2001). Osler's "a way of life" and other addresses, with commentary and annotations – Sir William Osler. Durham and London: Duke University Press.

16. Hoadley, B. (1980). Understanding wood. Newtown, Conn: the Taunton Press, Inc.

17. Horsley, V., & Clarke, R.H. (1908).The structure and functions of the cerebellum examined by a new method. Brain, 31, 45-125.

18. Hounsfield, G. N. (1973). Computerized transverse axial scanning (tomography): part 1. Description of system. Br. J. Radiology, 46, 1016-1022.

19. Jennett, B., & Teasdale, G. (1981). Management of head injuries. Philadelphia, Penn: F.A. Davis Co.

20. Johnson, A., & Sataline, S. (2010, April 2). WellPoint drops stellaris hospitals. Wall Street Journal, p. B-4.

21. Kalleya, A. (1993). Olympia. Athens: B. Giannikos – B. Kaldis.

22. Karpodini – Dimitriadi, E. (1997). The Peloponnese. Athens: Ekdotike Athenon S.A.

23. Kavas, S., & Struckmann, R. (1990). Important medical centres in the antiquity Epidaurus and Corinth. Athens: Editions Kasas.

24. Lasater, L. (1972). The Lasater philosophy of cattle raising. El Paso, Texas: Texas Western Press.

25. Leksell, L. (1949). A stereotaxic apparatus for intracerebral surgery. Acta chir. Scand., 99, 229-233.

26. Mapp, A. (1991). Thomas Jefferson passionate pilgrim. Lanham, Md: Madison Books.

27. Maroon, J. P. (1986). Presidential Address: from aequanimitas to Icarus. Clinical neurosurgery, 34, (pp. 3-15). Baltimore, Md: Williams and Wilkins.

28. McCaughey, B. (2009, August 27). Obama's health rationer-in-chief. Wall Street Journal, Opinion.

29. Mills, C. W. (1956, 2000). The Power Elite. New York, NY: Oxford University Press.

30. Palmer, B. J., Stams, V., Russell, T.R., Harken, A.H., & Britt, L. D. (2009). ACS promotes the six competencies of the Accreditation Council for Graduate Medical Education. Bulletin of the American College of Surgeons, 94(7), 16-22.

31. Peerless, S. J. (1985). Indications for the extracranial-intracranial arterial bypass in light of the EC-IC Bypass Study. Clinical neurosurgery, 33, (pp. 307-326) Baltimore, Md: Williams and Wilkins.

32. Pugh, M. B. (2000).Stedman's Medical Dictionary (27th Ed.). Baltimore, Md.: Lippincott William &Wilkens.

33. Russell, T. (2009). From my perspective. Bulletin of the American College of Surgeons, 94(10), 4-5.

34. Russell, T. (2009). From my perspective. Bulletin of the American College of Surgeons, 94(11), 4-7.

35. Section of Pediatric Neurosurgery of the American Association of Neurological Surgeons (1982). Pediatric neurosurgery. New York, NY: Grune and Stratton, Inc.

36. Siliotti, A. (1996). Egypt – splendors of an ancient civilization. New York, NY: Thames and Hudson Inc.

37. Souli, S. (1995). Greek Mythology. Athens: Michalis Toubis S A.

38. Spiegel, E.A., Wycis, H.T., Marks, M., & Lee, A.J. (1947). Stereotaxic apparatus for operations on the human brain. Science, 106, 349-350.

39. Stapp, J.P. (1967). The problem: biomechanics of injury The Prevention of Highway Injury, 159-164. Ann Arbor, Mich.: Highway Safety Research Institute.

40. Stein, B. M. (1988). Transcallosal approach to tumors of the third ventricle. Operative neurosurgical techniques – indications, methods and results, 1, (pp.381-387) Orlando, Fl.: Grune and Stratton.

41. Stephens, R. B., & Stilwell, D. L. (1969). Arteries and veins of the human brain. Springfield, Ill.: Charles C. Thomas.

42. Stookey, B., & Ransohoff, J. (1959). Trigeminal neuralgia: Its history and treatment. Springfield, Ill.: Charles C. Thomas.

43. Theodore Roosevelt Association (2001). Timeline. Life of Theodore Roosevelt. Retrieved Dec. 23, 2009, from http://www.theodoreroosevelt.org/life/timeline.htm.

44. Turner, G.M. (2010, March 17). The failure of Romney Care. Wall Street Journal, p.A-21.

45. White, R. (2010, August). Recent challenges to caps on non-economic damages. Cap Scan, 16, 20. Tallahassee, Fl: Capital Medical Society.

46. White, J., & Sweet, W. (1969). Pain and the neurosurgeon. Springfield, Ill.: Charles C. Thomas.

47. Wilkins, R., & Rengachary, S. (1985). Neurosurgery. New York, NY: McGraw-Hill.

48. Winstein, K. (2010, February 11). A simple health-care fix fizzles out. Wall Street Journal.

49. Yonab, M. A., & Shatzman, I. (1975). Illustrated Encyclopedia of the Classical World. New York, NY: Harper and Row.

Acknowledgements

~~~

Foremost, my appreciation goes out to all of those friends and relatives who have been such a great source of inspiration in encouraging me to write my memoirs. Special thanks go out to Dr. Charles E. Moore, the author of a book himself, who edited the manuscript and kindly provided the "Foreword." Dr. Frank M. Davis, my neurosurgical partner for so many years, kindly served as a secondary editor. His support and encouragement in this project provided me with added motivation for its successful completion. To Dr. Robert L. Doherty, a true scholar in so many fields of interest, including the law; I am indebted for his many valuable suggestions and contributions in addition to his final editing of the manuscript. To cite his own words after reviewing this work: "I have endeavored to count all of the sponges." Dr. Frank A. Melichar has been supportive in reviewing much of the scientific technical information regarding radiological imaging. Finally, I am most deeply appreciative to my loving wife, Elaine, without whose technical assistance this book would not have been possible.
~~~

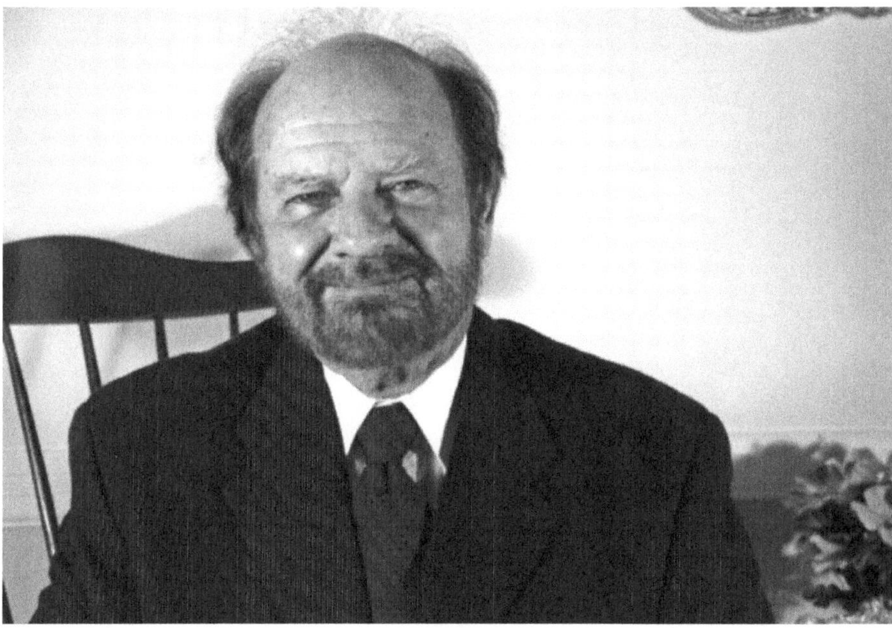

Author

CPSIA information can be obtained at www.ICGtesting.com
Printed in the USA
LVOW01*0812310515

440582LV00010B/100/P

9 780984 741809